Elbow Injuries and Treatment

Editor

JEFFREY R. DUGAS

CLINICS IN SPORTS MEDICINE

www.sportsmed.theclinics.com

Consulting Editor
MARK D. MILLER

July 2020 • Volume 39 • Number 3

ELSEVIER

1600 John F. Kennedy Boulevard • Suite 1800 • Philadelphia, Pennsylvania, 19103-2899

http://www.theclinics.com

CLINICS IN SPORTS MEDICINE Volume 39, Number 3
July 2020 ISSN 0278-5919, ISBN-13: 978-0-323-75519-1

Editor: Lauren Boyle
Developmental Editor: Donald Mumford

Clinics in Sports Medicine (ISSN 0278-5919) is published quarterly by Elsevier Inc., 360 Park Avenue South, New York, NY 10010-1710. Months of issue are January, April, July, and October. Business and Editorial Offices: 1600 John F. Kennedy Blvd., Ste. 1800, Philadelphia, PA 19103-2899. Customer Service Office: 3251 Riverport Lane, Maryland Heights, MO 63043. Periodicals postage paid at New York, NY and additional mailing offices. Subscription prices are $364.00 per year (US individuals), $733.00 per year (US institutions), $100.00 per year (US students), $405.00 per year (Canadian individuals), $904.00 per year (Canadian institutions), $100.00 (Canadian students), $475.00 per year (foreign individuals), $904.00 per year (foreign institutions), and $235.00 per year (foreign students). Foreign air speed delivery is included in all *Clinics* subscription prices. All prices are subject to change without notice. **POSTMASTER:** Send address changes to *Clinics in Sports Medicine*, Elsevier Health Sciences Division, Subscription Customer Service, 3251 Riverport Lane, Maryland Heights, MO 63043. Customer Service (orders, claims, online, change of address): Elsevier Health Sciences Division, Subscription Customer Service, 3251 Riverport Lane, Maryland Heights, MO 63043. **Tel: 1-800-654-2452 (U.S. and Canada); 314-447-8871 (outside U.S. and Canada). Fax: 314-447-8029. E-mail: journalscustomerservice-usa@elsevier.com (for print support); journalsonlinesupport-usa@ elsevier.com (for online support).**

Reprints. For copies of 100 or more of articles in this publication, please contact the Commercial Reprints Department, Elsevier Inc., 360 Park Avenue South, New York, NY 10010-1710. Tel.: 212-633-3874; Fax: 212-633-3820; E-mail: reprints@elsevier.com.

Clinics in Sports Medicine is covered in *MEDLINE/PubMed (Index Medicus) Current Contents/Clinical Medicine, Excerpta Medica,* and *ISI/Biomed.*

Contributors

CONSULTING EDITOR

MARK D. MILLER, MD
S. Ward Casscells Professor, Head, Department of Orthopaedic Surgery, Division of Sports Medicine, University of Virginia, Charlottesville, Virginia, USA; Team Physician, Miller Review Course, Harrisonburg, Virginia, USA

EDITOR

JEFFREY R. DUGAS, MD
Fellowship Director, American Sports Medicine Institute, Founder, Andrews Sports Medicine and Orthopedic Center, Birmingham, Alabama, USA

AUTHORS

CHRISTOPHER S. AHMAD, MD
Department of Orthopedic Surgery, Columbia University Irving Medical Center, New York, New York, USA

PAUL ALLEGRA, MD
University of Miami Sports Medicine Institute, Coral Gables, Florida, USA

RAMI GEORGE ALRABAA, MD
Department of Orthopedic Surgery, Columbia University Irving Medical Center, New York, New York, USA

CHRISTOPHER A. ARRIGO, MS, PT, ATC
Owner, Clinical Director, Advanced Rehabilitation, Tampa, Florida, USA; Special Consultant for Throwing Injuries, Lafayette Medical Director, MedStar Sports Medicine, Washington, DC, USA

JAMES P. BRADLEY, MD
Clinical Professor of Orthopaedic Surgery, University of Pittsburgh Medical Center, Head Team Physician, Pittsburgh Steelers, Burke and Bradley Orthopaedics, Pittsburgh, Pennsylvania, USA

EDWARD LYLE CAIN JR. MD
Andrews Sports Medicine and Orthopaedic Center, American Sports Medicine Institute, Birmingham, Alabama, USA

MICHAEL C. CICCOTTI, MD
Orthopaedic Sports Medicine Fellow, The Steadman Clinic, Steadman Philippon Research Institute, Vail, Colorado, USA

MICHAEL G. CICCOTTI, MD
Everett J. and Marian Gordon Professor of Orthopaedic Surgery, Chief, Division of Sports Medicine, The Rothman Institute at Thomas Jefferson University, Team Physician, Philadelphia Phillies and Saint Joseph's University, Philadelphia, Pennsylvania, USA

RICARDO E. COLBERG, MD
Physician, Andrews Sports Medicine and Orthopedic Center, American Sports Medicine Institute, Birmingham, Alabama, USA

NICHOLAS DANTZKER, MD
Department of Orthopedic Surgery, Columbia University Irving Medical Center, New York, New York, USA

HUNTER GARRETT, MD
Fellow, American Sports Medicine Institute, Birmingham, Alabama, USA

CHRISTOPHER P. EMERSON, MS
University of Miami Sports Medicine Institute, Coral Gables, Florida, USA

DYLAN N. GREIF, BA
University of Miami Sports Medicine Institute, Coral Gables, Florida, USA

SUNNY GUPTA, MD
Orthopedic Surgery Sports Medicine Fellow, Orlando Health, Orlando, Florida, USA

THOMAS R. HACKETT, MD
The Steadman Clinic, Steadman Philippon Research Institute, Vail, Colorado, USA

STEVE E. JORDAN, MD
Attending Surgeon, Andrews Institute, Andrews Research and Education Foundation, Pensacola, Florida, USA

LEE D. KAPLAN, MD
University of Miami Sports Medicine Institute, Coral Gables, Florida, USA

MATTHEW MEUNIER, MD
Clinical Professor, Orthopedic Surgery, UC San Diego Health System, San Diego, California, USA

KAARE S. MIDTGAARD, MD
The Steadman Clinic, Steadman Philippon Research Institute, Vail, Colorado, USA; Division of Orthopaedic Surgery, Oslo University Hospital, Oslo, Norway; Norwegian Armed Forces Joint Medical Services, Sessvollmoen, Norway

JOHN MILNER, BA
Candidate for Medical Degree 2021, Warren Alpert Medical School, Brown University, Providence, Rhode Island, USA

THOMAS JOHN NOONAN, MD
UCHealth Steadman Hawkins Clinic – Denver, Head Team Physician, Englewood, Colorado, USA; Assistant Professor, Department of Orthopedic Surgery, University of Colorado, Aurora, Colorado, USA

MICHAEL O'BRIEN, MD
Lee Schlessinger Professor of Othopaedic Surgery, Department of Orthopaedic Surgery, Tulane University, New Orleans, Louisiana, USA

MIMS G. OCHSNER III, MD
Andrews Sports Medicine and Orthopaedic Center, American Sports Medicine Institute, Birmingham, Alabama, USA

DARYL C. OSBAHR, MD
Chief of Sports Medicine, Attending Orthopedic Surgeon, Chief Medical Director, Orlando City Soccer Club, Orthopedic Consultant, Atlanta Braves, Orthopedic Consultant, WWE NXT, Orlando Health Orthopedic Institute, Orlando Health, Orlando, Florida, USA

GEORGE A. PALETTA Jr, MD, MBA
Head Team Orthopedic Surgeon, St. Louis Cardinals, The OrthopedicCenter of St. Louis, Chesterfield, Missouri, USA

NIMA REZAIE, MD
Orthopedic Surgery Resident, PGY-IV, Orlando Health, Orlando, Florida, USA

JOSEPH J. RUZBARSKY, MD
The Steadman Clinic, Steadman Philippon Research Institute, Vail, Colorado, USA

FELIX H. SAVOIE III, MD
Professor and Chair, Department of Orthopaedic Surgery, Tulane University, New Orleans, Louisiana, USA

MARK S. SCHICKENDANTZ, MD
Professor of Surgery and Director of Sports Medicine, Cleveland Clinic, Head Team Physician, Cleveland Indians, Garfield Heights, Ohio, USA

BENJAMIN C. SERVICE, MD
Attending Orthopedic Surgeon, Orlando Health, Orlando, Florida, USA

BRANDON J. SHALLOP, MD
University of Miami Sports Medicine Institute, Coral Gables, Florida, USA

CLEO D. STAFFORD II, MD, MS
Assistant Professor, Department of Orthopaedics and Rehabilitation Medicine, Emory University School of Medicine, Atlanta, Georgia, USA

FOTIOS PAUL TJOUMAKARIS, MD
Associate Professor, Orthopaedic Surgery, Sidney Kimmel College of Medicine, Thomas Jefferson University, Rothman Institute Orthopaedics, Egg Harbor Township, New Jersey, USA

RANDALL W. VIOLA, MD
The Steadman Clinic, Steadman Philippon Research Institute, Vail, Colorado, USA

CLARK MONROE WALKER, MD
UCHealth Steadman Hawkins Clinic – Denver, Englewood, Colorado, USA

KEVIN E. WILK, PT, DPT, FAPTA
Associate Clinical Director, Champion Sports Medicine-Physiotherapy Associates, Director of Rehabilitative Research, American Sports Medicine Institute, Birmingham, Alabama, USA

SERCAN YALCIN, MD
Clinical Research Fellow, Cleveland Clinic, Garfield Heights, Ohio, USA

Contents

examination. If the description suggests a postexertional compartment-like problem, consider having the patient throw before the examination, and the diagnosis becomes easier to either confirm or rule out. Once the diagnosis is established treatment includes rest or fasciotomy. Recovery is uncomplicated and athletes can return to throwing within a month.

 Video content accompanies this article at http://www.sportsmed. theclinics.com.

Sports-related peripheral neuropathies account for 6% of all peripheral neuropathies and most commonly involve the upper extremity. The routes of the median, radial, and ulnar nerves are positioned in arrangements of pulleys and sheaths to glide smoothly around the elbow. However, this anatomic relationship exposes each nerve to risk of compression. The underlying mechanisms of the athletic nerve injury are compression, ischemia, traction, and friction. Chronic athletic nerve compression may cause damage with moderate or low pressure for long or intermittent periods of time.

The elbow joint consists of the humeroulnar, humeroradial, and proximal radioulnar joints. Elbow stability is maintained by a combination of static and dynamic constraints. Elbow fractures are challenging to treat because the articular surfaces must be restored perfectly and associated soft tissue injuries must be recognized and appropriately managed. Most elbow fractures are best treated operatively with restoration of normal bony anatomy and rigid internal fixation and repair and/or reconstruction of the collateral ligaments. Advanced imaging, improved understanding of the complex anatomy of the elbow joint, and improved fixation techniques have contributed to improved elbow fracture outcomes.

This article is a brief overview of the elbow dislocations focusing on updates in treatment and rehabilitation protocols. The fight between obtaining elbow stability without leading to long-term elbow stiffness has been a continued focus in field of sports medicine. This article highlights advances made to help treat the injuries appropriately and obtain optimal patient outcomes.

Pain over the lateral aspect of the elbow without nerve injury or elbow instability often is diagnosed as lateral epicondylitis or, colloquially, tennis elbow. It is a common complaint, seen most frequently in women between ages 40 and 60, although it is common in men too. Typical presenting symptoms include pain with prolonged wrist extension activities, pain with resisted wrist or elbow extension, and pain at rest radiating from the elbow along the dorsum of the forearm.

Distal biceps tendon injuries typically occur from forced eccentric contraction against a heavy load and are more common in males than females. Most patients who rupture their distal biceps tendon undergo operative repair to minimize strength loss and fatigue. Single-incision and two-incision techniques have been developed in recent decades and achieve satisfactory outcomes. Cortical button and bone tunnel fixation demonstrate superior strength relative to suture anchors and interference screws for acute repairs. Patients who present late or who undergo surgery greater than 4 to 6 weeks from their injury are deemed chronic ruptures and may require autograft or allograft reconstruction.

Distal triceps ruptures are uncommon, usually caused by a fall on an outstretched hand or a direct blow. Factors linked to injury include eccentric loading of a contracting triceps, anabolic steroid use, weightlifting, and traumatic laceration. Risk factors include local steroid injection, hyperparathyroidism, and olecranon bursitis. Initial diagnosis can be complicated by pain and swelling, and a palpable defect is not always present. Plain radiographs can be helpful. MRI confirms the diagnosis and directs treatment. Incomplete tears can be treated nonsurgically; complete tears are best managed surgically. Good to excellent restoration of function has been shown with surgical repair.

Athletes are subject to traumatic and repetitive stress injuries at the elbow joint as a result of high levels of forces imparted across the elbow. Injuries can be acute to the point of tissue failure, or chronic as a result of repetitive overuse. Complete restoration of elbow function must be achieved to allow the athlete to return to their prior level of function. Systematic and progressive rehabilitation programs can help avoid overstressing healing tissues. Treatment programs are designed to restore full motion, muscular strength, endurance, and neuromuscular control. Multiphased rehabilitation programs are designed to restore function in the athlete's elbow.

Orthobiologics are exciting tools providing promising results for difficult orthopedic conditions. In the elbow there is high-level evidence for their use in lateral epicondylopathy and encouraging evidence for other elbow pathologies. This article provides an in-depth review of the current literature for the use of orthobiologics in elbow injuries.

CLINICS IN SPORTS MEDICINE

CLINICS IN SPORTS MEDICINE

SERIES OF RELATED INTEREST

Orthopedic Clinics
Foot and Ankle Clinics
Hand Clinics
Physical Medicine and Rehabilitation Clinics
Clinics in Pediatric Medicine and Surgery

THE CLINICS ARE AVAILABLE ONLINE!
Access your subscription at:
www.theclinics.com

Foreword
Elbowing Our Way Beyond Tommy John

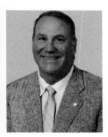

Mark D. Miller, MD
Consulting Editor

Dr Frank Jobe rocked the sports medicine world when he performed the first ulnar collateral ligament (UCL) reconstruction in 1974. Almost a half century later, we can reflect on the contributions of other sports medicine elbow pioneers, including Dr James Andrews, Dr Neal ElAttrache, and many of the authors of this issue of *Clinics in Sports Medicine*, including the Editor, Dr Jeff Dugas. This issue nicely summarizes the current state-of-the-art of sports-related elbow injuries to include not only the UCL but also other ligaments, tendons, fractures, dislocations, and nerve injuries involving this important joint. My sincere appreciation to Dr Jeff Dugas, who did a stellar job in putting together this issue. This is an excellent issue of *Clinics in Sports Medicine* that I encourage all to read and study.

Mark D. Miller, MD
Division of Sports Medicine
Department of Orthopaedic Surgery
University of Virginia
James Madison University
400 Ray C. Hunt Drive, Suite 330
Charlottesville, VA 22908-0159, USA

E-mail address:
mdm3p@virginia.edu

Clin Sports Med 39 (2020) xiii
https://doi.org/10.1016/j.csm.2020.04.003
0278-5919/20/© 2020 Published by Elsevier Inc.

Preface

The Athlete's Elbow: Not a "Bend in the Road"

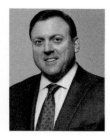

Jeffrey R. Dugas, MD
Editor

I would like to begin by thanking my friends and colleagues who have given of their time and talents to contribute to this issue of *Clinics in Sports Medicine*. These and other *very* talented physicians, surgeons, and therapists around the "elbow world" continue to raise the bar of the care of the athlete's elbow and collectively improve the outcomes in these patients.

Any physician practicing orthopedic sports medicine will inevitably have the opportunity to evaluate and treat elbow injuries in an athletic or active population. Regardless of the level of sport participation, injuries to the elbow can be debilitating from simply a quality-of-life perspective, if not managed in a timely and proper manner. In a typical sports medicine practice, elbow conditions tend to represent a smaller percentage of the total practice than the more common knee and shoulder injuries and conditions. For this reason alone, many clinicians choose to refer elbow injuries to subspecialists for their care. However, the vast majority of common elbow injuries can be successfully treated and result in return to normal activity and sports participation at rates similar to the more common injuries in those other joints. Although the elbow is the "bend" in the arm, it does not need to be a "bend in the road," beyond which the future is uncertain. In fact, return to sport rates following successful treatment in some elbow conditions are among the highest in all of sports medicine!

In this issue of *Clinics in Sports Medicine*, my colleagues and I hope to give the reader enough information to feel comfortable evaluating and caring for the most common conditions that affect the elbow in the athletic and active population, along with the most up-to-date techniques and biologic options to go along with those treatment options. Conditions commonly affecting the throwing athlete have been grouped together in the first part of this collection, with other common elbow injuries and conditions seen in athletics following those articles. The athlete's elbow is susceptible to a myriad of injuries ranging from simple tendinopathies to complex fractures and

Clin Sports Med 39 (2020) xv–xvi
https://doi.org/10.1016/j.csm.2020.04.002
0278-5919/20/© 2020 Published by Elsevier Inc.

sportsmed.theclinics.com

instability patterns. It is my hope that this issue of *Clinics in Sports Medicine* gives the reader a better ability to navigate the "bend" in the arm and find success in the treatment of these elbow injuries and conditions.

Jeffrey R. Dugas, MD
American Sports Medicine Institute
Andrews Sports Medicine and
Orthopedic Center
805 St. Vincent's Drive
Suite 100
Birmingham, AL 35205, USA

E-mail address:
Jeff.dugas@andrewssm.com

Ulnar Collateral Ligament Evaluation and Diagnostics

Michael C. Ciccotti, MD[a], Michael G. Ciccotti, MD[b],*

KEYWORDS

- Overhead throwing athlete • Baseball • Ulnar collateral ligament injury
- Physical examination • Diagnostic imaging • MRI • Stress ultrasound

KEY POINTS

- The overhead throwing motion results in a predictable pattern of stresses across the elbow joint (tension medially, compression laterally, and shear posteriorly), which may overwhelm the static and dynamic stabilizers and result in injury.
- In particular, the medial tensile stresses can exceed the tensile strength of the ulnar collateral ligament (UCL) and result in acute or chronic injury.
- History of UCL injury typically is acute or insidious decreased throwing effectiveness with symptoms exacerbated by the late cocking and early acceleration phases of throwing and localized directly to the course of the anterior band of the UCL.
- Physical examination is characterized by tenderness over the anterior band of the UCL with positive milking and moving valgus stress tests and can be confirmed with magnetic resonance imaging and stress ultrasound evaluation.
- The clinician caring for the overhead throwing athlete must combine a thorough history, comprehensive physical examination, and judicious diagnostic imaging to confirm UCL injury and rule out alternative or concomitant medial elbow pathology.

INTRODUCTION

The overhead throwing motion is a complex series of movements involving the lower extremity, core/trunk, and upper extremity, with the sequential transfer of energy through this kinetic chain toward the wrist and hand.[1,2] The stress transferred across the elbow joint during this activity can overwhelm the dynamic and static stabilizers of the elbow. As a result, throwers may incur a characteristic pattern of both acute and chronic elbow injuries, including ulnar collateral ligament (UCL) injury. Based on an understanding of the anatomy and biomechanics of the elbow joint and a thorough history and comprehensive physical examination, the clinician can distinguish UCL injury

[a] The Steadman Clinic and Steadman Philippon Research Institute, 181 W. Meadow Drive, 4th Floor, Vail, CO 81657, USA; [b] Division of Sports Medicine, The Rothman Institute at Thomas Jefferson University, 925 Chestnut Street, 5th Floor, Philadelphia, PA 19107, USA
* Corresponding author.
E-mail address: MICHAEL.CICCOTTI@ROTHMANORTHO.COM

Clin Sports Med 39 (2020) 503–522
https://doi.org/10.1016/j.csm.2020.02.002
0278-5919/20/© 2020 Elsevier Inc. All rights reserved.

sportsmed.theclinics.com

from other medial elbow pathology common among throwers. Once UCL injury is suspected, it can be confirmed by the judicious use of appropriately selected diagnostic imaging, thereby allowing the clinician to formulate a precise, evidence-based treatment strategy.

ANATOMY AND BIOMECHANICS

Proper diagnosis and treatment of elbow pathology in the throwing athlete require a firm understanding of the anatomy and biomechanics of the joint. The elbow joint is composed of 3 articulations: the proximal radioulnar joint, the ulnohumeral joint both anteromedially and posteriorly, and the radiocapitellar joint laterally. These articulations allow for both flexion/extension of the elbow and pronosupination of the forearm to occur and each may be a site of pathology in the overhead thrower. At low flexion angles (<20°), bony congruity of the joint provides primary stability as the coronoid process of the ulna articulates with the coronoid fossa of the humerus anteriorly and the olecranon process of the ulna articulates with the olecranon fossa posteriorly.[3–5] At higher flexion angles, stability is provided primarily by the static and dynamic soft tissue structures crossing the joint, including both muscles and ligaments. Between 20° and 120°, the primary stabilizer against valgus stresses is the anterior band of the UCL complex.[3,5,6] At flexion angles greater than 120°, stability is provided primarily by the posterior band of the UCL.[3,5] Most throwers maintain elbow flexion of approximately 80° to 110° during throwing, highlighting the critical importance of the anterior band of the UCL, which may be divided further into reciprocally tightening anterior and posterior bundles.[3,5] Additional secondary stability is provided by dynamic contraction of the flexor-pronator musculature originating from the medial epicondyle as well as the elbow joint capsule.[6] The clinician should furthermore be familiar with the course of the ulnar and medial antebrachial cutaneous nerves, because they may be associated with UCL injury and its treatment.

The throwing motion subjects the elbow to tremendous forces, which threaten to individually overwhelm the static and dynamic stabilizers, described previously. Fatigue and injury to 1 stabilizer may lead to a cascade of further injury to the joint. The throwing motion has been described based on the baseball pitch and traditionally has been divided into 6 phases that occur in less than 2 seconds.[7–9] Maximal forces across the elbow joint are experienced during the late cocking and early acceleration phases, where the elbow may achieve angular velocity of 3000° per second. A single pitch may result in a 64-N/m valgus torque, which is twice the ultimate strength of the anterior band of the UCL alone of 32 N/m, again highlighting the critical coordination of multiple stabilizers in preventing elbow injury during throwing.[6] These stresses result in a characteristic pattern of forces across the elbow, which can lead to the pattern of pathology subsequently seen: the medial elbow is subjected to tensile stresses, the lateral elbow to reciprocal compressive forces, and the posterior elbow experiences shear forces. As a result, the clinician must be cognizant of and closely examine each of these areas as a potential primary source of pathology in the throwing elbow.

HISTORY

The evaluation of an overhead throwing athlete with concern for UCL injury begins with a thorough history. That history should incorporate questions that are unique to throwers in order to confirm the presumptive diagnosis and rule out alternative or concomitant injuries. A majority of UCL injuries represent some combination of acute and chronic injury. These athletes describe preexisting or prior episodes of medial elbow pain that has worsened with a more recent event. A minority of athletes present with a clear history of a sudden, acute pop and medial elbow pain experienced with a single pitch. Depending on the acuity of injury, some throwers' chief complaint may not involve pain, because some athletes instead complain primarily of tightness or loss of effectiveness. Decreased effectiveness may occur as a result of diminished accuracy or declining velocity. The location, quality, and severity of symptoms should be identified as precisely as possible. The onset of symptoms, timing with respect to activity, and duration should be questioned and defined carefully. Timing with respective to activity should be defined as occurring immediate at the outset of throwing, insidiously over time, or after conclusion of throwing. Modifying factors (both aggravating and relieving), associated signs or symptoms, and prior treatments should be identified.

Additional questions unique to throwing athletes and their particular sport should supplement the standard history. Several points are of particular interest in throwers with concern for UCL injury. A patient's age with respect to skeletal maturity is critical because it may have an impact on the pattern of injury observed, whether failure occurs at the level of the physis or at the ligament itself. Hand dominance should be identified and whether or not it changes with throwing, batting, or activities of daily living in order to provide full functional context for injury. Frank instability and debilitating weakness are reported infrequently. The presence of neurovascular symptoms, including numbness, tingling, weakness, and temperature sensitivity/intolerance, also should be established for all athletes. Although UCL injury may be encountered more frequently in baseball pitchers, it also may be seen in other baseball players as well as softball players, javelin throwers, and American football quarterbacks. The clinician should know and understand the sport and position played by the athlete and their inherent demands. More specifically for pitchers, the discussion should include typical appearances per week (across all teams played for), number of pitches thrown, number of innings pitched, typical/target velocity, the types of pitches thrown, and which are associated with symptoms. The specific phase of throwing in which symptoms are experienced also is important for establishing an accurate diagnosis, and the patient can be encouraged to simulate the throwing motion if helpful. In order to formulate an appropriate treatment plan, the patient's level of competition (amateur, high school, collegiate, or elite/professional) should be discussed as well as desire to continue/future goals for activity. The timing with regards to an athlete's season or upcoming major competitions may inform this decision making further. Finally, any previous injuries or surgeries to the ipsilateral upper extremity as well as the remaining kinetic chain should be confirmed.

PHYSICAL EXAMINATION

With concern for UCL injury, physical examination of the throwing athlete should not be limited to the elbow alone. The athlete should be looked at holistically. A thorough and comprehensive examination should be undertaken, with the standard inclusion of inspection, palpation, range of motion, strength and sensation testing, and special provocative maneuvers. The entirety of the kinetic chain should be evaluated, including the lower extremities and core to identify any deficiencies, which may be contributing to the athlete's complaints.[10–12] The neck and cervical spine always should be evaluated, particularly if history reveals neurovascular complaints. Finally, both upper extremities should be examined. The authors advocate for examining the contralateral extremity first, to establish baselines while cognizant that throwing athletes may demonstrate asymptomatic/adaptive asymmetries. Both shoulders and scapulae should be evaluated comprehensively as if they were the source of the primary complaint with attention to range of motion, strength, and provocative maneuvers. Differences in range of motion at the shoulder are particularly common in throwers. Although throwers may demonstrate increased external rotation and decreased internal rotation in their throwing arm, total arc of motion should remain equivalent to the nonthrowing arm.[13] Pain or irregularity in any joint along the kinetic chain should prompt a full, thorough, comprehensive examination of that joint. The authors typically evaluate the painful elbow last, so as not to induce premature guarding while examining the remainder of the athlete's kinetic chain. The remainder of this section focuses on examination of the throwing elbow specifically, but the same principles should be applied to any joint of concern in the athlete with a throwing elbow complaint.

Inspection

An athlete should be inspected in shorts and free of sleeves or other clothing so that the entirety of the skin and the patient's station can be assessed clearly. In throwing athletes with elbow complaints and a concern for UCL injury, ecchymosis is uncommon and typically seen only with higher-energy, direct trauma to the limb. Similarly, swelling of the joint is uncommon but, if present, often may be best evaluated at the lateral soft spot in the triangle formed by the lateral epicondyle, olecranon, and radial head. If a patient reports a prior history of traumatic injury or surgery, the presence and location of any surgical scars should be noted so that they can be accounted for in any surgical planning.

Palpation

Palpation should be systematic, with the primary purpose of further localizing the thrower's chief complaint. The authors advocate careful palpation of the medial epicondyle, the flexor-pronator mass, the ulnohumeral joint/ course of the anterior band of the UCL from the sublime tubercle to the base of the medial epicondyle, the borders of the olecranon, and the radiocapitellar joint. Injury to any of these structures generates discomfort along the anatomic course of the structure. Crepitus, warmth, or tissue defects also should be noted wherever present. Precise localization of the point of maximal tenderness is critical to arriving at the correct diagnosis.

Range of Motion

Range of motion of the elbow should be compared with the contralateral extremity. Presence of a flexion contracture is common among high-level throwing athletes in their dominant, throwing arm and may be asymptomatic. There should be no pain, however, at the extremes of motion with a flexion contracture. Pain at terminal motion, in particular, posterior or posteromedial with terminal extension, may indicate posteromedial impingement, posterior loose bodies, or olecranon stress pathology. The forearm should be evaluated for pronosupination deficits or blocks in comparison to the contralateral limb, because this may be indicative of intra-articular pathology. The carrying angle of the elbow also should be assessed at this time. The normal elbow exhibits cubitus valgus of 5° to 15°, although variation has been reported between the dominant and nondominant extremities as well as between male athletes and female athletes.[14]

Strength

All muscles crossing the elbow joint should be assessed with standard manual muscle testing. Particular attention should be paid to the function of the musculature originating from the medial epicondyle and its role in reproducing the patient's chief complaint. Resisted finger/wrist flexion and forearm pronation should be evaluated carefully, because weakness and pain may indicate flexor-pronator pathology. Resisted finger/wrist extension, forearm supination, and elbow flexion and extension should be assessed as well to evaluate for concomitant pathology. Hand intrinsic strength should be evaluated as a means of identifying ulnar nerve pathology, although weakness typically is present only with advanced or chronic compression.

Neurovascular

Neurologic and vascular evaluations are necessary components of any elbow examination in the throwing athlete. Sensation to light touch should be assessed in the peripheral nerve distributions of the medial antebrachial cutaneous, lateral antebrachial cutaneous, radial, superficial radial, posterior interosseous, median, anterior interosseous, and ulnar nerves. Decreased sensation in the fifth and ulnar half of the fourth digits suggests ulnar nerve pathology. The ulnar and radial pulses also should be palpated and distal capillary refill in the nail beds of all digits should be evaluated to confirm adequate dual blood supply to the hand. Trophic changes should be noted if present. As discussed previously, the ulnar nerve often is given special consideration in throwers with medial elbow complaints. The presence of Tinel sign should be evaluated along the course of the ulnar nerve and its location documented. Finally, studies suggest that asymptomatic ulnar nerve subluxation can occur in the general population, but pain radiating distally with tingling in the fourth and fifth digits may suggest symptomatic subluxation.[15]

Special Provocative Maneuvers

Finally, several specific provocative maneuvers have been described aid in diagnosing pathology in the thrower's elbow. These maneuvers allow clinicians to hone their diagnosis more precisely and rule out concomitant or alternative pathology. Two maneuvers commonly are utilized for evaluation of the anterior band of the UCL: the milking test and moving valgus stress test. In the milking Test (**Fig. 1**), the patient's shoulder is abducted and externally rotated and the examiner grabs the ipsilateral thumb and milks it in order to place a valgus force across the elbow thereby replicating the stresses of throwing.[16] The complementary maneuver, the moving valgus stress test (**Fig. 2**), is performed by applying a valgus stress across the elbow in a similar fashion and dynamically flexing and extending the elbow between 30° and 120° of flexion in order to reproduce the late cocking and early acceleration phases of throwing.[17] These tests are positive if they elicit pain and apprehension that the patient localizes to the anterior band of the UCL and underlying ulnohumeral joint. Pain localized elsewhere should suggest alternative diagnoses. Furthermore, gross laxity of the joint is uncommon even in the presence of complete UCL injury and is not necessary for diagnosis of UCL injury. As discussed previously, the flexor-pronator musculature is evaluated specifically with resisted wrist flexion and forearm pronation, and flexor-pronator strain or injury generates maximum tenderness approximately 1 cm distal and anterior to the medial epicondyle. The articulation of the olecranon within the olecranon fossa, which may be a source of pain in valgus extension overload (VEO) with posteromedial impingement, can be evaluated by the arm bar test (**Fig. 3**).[18] The examiner pronates the patient's forearm, extends the elbow, and abducts and maximally internally rotates the shoulder all with the patient's involved extremity resting on the examiner's shoulder and the olecranon facing the ceiling. The examiner then applies a downward force on the distal humerus to produce maximal extension/hyperextension of the patient's elbow. A positive arm bar test is characterized by pain within

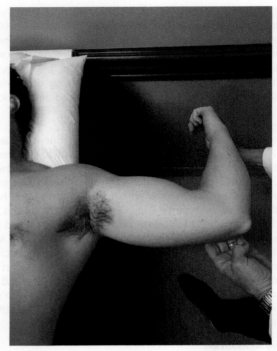

Fig. 1. Milking test.

the olecranon fossa/along the border of the olecranon, which replicates the athlete's complaint in the ball release/follow-through phases of throwing. Complaints localized to the radiocapitellar joint due to the compressive lateral forces of throwing can be assessed further with the active radiocapitellar compression test.[19] The examiner asks the patient to actively pronate and supinate the fully extended elbow. A positive test reproduces lateral symptoms of pain and crepitation. Finally, for patients with history or prior examination findings suggestive of ulnar neuropathy, the ulnar nerve may be evaluated further with the elbow flexion test (**Fig. 4**). The examiner positions the thrower's involved extremity in the fully abducted, externally rotated position while flexing the elbow, pronating the forearm, and extending the wrist. The position then is held in place for 30 seconds and a positive test is characterized by the reproduction of pain along the ulnar nerve and/or the reported development of sensory changes/paresthesias.

IMAGING OF THE THROWING ELBOW

Some diagnoses in the thrower may be made based on a thorough history and comprehensive physical examination; however, diagnostic imaging often is valuable to confirm the diagnosis and rule out concomitant pathology. As in most musculoskeletal complaints, plain radiography typically is the initial imaging study obtained. As in other joints, plain radiographs of the elbow can provide the clinician with significant information regarding loss of joint space, osteophyte formation, loose bodies, calcifications, *osteochondritis dissecans* lesions, cystic changes, and fractures.[20–24] Radiographs of the contralateral elbow often are valuable for comparison;

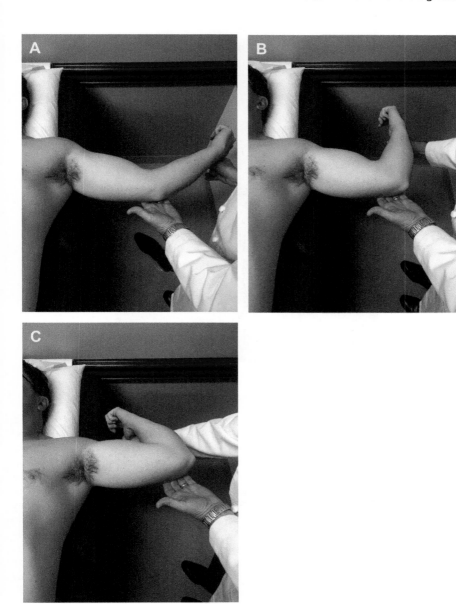

Fig. 2. (A–C) Moving valgus stress test at increasing flexion angles. A - 30 degrees; B - 90 degrees; C - 120 degrees.

as discussed previously, throwers may develop asymptomatic, adaptive changes in their dominant, throwing arm.[25] In skeletally immature throwers, all physes and epiphyses should be methodically evaluated for widening and fragmentation.[26] For some diagnoses, plain radiography may be sufficient. In other cases, however, advanced imaging in the form of stress radiographs, computed tomography (CT), magnetic resonance imaging (MRI), and ultrasound (US) play a critical role for management of the throwing athlete.

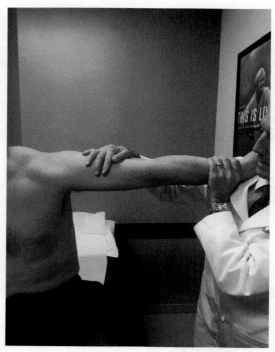

Fig. 3. Arm bar test.

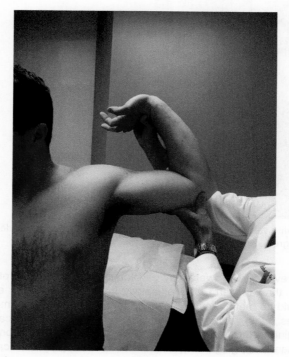

Fig. 4. Elbow flexion test.

The plain radiographs of UCL injury often are unremarkable but medial soft tissue calcifications, radiocapitellar joint chondrosis, and posteromedial osteophytes also may be observed (**Fig. 5**).[25,27] Given the role of the anterior band of the UCL as the primary stabilizer to valgus stress, valgus stress radiographs techniques have been described using anteroposterior (AP) radiographs while the elbow is stress in approximately 20° to 30° of flexion.[20,28,29] With stress radiography, 0.4 to 0.6 mm or greater of ulnohumeral joint opening with applied valgus stress has been reported to be indicative of UCL injury.[28,29] Stress imaging must be interpreted with care and correlated with the athlete's history and examination because some elite throwers have been shown to have asymptomatic, increased joint gapping in their throwing arm.[30] The gold standard for diagnosis of UCL injury is MRI with or without intra-articular gadolinium.[23,24,31–34] The anterior band of the UCL is best appreciated on coronal sequences running from the base of the medial epicondyle to the sublime tubercle of the ulna.[35–38] T2-weighted magnetic resonance (MR) sequences often best reveal UCL injury with discontinuous fibers, increased signal intensity within the ligament substance, and/or retraction of a completely ruptured ligament (**Figs. 6** and **7**).[38,39] Chronic injury may present as intraligamentous hyperintensity, ligament thickening, and plastic deformation, resulting in a redundant ligament with reduced functionality.[33,38] Intra-articular gadolinium has been reported to dramatically increased the accuracy, sensitivity, and specificity of MRI for the diagnosis of UCL injury, in particular, partial injuries.[31–34,40–42] Elite throwers may be resistant to the injection of contrast into their throwing elbow, and although unenhanced MRI has been reported to have extremely high sensitivity for full-thickness UCL tears, sensitivity for partial tears has been reported as low as 14%. MR classifications of UCL injury recently

A   **B**

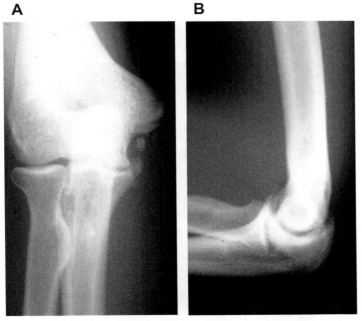

Fig. 5. Plain radiographs of the thrower's elbow: (*A*) AP view with osteophyte and medial calcification and (*B*) lateral view with posterior olecranon spurring.

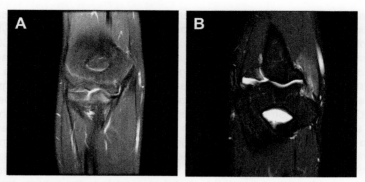

Fig. 6. MR arthrogram, coronal view: (*A*) normal UCL and (*B*) UCL midsubstance tear.

have been published by Joyner and colleagues,[43] Podesta and colleagues,[44] and Ramkumar and colleagues.[45] Although the clinical application and prognostic value of each of these systems remains undefined, they allow clinicians to describe both the severity and anatomic location of injury precisely in a common system. Ramkumar and colleagues classification has been reported to have high interobserver and intraobserver reliability.[45] Although invaluable to the clinician, MR does remain a static examination that can be expensive, invasive, and time consuming. In contrast, stress US (SUS) provides rapid, low-cost, noninvasive, nonradiating examination for UCL injury with the ability to dynamically stress the joint at a resolution that equals or exceeds that of MRI.[46] A proliferation of SUS-related literature has demonstrated the increasing role of this modality in the evaluation of patients with UCL injury.[5,24,40,46–52] Just as asymptomatic abnormalities may be appreciated on plain radiographs and MRI for throwers, ligament thickening, intraligament calcifications, and hypoechoic foci have been described for SUS.[46] Similar to MRI, UCL injury is diagnosed with ligament fiber

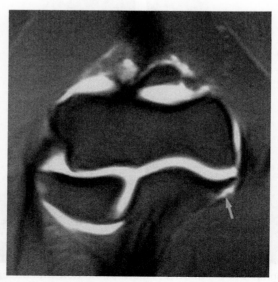

Fig. 7. MR arthrogram, T-sign at distal insertion of UCL on sublime tubercle of the ulna.

disruption, loss of ligament tension, and anechoic fluid within a tear. The significant added value of SUS is to dynamically assess the function of the UCL by measuring the ulnohumeral joint space with applied valgus stress at virtually any flexion angle. Furthermore, comparison to the contralateral arm easily can be obtained. Ulnohumeral joint space typically is measured in both arms with and without applied valgus stress. A growing body of literature and work performed at the authors' institution in a 10-year longitudinal study of 368 asymptomatic major league baseball pitchers as well as cadaveric work has led to using 1.5 mm of increased joint space with valgus stress as indicative of UCL injury (**Fig. 8**).[5,39,40,49–52] As with stress radiography, however, asymptomatic increased joint gapping exists among elite throwers and any imaging finding must be correlated with history and physical examination. Full-thickness UCL tears may result in even greater observed ulnohumeral instability, with mean increase of 3.3 mm in ulnohumeral joint space with valgus stress.[53] Roedl and colleagues[53] has reported that SUS can further increase the sensitivity, specificity, and accuracy of MRI for a host of medial elbow diagnoses common among throwing athletes, including UCL injury. SUS, particularly in combination with MRI, can be of particular value to the clinician in athletes presenting with partial UCL injury or recurrent UCL injury after prior reconstruction.

Flexor-pronator injury typically presents with unremarkable plain radiographs, although the same asymptomatic changes, described previously, may be seen in long-time throwers. MRI allows direct assessment of the soft tissues of the flexor-pronator musculotendinous unit, with common flexor thickening described on T1-weight sequences and edema present on T2-weighted sequences in the setting of injury.[54,55] In some cases, more diffuse inflammation may be observed in the surrounding soft tissues.[55] True flexor-pronator tears may demonstrate a fluid-filled gap, with displacement of the tendon from its origin on the medial epicondyle seen on MRI or US (**Fig. 9**). Integrity of the underlying UCL can be evaluated simultaneously.

VEO with posteromedial impingement typically demonstrates posteromedial olecranon spurring that is evident on plain radiographs with or without the concomitant presence of loose bodies in the posterior compartment. Although the sensitivity and specificity of plain radiography or CT has been reported as equivalent to MRI for the diagnosis of posteromedial impingement, MRI does allow alternative or concomitant diagnoses, such as UCL injury, to be simultaneously assessed. Posteromedial impingement is visualized on MRI as increased signal intensity of the medial surfaces

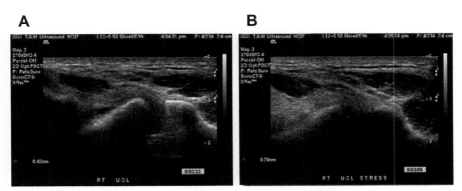

Fig. 8. SUS of the medial elbow: (*A*) unstressed and (*B*) stressed with joint gapping greater than 1.5-mm threshold.

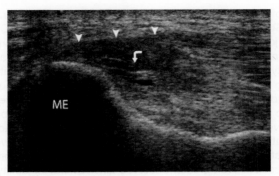

Fig. 9. US demonstrating flexor-pronator tendon tear from the medial epicondyle (ME). *Arrowheads* indicate common flexor, Pronator tendon. *Arrow* indicates tendon tearing.

of the olecranon and olecranon fossa on T2-weighted sequences (**Fig. 10**). In addition to osteophyte formation and increased intraosseous signal, synovitis of the surrounding posteromedial gutter may be seen with additional findings of medial triceps insertional tendinosis and loose bodies also reported.[56,57]

Olecranon stress fractures may be evaluated initially by plain radiograph but may not be evident depending on the severity of the stress response. Both CT and MRI have been used for further evaluation and both studies can clearly demonstrate olecranon stress fractures. On MRI, stress reaction appears as increased T2 signal intensity within the trabecular structure of the olecranon without a discrete fracture line (**Fig. 11**). Stress fractures are diagnosed when a fracture line is present, often best appreciated as a low signal intensity line on T1-weighted sequences. Furushima and colleagues[58] have published their classification of olecranon stress fractures: (1) physeal type—occurring in skeletally immature throwers with delayed closure or nonunion of the physis; (2) classic type—occurring in adults with an obliquely oriented

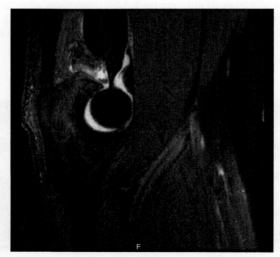

Fig. 10. MRI, sagittal view, showing VEO findings of local edema with increased signal intensity of the posterior medial articular surface on T2-weighted sequences.

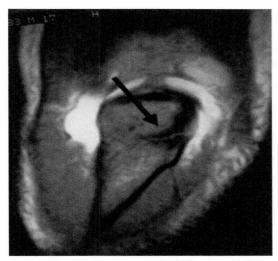

Fig. 11. MRI, coronal view, showing olecranon stress fracture (type 2) with low signal intensity fracture line on T1-weighted sequence. The *arrow* indicates the stress fracture.

fracture line; (3) transitional type—which combines the appearance of a physeal type on AP or coronal views with the appearance of a classic type on lateral or sagittal views; (4) sclerotic type—which has sclerosis without fracture on plain radiography, but a fracture, which can be appreciated on advanced imaging; and (5) distal type—with the fracture line originating from the cortical notch of the trochlear groove.

In throwers reporting neurologic symptoms or with physical examination findings concerning for ulnar nerve pathology, plain radiography can be obtained initially. Plain radiographs can identify deformity or osteophytes, which may be contributing to nerve compression but typically are unremarkable. As in the diagnoses discussed previously, MRI is valuable to rule out concomitant and alternative diagnoses, including UCL injury. The ulnar nerve typically is best visualized as a fat-encased structure posterior to the medial epicondyle on axial sequences.[59,60] Ulnar neuropathy may demonstrate thickening of the nerve, increased signal intensity, distortion of the fascicular structure, and perineural edema.[55,61] The presence of increased signal intensity on T2-weight sequences has a sensitivity of 83% and specificity of 85% for ulnar neuritis.[62] Nerve caliber has been further utilized to determine neuritis severity with a reported accuracy of 88%.[62] Although uncommon, advanced cases begin to demonstrate the effects of chronic compression, including increased signal intensity within muscle, fat infiltration of muscle, and finally muscle atrophy.[61,63] US can be extremely useful for dynamically assessing ulnar nerve stability and directly visualizing subluxation in patients for whom transposition may be considered (**Fig. 12**).[46] Finally, as discussed previously, electrodiagnostic studies should always be considered in patients with significant neurologic symptoms.

DIFFERENTIAL DIAGNOSIS

The differential diagnosis for medial elbow symptoms in a throwing athlete for whom UCL injury is suspected covers several alternative diagnoses (**Table 1**), some of which may occur concomitantly with UCL injury. The clinician's thorough history and comprehensive physical examination in addition to the judicious use of imaging

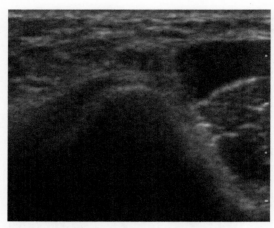

Fig. 12. SUS showing ulnar nerve subluxation with elbow flexion.

studies should be aimed at ruling out these alternative diagnoses. Although the history, physical examination, and imaging may encourage a clinician to focus on the elbow as the source of pathology, alternative diagnoses, such as shoulder pathology, thoracic outlet syndrome, and cervical spine pathology, certainly also should be considered and ruled out when appropriate. Medial elbow pathology in the throwing athlete should serve as the minimum differential and includes UCL injury, flexor-pronator injury, VEO/posteromedial impingement, olecranon stress fracture, and ulnar nerve pathology. In skeletally immature throwers with an open medial epicondyle physis, medial epicondyle apophysitis or medial epicondyle avulsion can be considered part of a spectrum of UCL injury, in which failure occurs at the level of the physis rather than the ligament.

The history associated with UCL injury most commonly is insidious loss of effectiveness/velocity/control with throwing, although some athletes may describe an audible or palpable pop with a single pitch.[64] Throwers complain of pain and tightness, less commonly complaining of gross instability. Symptoms typically are experienced with attempted throwing and less frequently with activities of daily living. When questioned regarding which phase of throwing causes maximal symptoms, throwers with UCL injury typically identify the late cocking and early acceleration phases. On physical examination, these athletes have maximal tenderness directly over the course of the anterior band of the UCL. They exhibit positive milking and moving valgus stress tests with the athlete localizing their symptoms to the same location. Although plain radiographs may provide indirect evidence, MRI, MR arthrography, and US help to confirm the presence and extent of injury to the UCL.

Flexor-pronator injury includes both tendinitis as well as tears. Tendinitis typically has an insidious onset whereas tears may occur abruptly. In contrast to UCL injury, the phase of throwing in which flexor-pronator injury symptoms typically are maximal is at ball release as the forearm pronates and wrist flexes. Maximal tenderness on examination is distal and anterior to the medial epicondyle and pronounced with resisted wrist flexion and forearm pronation. In acute tears, a defect may be palpable at the site of the tear. MRI/MR arthrogram as well as US allows direct assessment and extent of flexor-pronator injury.

VEO is a syndrome resulting from the combination of forces imposed on the elbow from the stress of throwing, consisting of medial tensile forces, lateral compressive forces, and posterior shear forces. The posterior shear commonly results in

Table 1
Differential diagnoses for the overhead throwing athlete

Diagnosis	History	Examination	Imaging
UCL injury	Symptoms maximal in late cocking/ early acceleration Decreased throwing effectiveness (control/velocity) Insidious vs acute pop	Tenderness directly over the UCL +Milking test +Moving valgus stress test	MR with UCL ligament disruption Stress radiographs and SUS with ligament disruption, increased joint space with valgus stress
Flexor-pronator injury	Insidious (tendinosis) vs acute (tear) Symptoms maximal at ball Release (wrist flexion, forearm pronation)	Tender distal and anterior to medial epicondyle +Pain with resisted wrist flexion and forearm pronation	MRI with flexor-pronator edema or full-thickness tear US with tendon disruption
VEO/posteromedial impingement	Insidious onset Symptoms maximal at ball release/ follow through (full extension)	Tenderness over/ along the olecranon +Arm bar test	Plain radiographs and MRI with olecranon osteophytes +/−Loose bodies
Olecranon stress fracture	Insidious onset Symptoms maximal at ball release/ follow through (full extension)	Tender over/along the olecranon	MRI with stress fracture or stress reaction across olecranon
Ulnar nerve pathology	Insidious-onset Numbness, tingling, temperature sensitivity, decreased grip Dull, achy, nonspecific medial elbow pain +/−Medial elbow popping/snapping with instability	+/−Tinel +/−Diminished sensation fourth and fifth digits +/−Diminished hand intrinsic strength +/−Visible/palpable ulnar nerve subluxation	MRI with thickening and edema SUS with ulnar nerve instability EMG/NCV with diminished NCVs

Abbreviations: +, positive; +/-, with or without.

posteromedial impingement of the olecranon against the olecranon fossa, resulting in osteophyte formation.[65] The history of throwers with VEO and posteromedial impingement typically involves symptoms exacerbated at ball release and follow-through as the elbow reaches full extension and the olecranon articulates with the olecranon fossa. On examination, tenderness often is appreciated along the posteromedial border of the olecranon and the arm bar test should be positive. Plain radiography, CT, and MR all provide evidence for diagnosing VEO.

Olecranon stress fractures are a challenging entity for both athlete and provider because they frequently are slow and resistant to healing and recur with relative ease. Similar to VEO and posteromedial impingement, symptoms typically are worst at terminal extension in the release and follow-through phases of throwing. On examination, tenderness to palpation often is present directly over the olecranon, although the precise location may be dependent on the pattern of fracture and, in some cases, may be difficult to distinguish on history and examination alone from posteromedial impingement. Different patterns of stress fracture have been described and alternative mechanisms proposed; however, skeletally immature patients typically manifest a stress fracture due to distraction of the immature olecranon physis by contraction of the triceps during elbow extension, whereas adults may represent more of a spectrum of injury with VEO.[20,66–72] Both CT and MRI studies can be of use for definitively diagnosing olecranon stress fractures.

Ulnar nerve pathology may occur as the medial tensile forces of throwing result in stretching and traction of the ulnar nerve. Throwers with ulnar nerve pathology typically complain primarily of sensory symptoms, with true weakness uncommon. These sensory symptoms may interfere with a thrower's ability to grip the ball, however, and the clinician always should question the athlete carefully regarding the presence of numbness, tingling, dysesthesia, and altered temperature sensation. Pain is often more vague than in alternative diagnoses and may present anywhere along the course of the ulnar nerve or in its distal distribution. Examination may reveal a positive Tinel sign and this should be localized as best as possible to identify the area of greatest compression, particularly if a decompression is warranted. Furthermore, athletes should be questioned regarding subluxation and snapping, and these should be assessed during passive motion to determine if transposition may be warranted as well.[73] In cases of more pronounced or longer standing sensory symptoms or weakness on examination, electrodiagnostic testing, including both electromyography (EMG) and nerve conduction velocities (NCVs), should be considered. This allows confirmation of the diagnosis as well as providing a baseline with which future testing can be compared. MRI can identify changes consistent with ulnar neuritis, while US can demonstrate the presence of ulnar nerve subluxation.

SUMMARY

The overhead throwing motion subjects the elbow to a predictable pattern of forces, including medial tension, lateral compression, and posterior shear that in turn results in a predictable pattern of injury. This pattern serves as the principle differential diagnosis for clinicians caring for an overhead throwing athlete with medial elbow symptoms. Amongst this differential, careful history, physical examination, and diagnostic imaging allow the clinician to correctly identify UCL injury. Athletes with UCL injury complain of acute or chronic medial elbow injury resulting in decreased throwing effectiveness, with loss of control and/or velocity. Symptoms usually are localized directly over the course of the anterior band of the UCL and exacerbated by the late cocking and early acceleration phases of throwing. Milking and moving valgus stress tests can be used as adjuncts to help localize injury to the UCL. MRI is the gold standard for diagnosis, but SUS rapidly is becoming an important imaging modality, particularly in diagnostically challenging situations like partial injury or recurrent injury after reconstruction. Thorough history, comprehensive physical examination, and judicious use of imaging studies allow clinicians to precisely diagnose UCL injury in the throwing athlete.

DISCLOSURE

The authors have nothing to disclose.

REFERENCES

1. Kibler WB, McMullen J, Uhl T. Shoulder rehabilitation strategies, guidelines, and practice. Orthop Clin North Am 2001;32(3):527–38.
2. Rubin BD, Kibler WB. Fundamental principles of shoulder rehabilitation: conservative to postoperative management. Arthroscopy 2002;18(9 Suppl 2):29–39.
3. Morrey B, Tanaka S, An K-N. Valgus stability of the elbow: a definition of primary and secondary constraints. Clin Orthop 1991;(265):187–95.
4. Erickson BJ, Romeo AA. The ulnar collateral ligament injury: evaluation and treatment. J Bone Joint Surg Am 2017;99(1):76–86.
5. Ciccotti MC, Hammoud S, Dodson CC, et al. Stress ultrasound evaluation of medial elbow instability in a cadaveric model. Am J Sports Med 2014;42(10):2463–9.
6. Park MC, Ahmad CS. Dynamic contributions of the flexor-pronator mass to elbow valgus stability. J Bone Joint Surg Am 2004;86-A(10):2268–74.
7. Dillman C, Fleisig G, Andrews J. Biomechanics of pitching with emphasis upon shoulder kinematics. J Orthop Sports Phys Ther 1993;18(2):402–8.
8. Fleisig GS, Andrews JR, Dillman CJ, et al. Kinetics of baseball pitching with implications about injury mechanisms. Am J Sports Med 1995;23(2):233–9.
9. Pappas AM, Zawacki RM, Sullivan TJ. Biomechanics of baseball pitching: a preliminary report. Am J Sports Med 1985;13(4):216–22.
10. Kibler WB, Sciascia A. Kinetic chain contributions to elbow function and dysfunction in sports. Clin Sports Med 2004;23(4):545–52.
11. Kibler WB, Wilkes T, Sciascia A. Mechanics and pathomechanics in the overhead athlete. Clin Sports Med 2013;32(4):637–51.
12. Chu SK, Jayabalan P, Kibler WB, et al. The kinetic chain revisited: new concepts on throwing mechanics and injury. PM R 2016;8(3, Supplement):S69–77.
13. Wilk KE, Macrina LC, Fleisig GS, et al. Correlation of glenohumeral internal rotation deficit and total rotational motion to shoulder injuries in professional baseball pitchers. Am J Sports Med 2011;39(2):329–35.
14. Paraskevas G, Papadopoulos A, Papaziogas B, et al. Study of the carrying angle of the human elbow joint in full extension: a morphometric analysis. Surg Radiol Anat 2004;26(1):19–23.
15. Van Den Berg PJ, Pompe SM, Beekman R, et al. Sonographic incidence of ulnar nerve (sub)luxation and its associated clinical and electrodiagnostic characteristics. Muscle Nerve 2013;47(6):849–55.
16. Veltri DM, O'Brien SJ, Field LD, et al. The milking manuever-a new test to evaluate the MCL of the elbow in the throwing athlete. J Shoulder Elbow Surg 1995;4:S10.
17. O'Driscoll SWM, Lawton RL, Smith AM. The "moving valgus stress test" for medial collateral ligament tears of the elbow. Am J Sports Med 2005;33(2):231–9.
18. O'Driscoll SW. Valgus extension overload and plica. In: Levine WN, editor. The athlete's elbow. Rosemont (IL): American Academy of Orthopaedic Surgeons; 2008. p. 71–83.
19. Buehler M, Thayer D. The elbow flexion test: a clinical test for the cubital tunnel syndrome. Clin Orthop 1988;(233):213–6.
20. Cain EL, Dugas JR, Wolf RS, et al. Elbow injuries in throwing athletes: a current concepts review. Am J Sports Med 2003;31(4):621–35.
21. Patel RM, Lynch TS, Amin NH, et al. The Thrower's elbow. Orthop Clin North Am 2014;45(3):355–76.
22. Bowerman JW, McDonnell EJ. Radiology of athletic injuries: baseball. Radiology 1975;116(3):611–5.

23. Mulligan SA, Schwartz ML, Broussard MF, et al. Heterotopic calcification and tears of the ulnar collateral ligament. Am J Roentgenol 2000;175(4):1099–102.

24. Popovic N, Ferrara MA, Daenen B, et al. Imaging overuse injury of the elbow in professional team handball players: a bilateral comparison using plain films, stress radiography, ultrasound, and magnetic resonance imaging. Int J Sports Med 2002;22(01):60–7.

25. Gustas CN, Lee KS. Multimodality imaging of the painful elbow: current imaging concepts and image-guided treatments for the injured thrower's elbow. Radiol Clin North Am 2016;54(5):817–39.

26. Saltzman BM, Chalmers PN, Mascarenhas R, et al. Upper extremity physeal injury in young baseball pitchers. Phys Sportsmed 2014;42(3):100–11.

27. Dugas JR. Valgus extension overload: diagnosis and treatment. Clin Sports Med 2010;29(4):645–54.

28. Rijke AM, Goitz HT, McCue FC, et al. Stress radiography of the medial elbow ligaments. Radiology 1994;191(1):213–6.

29. Bruce JR, Hess R, Joyner P, et al. How much valgus instability can be expected with ulnar collateral ligament (UCL) injuries? A review of 273 baseball players with UCL injuries. J Shoulder Elbow Surg 2014;23(10):1521–6.

30. Ellenbecker TS, Mattalino AJ, Elam EA, et al. Medial elbow joint laxity in professional baseball pitchers. Am J Sports Med 1998;26(3):420–4.

31. Brunton LM, Anderson MW, Pannunzio ME, et al. Magnetic resonance imaging of the elbow: update on current techniques and indications. J Hand Surg 2006; 31(6):1001–11.

32. Cotten A, Jacobson J, Brossmann J, et al. Collateral ligaments of the elbow: conventional MR imaging and MR arthrography with coronal oblique plane and elbow flexion. Radiology 1997;204(3):806–12.

33. Kaplan LJ, Potter HG. MR imaging of ligament injuries to the elbow. Radiol Clin North Am 2006;44(4):583–94.

34. Schwartz ML, al-Zahrani S, Morwessel RM, et al. Ulnar collateral ligament injury in the throwing athlete: evaluation with saline-enhanced MR arthrography. Radiology 1995;197(1):297–9.

35. Regan WD. Biomechanical study of ligaments around the elbow joint. Clin Orthop 1991;(271):170–9.

36. Dewan A, Chhabra A, Khanna A, et al. MRI of the Elbow: Techniques and Spectrum of Disease: AAOS Exhibit Selection. J Bone Joint Surg Am 2013;95(14): e99, 1-13.

37. Hill NB Jr, Bucchieri JS, Shon F, et al. Magnetic resonance imaging of injury to the medial collateral ligament of the elbow: a cadaver model. J Shoulder Elbow Surg 2000;9(5):418–22.

38. Mirowitz SA, London SL. Ulnar collateral ligament injury in baseball pitchers: MR imaging evaluation. Radiology 1992;185(2):573–6.

39. De Smet AA, Winter TC, Best TM, et al. Dynamic sonography with valgus stress to assess elbow ulnar collateral ligament injury in baseball pitchers. Skeletal Radiol 2002;31(11):671–6.

40. Nazarian LN, McShane JM, Ciccotti MG, et al. Dynamic US of the anterior band of the ulnar collateral ligament of the elbow in asymptomatic major league baseball pitchers. Radiology 2003;227(1):149–54.

41. Timmerman LA, Schwartz ML, Andrews JR. Preoperative evaluation of the ulnar collateral ligament by magnetic resonance imaging and computed tomography arthrography. Am J Sports Med 1994;22(1):26–32.

42. Fritz RC. MR imaging of the elbow. An update. Radiol Clin North Am 1997;35(1): 117–44.
43. Joyner PW, Bruce J, Hess R, et al. Magnetic resonance imaging–based classification for ulnar collateral ligament injuries of the elbow. J Shoulder Elbow Surg 2016;25(10):1710–6.
44. Podesta L, Crow SA, Volkmer D, et al. Treatment of partial ulnar collateral ligament tears in the elbow with platelet-rich plasma. Am J Sports Med 2013;41(7): 1689–94.
45. Ramkumar PN, Frangiamore SJ, Navarro SM, et al. Interobserver and intraobserver reliability of an MRI-based classification system for injuries to the ulnar collateral ligament. Am J Sports Med 2018;46(11):2755–60.
46. Ciccotti M, Nazarian L, Ciccotti M. Ultrasound imaging of UCL injury. In: Dines J, Altchek DW, editors. Ulnar collateral ligament injury: a guide to diagnosis and treatment. New York: Springer; 2015. p. 79–91.
47. Jacobson JA, Propeck T, Jamadar DA, et al. US of the anterior bundle of the ulnar collateral ligament: findings in five cadaver elbows with MR arthrographic and anatomic comparison—initial observations. Radiology 2003;227(2):561–6.
48. Sasaki J, Takahara M, Ogino T, et al. Ultrasonographic assessment of the ulnar collateral ligament and medial elbow laxity in college baseball players. J Bone Joint Surg Am 2002;84(4):525–31.
49. Wood N, Konin JG, Nofsinger C. Diagnosis of an ulnar collateral ligament tear using musculoskeletal ultrasound in a collegiate baseball pitcher: a case report. N Am J Sports Phys Ther 2010;5(4):227–33.
50. Atanda A, Buckley PS, Hammoud S, et al. Early anatomic changes of the ulnar collateral ligament identified by stress ultrasound of the elbow in young professional baseball pitchers. Am J Sports Med 2015;43(12):2943–9.
51. Atanda A, Averill LW, Wallace M, et al. Factors related to increased ulnar collateral ligament thickness on stress sonography of the elbow in asymptomatic youth and adolescent baseball pitchers. Am J Sports Med 2016;44(12):3179–87.
52. Ciccotti MG, Atanda A, Nazarian LN, et al. Stress sonography of the ulnar collateral ligament of the elbow in professional baseball pitchers. Am J Sports Med 2014;42(3):544–51.
53. Roedl JB, Gonzalez FM, Zoga AC, et al. Potential utility of a combined approach with US and MR arthrography to image medial elbow pain in baseball players. Radiology 2016;279(3):827–37.
54. Stevens KJ, McNally EG. Magnetic resonance imaging of the elbow in athletes. Clin Sports Med 2010;29(4):521–53.
55. Kijowski R, Tuite M, Sanford M. Magnetic resonance imaging of the elbow. Part II: Abnormalities of the ligaments, tendons, and nerves. Skeletal Radiol 2005; 34(1):1–18.
56. Cohen SB, Valko C, Zoga A, et al. Posteromedial elbow impingement: magnetic resonance imaging findings in overhead throwing athletes and results of arthroscopic treatment. Arthroscopy 2011;27(10):1364–70.
57. Bianchi S, Martinoli C. Detection of loose bodies in joints. Radiol Clin North Am 1999;37(4):679–90.
58. Furushima K, Itoh Y, Iwabu S, et al. Classification of olecranon stress fractures in baseball players. Am J Sports Med 2014;42(6):1343–51.
59. Ouellette H, Kassarjian A, Tretreault P, et al. Imaging of the overhead throwing athlete. Semin Musculoskelet Radiol 2005;09(04):316–33.
60. Ouellette H, Bredella M, Labis J, et al. MR imaging of the elbow in baseball pitchers. Skeletal Radiol 2008;37(2):115–21.

61. Kijowski R, Tuite M, Sanford M. Magnetic resonance imaging of the elbow. Part I: Normal anatomy, imaging technique, and osseous abnormalities. Skeletal Radiol 2004;33(12):685–97.
62. Bäumer P, Dombert T, Staub F, et al. Ulnar neuropathy at the elbow: MR neurography—Nerve T2 signal increase and caliber. Radiology 2011;260(1):199–206.
63. Bordalo-Rodrigues M, Rosenberg ZS. MR imaging of entrapment neuropathies at the elbow. Magn Reson Imaging Clin N Am 2004;12(2):247–63.
64. Hariri S, Safran MR. Ulnar collateral ligament injury in the overhead athlete. Clin Sports Med 2010;29(4):619–44.
65. Andrews JR, Timmerman LA. Outcome of elbow surgery in professional baseball players. Am J Sports Med 1995;23(4):407–13.
66. King J, Brelsford H, Tullos H. Analysis of the pitching arm of the professional baseball pitcher. Clin Orthop 1969;67:116–23.
67. Ahmad CS, ElAttrache NS. Valgus extension overload syndrome and stress injury of the olecranon. Clin Sports Med 2004;23(4):665–76, x.
68. Nuber GW, Diment MT. Olecranon stress fractures in throwers. A report of two cases and a review of the literature. Clin Orthop 1992;278:58–61.
69. Schickendantz MS, Ho CP, Koh J. Stress injury of the proximal ulna in professional baseball players. Am J Sports Med 2002;30(5):737–41.
70. Slocum DB. Classification of elbow injuries from baseball pitching. Tex Med 1968; 64(3):48–53.
71. Suzuki K, Minami A, Suenaga N, et al. Oblique stress fracture of the olecranon in baseball pitchers. J Shoulder Elbow Surg 1997;6(5):491–4.
72. Torg JS, Moyer RA. Non-union of a stress fracture through the olecranon epiphyseal plate observed in an adolescent baseball pitcher. A case report. J Bone Joint Surg Am 1977;59(2):264–5.
73. Childress HM. Recurrent ulnar-nerve dislocation at the elbow. Clin Orthop 1975; 108:168–73.

Ulnar Collateral Ligament Reconstruction

Edward Lyle Cain Jr, MD*, Mims G. Ochsner III, MD

KEYWORDS

- UCL • UCL reconstruction • UCL tear • UCL reconstruction techniques
- Return to play after UCL reconstruction • UCL complications

KEY POINTS

- Increased involvement, poorly defined pitch counts, and year-round play are risk factors contributing to the rising frequency of ulnar collateral ligament (UCL) tears in young athletes.
- History, physical examination, and appropriate imaging are required to appropriately diagnose a UCL tear.
- There are multiple surgical techniques for UCL reconstruction that have successfully returned overhead athletes to their sport.
- The most common complication following UCL reconstruction is transient ulnar neuritis.
- Revision UCL reconstruction has poorer outcomes with a higher complication rate when compared with the index procedure.

INTRODUCTION

Atraumatic ulnar collateral ligament (UCL) injuries most commonly occur in overhead athletes. The player with a UCL injury often presents with loss of throwing speed and control. There is a spectrum of clinical presentation, ranging from acute injuries to a more gradual onset of progressive pain with throwing and diminished performance. Although rest and rehabilitation are a reasonable option when treating UCL injuries, ligament reconstruction has resulted in return to prior competition level for most athletes.[1]

ANATOMY

The UCL consists of 3 substructures: the anterior, posterior, and oblique bundles.[2] The anterior bundle primarily resists valgus stress from 30° to 120° of flexion and is the most important restraint to valgus during a pitcher's throwing motion.[3] The posterior bundle is fan shaped and provides minimal stability to the elbow.[4] In a cadaveric

Andrews Sports Medicine and Orthopaedic Center, American Sports Medicine Institute, 805 St. Vincent's Drive, Suite 100, Birmingham, AL 35205, USA
* Corresponding author.
E-mail address: Lyle.Cain@andrewssm.com

Clin Sports Med 39 (2020) 523–536
https://doi.org/10.1016/j.csm.2020.02.003
0278-5919/20/© 2020 Elsevier Inc. All rights reserved.

study, Dugas and colleagues[3] examined the origin and insertion of the anterior bundle of the UCL. The anterior bundle originates at the anteroinferior aspect of the medial humeral epicondyle with an average footprint of 45.5 mm^2. The insertion is located 2.8 mm^2 distal to the ulnohumeral joint on the sublime tubercle with an average footprint of 29.2 mm^2. Within the sublime tubercle exists a ridge, which further divides the anterior bundle into an anterior and posterior band. Successful surgical reconstruction relies on repair of the anterior band, which provides most of the valgus restraint at 60° to 90° of flexion. The posterior band is a secondary valgus restraint at 90° to 120° of elbow flexion.[4]

CLINICAL PRESENTATION
Risk Factors

Several risk factors for UCL injury exist. Younger throwers are at an increased risk for UCL injury. In fact, throwers 15 to 19 years in age account for most surgical reconstructions and are the fastest growing group undergoing surgical intervention.[5] The higher prevalence of UCL injuries in younger patients has garnished recent attention. Olsen and colleagues[6] found a correlation between increased pitch count and injury in adolescent baseball players. The study participants were also taller, heavier, participated in showcases, played for multiple teams, and pitched while in a fatigued state. Fleisig and colleagues[7] also identified increased pitch volume, longer seasons, year-round participation, and pitching while fatigued as risk factors for UCL injury. In addition, they identified athletes who play both catcher and pitcher are at even more risk, given that they have more total throws than pitchers alone.

History

A thorough history is crucial when examining the athlete with a suspected UCL injury. In overhead athletes, it is important to determine what point during a throwing motion elicits pain. Of individuals with a UCL injury, 96% report pain during late cocking and early acceleration.[1] The onset of symptoms may be variable. Cain and colleagues[1] reported that 47% of patients experience an acute onset of pain, whereas the remaining 53% of patients experienced a gradual onset of symptoms. Three out of 4 athletes were injured during competition, and of those with an injury, almost a quarter experienced ulnar nerve paresthesias during the throwing motion.

Physical Examination

Most athletes with a UCL injury present without visual signs of trauma or swelling. A small deficit of elbow range of motion (ROM) may exist. Upon palpation, subjects may be tender over the humeral medial epicondyle or ulnar sublime tubercle. A thorough examination of all palpable landmarks of the elbow precludes missing a coexisting injury. Specific physical examination maneuvers help facilitate diagnosing a UCL injury. The *moving valgus stress test* (**Fig. 1**) is performed with the forearm supinated and elbow fully flexed. A valgus force is applied as the elbow is extended. Elicitation of medial pain as the elbow is moved from 120° to 70° of flexion is considered a positive test.[8] The *milking maneuver* (**Fig. 2**) tests for UCL injury with the elbow in the overhead throwing position. The shoulder is abducted to 90° and the elbow is flexed to 90° with the forearm in a supinated position. The examiner pulls the subject's thumb posteriorly, eliciting pain or apprehension. Evaluation of the elbow at 30° of flexion allows for the assessment of increased valgus instability. Instability is difficult to detect clinically, even when dealing with complete UCL tears, because only 1 to 2 mm of laxity is typically present.[9] Overhead athletes sometimes develop a painful posteromedial

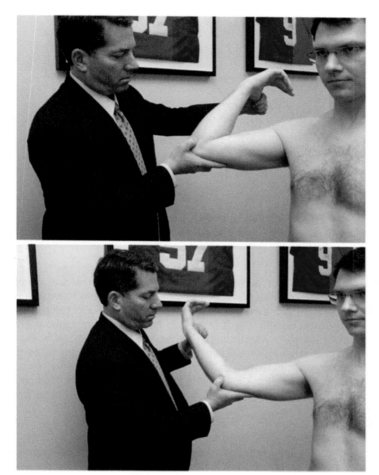

Fig. 1. The moving valgus stress test. Pain is elicited from 120° to 70° of elbow flexion as the examiner applies a valgus stress.

olecranon osteophyte as a result of repetitive throwing. The *valgus extension overload test*[9] identifies the presence of this osteophyte by passively extending the elbow quickly with a valgus force. Elicitation of posteromedial elbow pain with this examination maneuver is a positive test, and the surgeon may remove this osteophyte during reconstruction of the ulnar collateral ligament (UCL-R).[9] The examiner must perform a neurovascular assessment of the upper extremity, with a diligent evaluation of ulnar nerve function. Oftentimes, players with ulnar nerve pathologic condition will have a positive Tinel test at the cubital tunnel. It is imperative to document strength and ROM of the shoulder and wrist because pathologic condition of these structures can occur concomitantly with UCL injuries.

RADIOGRAPHIC EVALUATION

Radiographs including anteroposterior, lateral, medial, and lateral obliques and axial olecranon views are typically obtained when evaluating the thrower's elbow. More

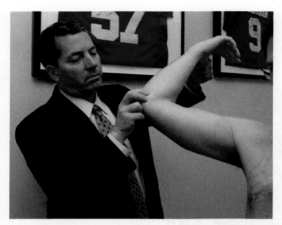

Fig. 2. The milking maneuver. With the arm in the throwing position, the examiner creates a valgus stress by pulling on the patient's thumb, producing pain.

than half of patients with UCL pathologic condition have abnormal radiographs, either in the form of a posteromedial olecranon osteophyte or ossicle formation within the UCL.[1] Valgus stress radiographs may be performed, but are uncomfortable and provide limited diagnostic benefit. Ellenbecker and colleagues[10] reported a baseline increase in medial joint laxity when comparing the stress radiographs of the throwing arm to nondominant arm in professional pitchers. MRI arthrography is the gold standard for diagnosing a suspected UCL tear. When compared with noncontrasted studies, the addition of contrast fluid helps better visualize partial-thickness undersided tears. Schwartz and colleagues[11] successfully identified 83% of partial UCL tears when using a contrasted MRI study, compared with only 14% when using a noncontrast MRI (**Fig. 3**). Timmerman and colleagues[12] coined the term *T sign* (**Fig. 4**) for this tear pattern, originally describing it in computed tomographic (CT) arthrography. However, MRI arthrography is routinely performed in lieu of CT arthrography given the superior visualization of soft tissue structures and lower radiation doses required.

NONSURGICAL MANAGEMENT

There is no consensus algorithm for operative versus nonoperative management of UCL injuries. Those athletes who are not adamant about returning to play a sport requiring valgus stability have radiographic indications of ulnohumeral arthritis, or those who are unwilling to comply with the UCL-R rehabilitation protocol are often better suited for nonoperative management.[13] Even if surgical reconstruction is ultimately chosen, the athlete generally should attempt 3 months of conservative therapy before an operation. However, elite athletes often experience a shorter trial of nonsurgical management to meet season schedules and time-sensitive requirements. Nonoperative management begins with 3 months of rest from overhead throwing. During this timeframe, the patient undergoes shoulder- and elbow-directed rehabilitation. At the 3-month mark, the asymptomatic player begins a gradual throwing protocol, and upon completion, may return to play.

Historically, conservative treatment of UCL injuries has resulted in poor outcomes. Rettig and colleagues[14] described a 42% success rate with 6 months of rest and rehabilitation. Conversely, Ford and colleagues[15] reported an 84% success rate with

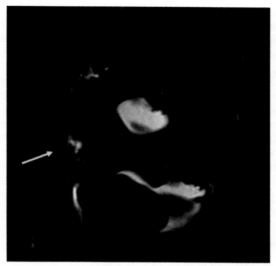

Fig. 3. MRI arthrogram of the elbow demonstrating a complete tear of the UCL from the humeral origin (*arrow*).

nonoperative management of 31 partial-thickness UCL injuries in professional baseball players. However, if a patient failed to respond to rehabilitation at 6 to 8 weeks, the investigators recommended surgical reconstruction. Cascia and colleagues[15] performed a systematic review examining the nonsurgical treatment of UCL injuries in overhead athletes. They reported a range from 42% to 100% return to play (mean 78% ± 20%).[15]

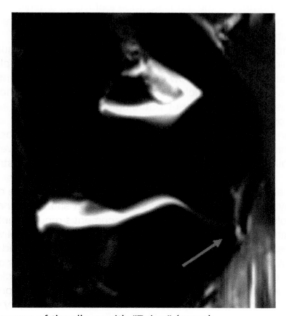

Fig. 4. MRI arthrogram of the elbow with "T sign" (*arrow*).

Tear location may also play a role in the success of nonoperative treatment. Frangiamore and colleagues[16] identified higher failure rates in ulnar insertional injuries (82%) when compared with humeral-sided injuries (19%). These findings argue for aggressive operative intervention when managing ulnar-sided tears versus humeral tears.[16]

Orthobiologics have recently shown promise as a potential adjuvant to nonoperative management of partial UCL injuries. Platelet-rich plasma (PRP) is an orthobiologic that promotes angiogenesis and endothelial proliferation. It is an autologous blood product that contains several growth factors, like vascular endothelial growth factor, transforming growth factor-beta, and platelet-derived growth factor. Podesta and colleagues[17] examined overhead athletes who received an ultrasound-guided injection of PRP after failing a trial of nonoperative treatment of partial-thickness UCL tears. Of these athletes, 88% were able to return to play at an average of 12 weeks after injection. Although promising, better evidence, including randomized controlled trials, is needed to solidify the role of PRP in managing UCL injuries.

OPERATIVE MANAGEMENT

The most commonly selected graft for UCL-R is the palmaris longus tendon. The clinician must evaluate the presence of this structure in the preoperative setting because 16% of individuals have a unilateral congenital absence, and 9% have bilateral absence.[18] Identification of the tendon's presence is performed by having the patient oppose the thumb and small finger during resisted wrist flexion. In preparation for surgical harvest, the course of the tendon should be marked with a marking pen in the preoperative holding bay (**Fig. 5**). If palmaris longus is absent, or if there is a bony ossicle within the ligament, the gracilis tendon may be used.[19] The authors prefer the contralateral gracilis tendon for ease of surgeon position during graft harvest. Other graft options include toe extensors, the plantaris tendon, a portion of the Achilles tendon, and allograft. For the modified Jobe technique, a minimum graft length of 13 cm is required to successfully pass through the ulnar and humeral tunnels and to ensure good fixation.

With regards to elbow arthroscopy and UCL-R, Cain and colleagues[1] recognized that arthroscopic evaluation rarely changes the preoperative plan. Therefore, arthroscopic evaluation of the elbow is indicated only if there is anterior compartment pathologic condition, such as loose bodies or osteochondral defects. Concomitant posterior compartment pathologic condition, such as loose bodies or olecranon osteophytes, may be addressed by making an arthrotomy during dissection, although some surgeons prefer concurrent arthroscopic removal. Removal of osteophytes must be done with caution to avoid overresection and potential destabilization of the ulnohumeral joint with additional stress applied to the UCL.

Several surgical techniques have been developed for UCL-R. The original procedure described by Jobe and colleagues[20] in 1986 involved ulnar nerve transposition (UNT) and complete flexor pronator mass detachment from the medial epicondyle to allow visualization of the native ligament. A Y-shaped bone tunnel was then drilled through the humeral medial epicondyle and a V-shaped tunnel around the sublime tubercle of the ulna in order to re-create the anterior band of the anterior bundle of the native UCL.[3] The graft was passed from ulna to humerus and tied back onto itself with the elbow tensioned in varus, creating a figure-of-8 graft configuration. Of the subjects in Jobe's study, 63% returned to sport at the same level before injury, and 20% of all subjects experienced ulnar nerve complications.[20]

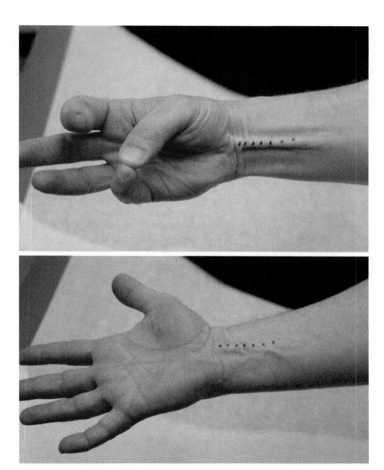

Fig. 5. The palmaris longus tendon. Identified by opposing the thumb and small finger with resisted wrist flexion. The distal course of the tendon is then marked to assist with intraoperative identification.

Less invasive modifications to the original Jobe technique (modified Jobe) have since been developed. With the modified Jobe technique, anterior elevation of the flexor pronator mass also allows access to the UCL without flexor pronator mass transection, but requires UNT[21] (**Fig. 6**). Rather than transection and later reattachment of the flexor pronator mass, a muscle-splitting approach may be used to access the UCL. This technique modification exploits the interneural plane between the flexor carpi ulnaris and anterior flexor pronator muscle mass, avoiding the need for UNT.[22]

The decision to transpose the ulnar nerve is controversial. Cain and colleagues[1] elevated the flexor pronator mass and performed subcutaneous UNT in all 743 of their subjects who underwent UCL-R, reporting a 16% incidence of ulnar nerve paresthesias that ultimately resolved (**Fig. 7**). In another study, Thompson and colleagues[23] performed a muscle-splitting approach without UNT that resulted in a 5% incidence of transient ulnar nerve paresthesias. Although ulnar nerve paresthesias can occur in both techniques, symptoms typically resolve with time.

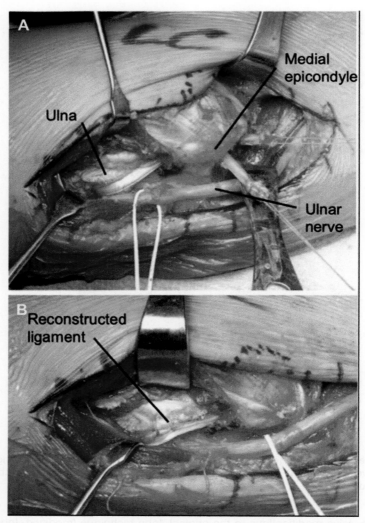

Fig. 6. American Sports Medicine Institute–modified Jobe technique. The 2 limbs of the graft are first passed through a U-shaped ulnar tunnel and then crossed in a figure-of-8 fashion into a Y-shaped humeral tunnel (*A*). The graft is then sewn into the native ligament between the humerus and ulna (*B*).

The docking technique[24] is another popular option for UCL-R. It was developed to address concerns regarding the Jobe technique, including excessive handling of the ulnar nerve, adequate graft tensioning, potential complications associated with flexor pronator mass detachment and repair, and the requirement for 2 large bone tunnels in the humeral medial epicondyle. The docking technique uses a muscle-splitting approach without UNT. The ulnar bone tunnels are drilled in the same fashion as the modified Jobe technique. A Y-shaped tunnel is drilled for the humerus with smaller proximal exit holes when compared with the modified Jobe technique. Instead of passing the graft out of the 2 proximal exit holes, the 2 free ends are "docked" in the humerus, and the sutures are tied over a bone bridge.[24,25]

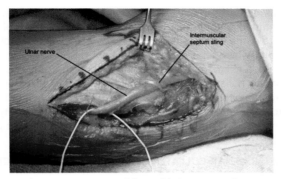

Fig. 7. Subcutaneous ulnar nerve transposition with intermuscular septum sling.

UCL-R with interference screw fixation has also been described. This technique requires 2 drill holes at the sites of the native ligament origin and insertion. Given that there are only 2 osseous tunnels drilled, there is a theoretic decreased risk for ulnar and humeral tunnel fracture. Graft tensioning using this technique is easier than osseous tunnel techniques. There is also a decreased risk of ulnar nerve injury because the posterior-directed humeral tunnel is not used.[26]

The DANE TJ (David Altchek and Neal ElAttrache for Tommy John)[27] procedure incorporates a combination of fixation techniques, using interference screw fixation at the insertion of the UCL on the ulna, and the docking technique for the humerus. This procedure limits the risk for ulnar bone tunnel and may be a good option in the revision setting where there are limited options for bony fixation.[27]

Additional techniques include cortical button suspensory fixation or other combinations of humerus and ulna techniques. Watson and colleagues[28] performed a systematic review comparing all of the above-mentioned techniques. The Jobe technique had the highest complication rate (29.2%), and the modified docking technique had the lowest complication rate (4.3%). Overall, the ability to return to prior level of play was 78.9%, and the investigators found that no reported surgical technique was superior; therefore, the surgeon should use the reconstruction that is most familiar.

POSTOPERATIVE REHABILITATION

Most UCL-R rehabilitation protocols involve an initial immobilization period of 5 to 7 days to allow for wound healing, and this is accomplished with either a splint or a brace locked at 90° of flexion. Isometric biceps and shoulder exercises are allowed. At the end of the initial immobilization period, elbow ROM increases at weekly increments with a goal of full ROM by week 6.[29–31] Individual patient presurgical ROM should be noted, because many throwing athletes have a developmental flexion contracture and resulting extension loss before injury. After attaining full preinjury motion, rehabilitation focuses on a progressive isotonic strengthening program. Shoulder ROM and strengthening exercises as well as The Thrower's Ten Exercise Program are initiated. At this point, any strength deficits are addressed. By week 13, the patient begins a sport-specific exercise program and initiates isotonic upper-extremity weight-lifting and throwing plyometrics. For the overhead athlete, an interval throwing program begins between 16 and 20 weeks postoperatively.[29–31] Most throwing programs contain 2 phases. The first phase applies to all player positions and progresses in distance and repetition number up to 180 to 300 feet, based on the player's preinjury routine. If pain is encountered at any point, the program is dialed back to a shorter distance and then resumed as tolerated. Upon completion of phase I, players other than pitchers progress to game time simulations and advance to play as tolerated. Pitchers progress to phase II, which involves throwing from the mound. Pitchers begin with fastballs that progress in quantity and velocity. Once the pitcher's fastball obtains full intensity, breaking balls and off-speed pitches are incorporated. Phase II ends with simulated in-game pitching. The player begins with 15 simulated throws and progresses by 15 throws per outing. With this protocol, position players typically return to play at 6 to 7 months and pitchers return to play at 10 to 14 months postoperatively.

PERFORMANCE AFTER ULNAR COLLATERAL LIGAMENT RECONSTRUCTION

Postsurgical success depends on an athlete's ability to return to the same or higher level of performance obtained before injury. Generally, results following UCL-R have been good. Cain and colleagues[1] reported an 83% return to sport in 743 athletes undergoing UCL-R with minimum 2-year follow-up. Of the subjects, 95% were baseball players, and 89% were pitchers. The same cohort was later reassessed with an average of 12.6 years follow-up. Of the 256 athletes within the follow-up study, 93% reported they were satisfied with their reconstruction. The average career after surgery was 3.6 years, with 2.9 years of play at or above preinjury level. The vast majority (86%) of athletes reported shoulder, not elbow pathologic condition as the main reason for retirement.[32]

A systematic review of 20 studies on UCL-R reported an 86.2% return to play rate. Of these patients, 90% reported an excellent or good outcome (82% excellent, 8% good). Collegiate athletes followed by high school and professional athletes had the highest return to play rates at 95%, 89%, and 86%, respectively.[33]

Outcomes following UCL-R in professional baseball players have been studied extensively. Keller and colleagues[34] performed a retrospective case-control study on Major League Baseball (MLB) pitchers (n = 168). The investigators reported 87% return to play, but pitchers after UCL-R had poorer performance with regards to earned run average, walks, and hits per inning. Another retrospective study evaluating 147 MLB pitchers found only a 67% return to play defined as playing 10 or more games in a season. Of the patients in the study, 50% returned to the disabled list, although this rate was less than the incidence presurgery.[35] In contrast, Erickson and colleagues[36] performed a retrospective epidemiologic study on 790 MLB pitchers that revealed pitchers after UCL-R had fewer losses, lower earned run average, fewer walks, and fewer hits and runs allowed, arguing for improved performance after reconstruction.

The effect of UCL-R on pitch velocity in MLB players has also been studied. One study evaluated 80 MLB pitchers after reconstruction, noting a decrease in fastball speed from 91.3 to 90.6 mph, although UCL-R did not significantly affect pitch speed for any other types of pitches.[37] Other studies have evaluated pitch velocity in pitchers after UCL-R, comparing them with age-matched cohorts. Again, a small, but significant decrease in ball speed was noted; however, when compared with age-matched controls, there was no difference with regards to pitch velocity for all pitch types.[35,38,39]

Despite the overall success of UCL-R in returning a player to sport, there may be a general misconception within the public that it enhances a player's overall performance. Ahmad and colleagues[40] reported 30% of coaches, 37% of parents, 51% of high school athletes, and 26% of collegiate athletes believed UCL-R should be performed to enhance an uninjured player's performance.

RETURN TO PLAY FOLLOWING ULNAR COLLATERAL LIGAMENT RECONSTRUCTION

The timeline to return to play following UCL-R varies within the literature. Cain and colleagues[1] reported an average return to play of 11.6 months. Return to play may vary from 12 to 30 months in adolescent, collegiate, and professional athletes. This broad timeline potentially reflects a diversity of rehabilitation protocols, but may also illustrate a discrepancy in rehabilitation resources between high school and collegiate/professional players.[1,36,39,41–43]

Advanced player age may play a role in return to play after UCL-R. Osbahr and colleagues[44] reported that pitchers over the age of 30 are at a higher risk for developing flexor/pronator injuries in conjunction with UCL injury, thus increasing the recovery time and complication rate seen.[45]

REVISION ULNAR COLLATERAL LIGAMENT RECONSTRUCTION

The incidence of graft failure following UCL-R has increased as a result of the growing popularity of the procedure in overhead athletes. In the largest single-institution study to date, Cain and colleagues[1] reported a 1% revision rate. Camp and colleagues[46] recently evaluated 1429 cases of UCL-R in professional baseball players. The investigators reported a 9.4% revision rate in major league players, a 5.2% rate in minor league players, and an overall 6.7% revision rate for the entire subject group.

Performance and return to play after revision UCL-R indicate poorer outcomes when compared with the index procedure. When compared with control pitchers, those MLB pitchers who underwent revision UCL-R had careers that were 0.8 to 2.4 years shorter. Furthermore, these individuals only returned to sport 65% of the time.[46–49] Jones and colleagues[50] retrospectively evaluated functional outcomes of both starting and relief MLB pitchers who underwent revision UCL-R. Starting pitchers maintained 35% of their previous workload, whereas relief pitchers maintained 50%. Although 78% of all pitchers in the study returned to sport, this study illustrates the possibility that starting pitchers are at a higher risk for poor results with revision UCL-R given their higher pitch-count demands.

Transient ulnar neuritis is the most common complication following UCL-R, occurring in 7.9% of patients.[48] Of UCL-R complications, 13% are related to graft donor site and include wound dehiscence, weakness, and persistent pain.[48] Major complications following UCL-R are rare and include need for subsequent elbow surgery, most commonly ulnar tunnel fracture and medial epicondyle avulsion fracture.[1]

DISCLOSURE

The authors have nothing to disclose.

REFERENCES

1. Cain EL, Andrews JR, Dugas JR, et al. Outcome of ulnar collateral ligament reconstruction of the elbow in 1281 athletes results in 743 athletes with minimum 2-year follow-up. Am J Sports Med 2010;38(12):2426–34.
2. Fuss FK. The ulnar collateral ligament of the human elbow joint. Anatomy, function and biomechanics. J Anat 1991;175:203.
3. Dugas JR, Ostrander RV, Cain EL, et al. Anatomy of the anterior bundle of the ulnar collateral ligament. J Shoulder Elbow Surg 2007;16(5):657–60.
4. Floris S, Olsen BS, Dalstra M, et al. The medial collateral ligament of the elbow joint: anatomy and kinematics. J Shoulder Elbow Surg 1998;7(4):345–51.

5. Erickson BJ, Nwachukwu BU, Rosas S, et al. Trends in medial ulnar collateral ligament reconstruction in the United States: a retrospective review of a large private-payer database from 2007 to 2011. Am J Sports Med 2015;43(7):1770–4.

6. Olsen SJ, Fleisig GS, Dun S, et al. Risk factors for shoulder and elbow injuries in adolescent baseball pitchers. Am J Sports Med 2006;34(6):905–12.

7. Fleisig GS, Andrews JR, Dillman CJ. Kinetics of baseball pitching with implications about injury mechanism. Am J Sports Med 1995;23:233–9.

8. O'Driscoll SW, Lawton RL, Smith AM. The "moving valgus stress test" for medial collateral ligament tears of the elbow. Am J Sports Med 2005;33(2):231–9.

9. Bruce JR, Andrews JR. Ulnar collateral ligament injuries in the throwing athlete. J Am Acad Orthop Surg 2014;22(5):315–25.

10. Ellenbecker TS, Mattalino AJ, Elam EA, et al. Medial elbow joint laxity in professional baseball pitchers: a bilateral comparison using stress radiography. Am J Sports Med 1998;26(3):420–4.

11. Schwartz ML, Al-Zahrani S, Morwessel RM, et al. Ulnar collateral ligament injury in the throwing athlete: evaluation with saline-enhanced MR arthrography. Radiology 1995;197(1):297–9.

12. Timmerman LA, Schwartz ML, Andrews JR. Preoperative evaluation of the ulnar collateral ligament by magnetic resonance imaging and computed tomography arthrography evaluation in 25 baseball players with surgical confirmation. Am J Sports Med 1994;22(1):26–32.

13. Hurwit DJ, Garcia GH, Liu J, et al. Management of ulnar collateral ligament injury in throwing athletes: a survey of the American Shoulder and Elbow Surgeons. J Shoulder Elbow Surg 2017;26(11):2023–8.

14. Rettig AC, Sherrill C, Snead DS, et al. Nonoperative treatment of ulnar collateral ligament injuries in throwing athletes. Am J Sports Med 2001;29(1):15–7.

15. Ford GM, Genuario J, Kinkartz J, et al. Return-to-play outcomes in professional baseball players after medial ulnar collateral ligament injuries: comparison of operative versus nonoperative treatment based on magnetic resonance imaging findings. Am J Sports Med 2016;44(3):723–8.

16. Frangiamore SJ, Lynch TS, Vaughn MD, et al. Magnetic resonance imaging predictors of failure in the nonoperative management of ulnar collateral ligament injuries in professional baseball pitchers. Am J Sports Med 2017;45(8):1783–9.

17. Podesta L, Crow SA, Volkmer D, et al. Treatment of partial ulnar collateral ligament tears in the elbow with platelet-rich plasma. Am J Sports Med 2013;41(7):1689–94.

18. Thompson NW, Mockford BJ, Cran GW. Absence of the palmaris longus muscle: a population study. Ulster Med J 2001;70(1):22.

19. Dugas JR, Bilotta J, Watts CD, et al. Ulnar collateral ligament reconstruction with gracilis tendon in athletes with intraligamentous bony excision technique and results. Am J Sports Med 2012;40(7):1578–82.

20. Jobe FW, Stark H, Lombardo SJ. Reconstruction of the ulnar collateral ligament in athletes. J Bone Joint Surg Am 1986;68(8):1158–63.

21. Azar FM, Andrews JR, Wilk KE, et al. Operative treatment of ulnar collateral ligament injuries of the elbow in athletes. Am J Sports Med 2000;28(1):16–23.

22. Smith GR, Altchek DW, Pagnani MJ, et al. A muscle-splitting approach to the ulnar collateral ligament of the elbow. Neuroanatomy and operative technique. Am J Sports Med 1996;24(5):575–80.

23. Thompson WH, Jobe FW, Yocum LA, et al. Ulnar collateral ligament reconstruction in athletes: muscle-splitting approach without transposition of the ulnar nerve. J Shoulder Elbow Surg 2001;10(2):152–7.

24. Rohrbough JT, Altchek DW, Hyman J, et al. Medial collateral ligament reconstruction of the elbow using the docking technique. Am J Sports Med 2002;30(4): 541–8.
25. Dodson CC, Thomas A, Dines JS, et al. Medial ulnar collateral ligament reconstruction of the elbow in throwing athletes. Am J Sports Med 2006;34(12): 1926–32.
26. Ahmad CS, Lee TQ, ElAttrache NS. Biomechanical evaluation of a new ulnar collateral ligament reconstruction technique with interference screw fixation. Am J Sports Med 2003;31(3):332–7.
27. Conway JE. The DANE TJ procedure for elbow medial ulnar collateral ligament insufficiency. Tech Shoulder Elbow Surg 2006;7(1):36–43.
28. Watson JN, McQueen P, Hutchinson MR. A systematic review of ulnar collateral ligament reconstruction techniques. Am J Sports Med 2014;42:2510–6.
29. Wilk KE, Arrigo CA, Andrews JR. Rehabilitation of the elbow in the throwing athlete. J Orthop Sports Phys Ther 1993;17:305–17.
30. Wilk KE, Arrigo CA, Andrews JR, et al. Rehabilitation following elbow surgery in the throwing athlete. Oper Tech Sports Med 1996;4:114–32.
31. Wilk KE, Arrigo CA, Andrews JR, et al. Preventative and rehabilitation exercises for the shoulder and elbow. 4th edition. Birmingham (AL): American Sports Medicine Institute; 1996.
32. Osbahr DC, Cain EL, Raines BT, et al. Long-term outcomes after ulnar collateral ligament reconstruction in competitive baseball players: minimum 10-year follow-up. Am J Sports Med 2014;42(6):1333–42.
33. Erickson BJ, Chalmers PN, Bush-Joseph CA, et al. Ulnar collateral ligament reconstruction of the elbow: a systematic review of the literature. Orthop J Sports Med 2015;3(12). 2325967115618914.
34. Keller RA, Steffes MJ, Zhuo D, et al. The effects of medial ulnar collateral ligament reconstruction on major league pitching performance. J Shoulder Elbow Surg 2014;23:1591–8.
35. Makhni EC, Lee RW, Morrow ZS, et al. Performance, return to competition, and reinjury after Tommy John surgery in Major League Baseball pitchers: a review of 147 cases. Am J Sports Med 2014;42:1323–32.
36. Erickson BJ, Gupta AK, Harris JD, et al. Rate of return to pitching and performance after Tommy John surgery in Major League Baseball pitchers. Am J Sports Med 2014;42:536–43.
37. Lansdown DA, Feeley BT. The effect of ulnar collateral ligament reconstruction on pitch velocity in Major League Baseball pitchers. Orthop J Sports Med 2014;2(2). 2325967114522592.
38. Jiang JJ, Leland JM. Analysis of pitching velocity in Major League Baseball players before and after ulnar collateral ligament reconstruction. Am J Sports Med 2014;42(4):880–5.
39. Marshall NE, Keller RA, Limpisvasti O, et al. Pitching performance after ulnar collateral ligament reconstruction at a single institution in Major League Baseball pitchers. Am J Sports Med 2018;46:3245–53.
40. Ahmad CS, Grantham WJ, Greiwe RM. Public perceptions of Tommy John surgery. Phys Sportsmed 2012;40:64–72.
41. Gibson BW, Webner D, Huffman GR, et al. Ulnar collateral ligament reconstruction in Major League Baseball pitchers. Am J Sports Med 2007;35:575–81.
42. O'Brien DF, O'Hagan T, Stewart R, et al. Outcomes for ulnar collateral ligament reconstruction: a retrospective review using the KJOC assessment score with

two-year follow-up in an overhead throwing population. J Shoulder Elbow Surg 2015;24:934–40.

43. Jones KJ, Dines JS, Rebolledo BJ, et al. Operative management of ulnar collateral ligament insufficiency in adolescent athletes. Am J Sports Med 2014;42: 117–21.

44. Osbahr DC, Swaminathan SS, Allen AA, et al. Combined flexor-pronator mass and ulnar collateral ligament injuries in the elbows of older baseball players. Am J Sports Med 2010;38:733–9.

45. Hodgins JL, Trofa DP, Donohue S, et al. Forearm flexor injuries among Major League Baseball players: epidemiology, performance, and associated injuries. Am J Sports Med 2018;46:2154–60.

46. Camp CL, Conte S, D'Angelo J, et al. Epidemiology of ulnar collateral ligament reconstruction in Major and Minor League Baseball pitchers: comprehensive report of 1429 cases. J Shoulder Elbow Surg 2018;27:871–8.

47. Dines JS, Yocum LA, Frank JB, et al. Revision surgery for failed elbow medial collateral ligament reconstruction. Am J Sports Med 2008;36:1061–5.

48. Wilson AT, Pidgeon TS, Morrell NT, et al. Trends in revision elbow ulnar collateral ligament reconstruction in professional baseball pitchers. J Hand Surg Am 2015; 40:2249–54.

49. Marshall NE, Keller RA, Lynch JR, et al. Pitching performance and longevity after revision ulnar collateral ligament reconstruction in Major League Baseball pitchers. Am J Sports Med 2015;43:1051–6.

50. Jones KJ, Conte S, Patterson N, et al. Functional outcomes following revision ulnar collateral ligament reconstruction in Major League Baseball pitchers. J Shoulder Elbow Surg 2013;22:642–6.

Repair and InternalBrace Augmentation of the Medial Ulnar Collateral Ligament

George A. Paletta Jr, MD, MBA[a],*, John Milner, BA[b]

KEYWORDS

- Ulnar collateral ligament • InternalBrace • Repair • Primary Repair Reconstruction

KEY POINTS

- In summary, primary repair of the ulnar collateral ligament (UCL) using InternalBrace augmentation seems to have a predictably high rate of clinical success in properly selected patients.
- The ideal candidates for primary repair are generally younger athletes with high-grade avulsion type injuries of the proximal or distal portion of the ligament and without evidence of attritional or more diffuse ligament involvement.
- Continued long-term follow-up is necessary, but short-term results are on par with the results for traditional UCL reconstruction techniques but with shorter return to play times.

THE RISE OF ULNAR COLLATERAL LIGAMENT RECONSTRUCTION AND THE FALL OF ULNAR COLLATERAL LIGAMENT REPAIR

On July 25, 1974, Dr Frank Jobe performed the first ulnar collateral ligament (UCL) reconstruction on Los Angeles Dodgers pitcher Tommy John (**Fig. 1**). The success of that surgery resulted in it being called the Tommy John procedure. Jobe and colleagues[1] first reported his technique and initial results in 1986. Before he reported his groundbreaking technique and initial results, most patients with UCL tears were treated by repair of the native ligament. The first reported cases of repair of the UCL were by Norwood and colleagues,[2] in 1981. In the small series of 4 patients, 4 of 4 patients regained full elbow motion and had no residual instability at 2 years after surgical repair but only 2 of 4 were able to return to full participation. None of the patients in the study were overhead athletes. Because of the poor outcomes with repair, injuries of the UCL were considered career ending before Jobe's landmark technique.

Jobe's original article described the surgical technique of reconstruction using a palmaris longus tendon autograft.[1] He also described the postoperative rehabilitation protocol. Initial outcomes were reported in 16 throwing athletes, including the

[a] The Orthopedic Center of St. Louis, 14825 North Outer 40 Road, Chesterfield, MO 63017, USA;
[b] Brown University School of Medicine, 222 Richmond Street, Providence, RI 02903, USA
* Corresponding author.
E-mail address: gpaletta@toc-stl.com

Clin Sports Med 39 (2020) 537–548
https://doi.org/10.1016/j.csm.2020.04.001
0278-5919/20/© 2020 Elsevier Inc. All rights reserved.
sportsmed.theclinics.com

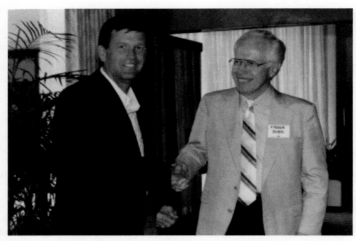

Fig. 1. Tommy John and Dr Frank Jobe in 2004 reflecting on the 30th Anniversary of the historic procedure.

procedure's namesake, Tommy John. Jobe reported good to excellent results in 10 of the 16 patients who returned to their previous level of participation in sports, one patient returned to a lower level of participation and 5 patients retired from professional athletics due to reasons not related to the UCL surgery. In 1992, Conway and colleagues[3] reported on a larger series of 70 patients treated by Dr Jobe who had undergone UCL surgery between 1974 and 1987. In that series, 56 patients had undergone reconstruction using the Tommy John reconstruction technique and 14 patients had undergone direct repair of the ligament to bone without graft reconstruction. The investigators reported good to excellent results in 80% off the reconstructions and 71% of the repairs. However, only 50% of the patients undergoing repair returned to the same level of play as compared with 68% of patients with reconstructions who returned to the same level. Even more damning was the return to play among Major League Baseball (MLB) players, as only 29% of MLB players undergoing repair return to the same level of play compared with 75% of those with reconstructions. Similarly, Andrews and colleagest[4] in 1995 and Azar and colleagues[5] in 2000 also reported poor outcomes of primary repair of the UCL as compared with reconstruction, which effectively signaled the death of UCL repair. Reconstruction using the Tommy John technique became the standard of care for the next 2 decades.

INDIVIDUALIZING TREATMENT OF THE ULNAR COLLATERAL LIGAMENT–INJURED ATHLETE

Since Dr Jobe's 2 landmark publications, virtually all UCL-injured athletes had been treated with some form of UCL reconstruction regardless of injury pattern, player age, or level of participation. Although physicians attempted to individualize treatment based on factors such as player age, player level, position played, time of season when injury occurred, baseball career expectations, and other sports participation, treatment was not individualized based on the pattern of ligament injury. Despite the fact that clinicians recognized and sought to classify injury patterns[6] as acute or chronic tears; partial or complete tears; high- or low-grade partial tears; or proximal, midsubstance or distal tears, the same surgical treatment option was applied to all tears, which is surgical reconstruction.

Researchers studying the success rates of nonsurgical treatment of different injury patterns noted that more distal tears, high-grade partial tears, and complete tears tended to do worse with nonoperative treatment and had a higher conversion rate to reconstruction.[7]

Clinicians who frequently treated athletes with elbow UCL injuries began asking if perhaps reconstruction of the UCL was too much surgery for certain injury patterns. This gave rise to a reemerging interest in the possibility of primary repair of the UCL in certain injury patterns, specifically acute proximal or distal avulsion type injuries without chronic ligament changes.

PRIMARY ULNAR COLLATERAL LIGAMENT REPAIR REVISITED

In 2006, Argo and colleagues[8] reported on a series of 18 patients undergoing primary repair of the UCL using a variety of primary repair techniques. All patients were female athletes competing in a variety of sports. There were 14 softball players (1 pitcher), gymnasts, and tennis player. It was a relatively young group with mean age of 22 years (range, 15.1–37.2 years). The mean follow-up was 38.8 months (range, 12.4–68.6 months). Repair techniques include plication (n = 6), repair to bone using anchors (n = 11), or drill holes (n = 1). The mean Andrews and Carson Elbow Outcome Score increased from a preoperative score of 120 to 191 postoperatively ($P < .0001$). Seventeen of eighteen athletes returned to their sport at a mean of 2.5 months postoperatively.

Two years later in 2008, Richard and colleagues[9] reported on a series of 11 athletes undergoing repair of acute tears of the proximal portion of the UCL at an average of 20 days after injury. All 11 athletes had suffered acute rupture of the medial UCL via traumatic injury but had not sustained an elbow dislocation. Valgus instability was present in 11 of 11 athletes, and MRI scans confirmed complete avulsion of the proximal UCL in all cases. All patients also had avulsion of the flexor-pronator origin from the medial epicondyle. Nine of eleven patients underwent direct repair of the avulsed UCL to the footprint of the medial epicondyle using a suture repair technique and 2 of 11 underwent repair using suture anchors. The investigators reported good outcomes with 9 or 11 returning to collegiate athletics by 6 months postop.

Savoie and colleagues[10] expanded on their initial work as reported by Argo and colleagues[8] by reporting on a much larger series of athletes undergoing primary repair of the UCL. Their study cohort included 60 young throwing athletes (mean age 17.2 years) undergoing repair of proximal or distal UCL avulsion injuries in young throwing athletes. The surgical techniques include 9 repaired by suture through bone tunnels and 51 repaired using single-suture anchors. At an average follow-up of 59.2 months, the investigators reported that 58 of 60 athletes returned to sport at the same level or higher within 6 months. They again used the Andrews and Carson Elbow Outcome Score and reported an increase from a preoperative score of 132 to a postoperative score of 188 ($P < .0001$). Good to excellent results were reported in 93% of patients and 58 of 60 were able to return to their same or higher level of sports participation by 6 months postoperatively. There were only 2 early failures.

These improved outcomes of primary repair of the UCL in select avulsion type injury patterns in young athletes served as the spark that reignited interest in the viability of UCL repair for a larger subset of UCL injured athletes. Combined with new technological advances in suture material and anchors, a repair revolution was about to take hold.

THE ROLE OF THE InternalBrace

Recent advances in technology have included the development of braided tapes and so-called super sutures as well as a plethora of nonmetallic and knotless suture anchors. One of these recent developments is the InternalBrace (Arthrex, Naples FL) (**Fig. 2**), which is spanning suture tape anchored on each end and used to augment ligament repair. It is composed of a FiberTape (Arthrex, Naples, FL) and 2 BiocompositeSwiveLock anchors (Arthrex, Naples, FL). The concept of the InternalBrace was first conceived and clinically used by Professor Gordon Mackay of Scotland.[11,12] He initially reported favorable clinical results using the InternalBrace in the repair of lateral ligament injuries as an augment to the classic Brostrom procedure as well as in ligament repairs of the knee including the anterior cruciate ligament and medial collateral ligament. Biomechanical studies[13–16] have validated the biomechanical advantages of internal bracing over primary repair using sutures or anchors alone.

Piggybacking off the initial clinical success of the InternalBrace in knee medial collateral ligament repair, Dugas and colleagues[17] extended the application of the InternalBrace to a biomechanical study of its potential use in repair of the medial UCL of the elbow. In a cadaveric study using 9 matched pairs of cadaveric elbows, the researchers compared the biomechanical, time zero properties of augmented UCL repair with the typical modified Jobe technique for UCL reconstruction. Using a cyclical valgus rotational torque applied to the humerus followed by a torque to failure, the intact state was compared with the UCL insufficient state by creating a surgical lesion of the UCL. Each matched pair specimen then underwent either augmented UCL repair or reconstruction. Gap formation, torsional stiffness, and maximum torque at failure were measured. After the repair or reconstruction procedures, the repair group showed less gapping during cyclical testing than the reconstruction group. There was no difference between the 2 groups for torsional stiffness or maximum torque to failure. The investigators concluded that the time-zero failure properties of the augmented repair technique were at least with those of the traditional modified Jobe reconstruction technique even after 500 cycles of valgus loading.

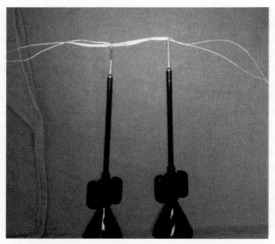

Fig. 2. InternalBrace (Arthrex, Naples FL) (**see Fig. 3**), which is spanning suture tape anchored on each end and used to augment ligament repair. It is composed of a 2-mm Fiber-Tape (Arthrex, Naples, FL) and two 3.5-mm BiocompositeSwiveLock anchors (Arthrex, Naples, FL). (*Courtesy of* Arthrex, Inc., Naples, FL.)

SURGICAL TECHNIQUE OF AUGMENTED REPAIR OF THE ULNAR COLLATERAL LIGAMENT

With the biomechanical study as a basis supporting the potential clinical application of augmented UCL repair, Dugas introduced a novel ligament repair technique using the InternalBrace. The goal of the technique was to restore valgus stability, decrease soft tissue dissection, preserve bone, and allow a faster return to play.

Ulnar Collateral Ligament Repair Technique

The current indications for primary repair of the UCL include younger patients (<age 25 years) with high-grade proximal or distal avulsion type injuries of the UCL without evidence of more diffuse ligament injury or attritional tearing.

A standard medial approach is used with an 8- to 10-cm incision extending distally from the medial epicondyle. Skin flaps are raised anteriorly and posteriorly, and any crossing superficial vessels are cauterized. The medial antebrachial cutaneous nerve and any of its branches are identified and preserved. The branches are usually found anterior and distal to the medial epicondyle and often cross the surgical field. Because muscle-splitting approach is used, the flexor-pronator mass is split between the anterior one-third and posterior two-thirds. There is often a raphe of the flexor carpe ulnaris fascia that can be identified and exploited for this muscle split. A periosteal elevator is used to split the muscle fibers and dissect down to the underlying UCL (**Fig. 3**). In many cases, the superficial fibers of the ligament may seem entirely normal except in cases of acute, full-thickness tears that are treated very soon after initial injury (**Figs. 4**A, 4B). The UCL is incised longitudinally from the sublime tubercle to the medial epicondyle. This is done to allow exposure of the underlying joint, inspection of the deep fibers, identification of the tear, and assessment of the overall ligament quality. If the UCL has signs of diffuse or attritional disease, repair is abandoned and reconstruction is performed. If the ligament injury pattern matches the MRI findings and is consistent with a high-grade or complete avulsion type tear of the proximal or distal portion of the ligament and the remainder of the ligament seems grossly normal without attritional changes, then repair is undertaken. Once the ligament is incised and the patient is deemed to be a candidate for repair, the site of the ligament tear, proximal or distal, is identified. For distal tears, debridement of periosteum and soft tissue from footprint of the UCL at the sublime tubercle is undertaken. For proximal tears, debridement of any fibrous tissue at the medial epicondyle origin of the

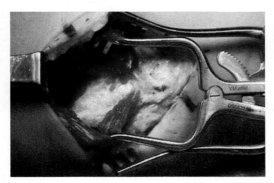

Fig. 3. Muscle splitting approach with exposure of the underlying UCL. Note the normal appearance of the superficial fibers.

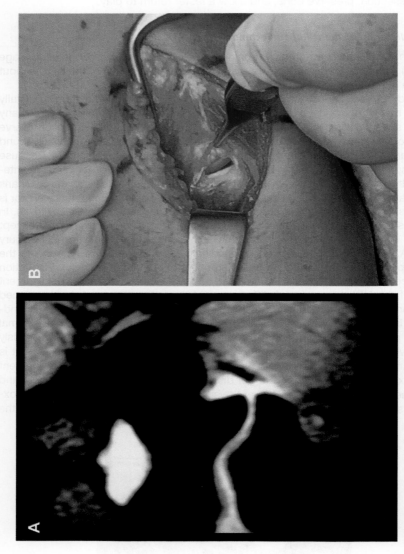

Fig. 4. (*A*, *B*) Complete tear of the distal UCL at the sublime tubercle. (*A*) MRI scan demonstrating complete tear of the distal ligament. (*B*) Intraoperative appearance of the tear.

ligament is debrided. In either case, the ulnar nerve should be identified and protected, especially during drilling. The first 3.5-mm nonabsorbable suture anchor (SwiveLock, Arthrex, Naples, FL) is placed on the side of the ligament tear. For distal tears, the anatomic UCL origin on the sublime tubercle is drilled and tapped. For proximal tears, the center of the origin of the UCL at the medial epicondyle is drilled and tapped. This anchor is loaded with 2-mm FiberTape (Arthrex) that is collagen-coated and second high-tensile nonabsorbable suture. For distal tears, a #0 high-tensile nonabsorbable suture is used. For proximal tears, a #1 high-tensile nonabsorbable suture is used. After the first anchor is placed (**Fig. 5**), the individual limbs of the high-tensile nonabsorbable suture are passed through the anterior and posterior limbs of the split ligament (**Fig. 6**). The elbow is placed in 60° of flexion, and varus load is applied to close down the medial joint. The sutures are then tied, thereby repairing the native ligament directly to bone at the site of the avulsion. The longitudinal split in the ligament is repaired from distal to proximal with size 0 Vicryl suture placed in mattress fashion. These sutures should be passed using the needle from posterior limb of the ligament through the anterior to the ulna nerve. These sutures are left untied until after the InternalBrace has been tensioned and fixed.

Attention is now directed to the opposite side of the ligament. For distal tears, the isometric point of the UCL at the medial epicondyle is determined. This is done by tensioning the FiberTape on the medial epicondyle and adjusting its position so that it does not change length with elbow flexion and extension (**Fig. 7**). For proximal tears, the distal footprint of the UCL is identified directly by both visualization and palpation. A drill hole is created and tapped and the second 3.5-mm SwiveLock suture anchor is placed (**Fig. 8**). All of the simple sutures used for the primary repair are tied except for the most proximal one. The FiberTape now spans the length of the native ligament. It is tensioned as the second anchor is placed. This is done with the arm in 60° of flexion and reduced in varus with the forearm supinated.

After the second anchor is inserted, the mattress sutures that had been placed in the native ligament are tied over the FiberTape to tack it down to the native ligament together (**Fig. 9**). Elbow motion is assessed to insure the joint has not been captured. The flexor-pronator fascial split is closed, and the remainder of the wound is closed in layers. The arm is immobilized in a posterior plaster splint with the elbow at 80° of flexion and the forearm in neutral rotation.

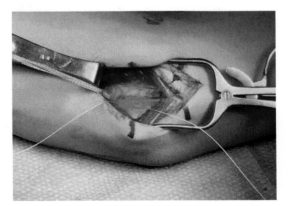

Fig. 5. Placement of the first anchor at the sublime tubercle for a distal tear. Note the FiberTape (Arthrex, Inc., Naples, FL) suture tape and the accessory nonabsorbable high-tensile strength suture. (*Courtesy of* Arthrex, Inc., Naples, FL.)

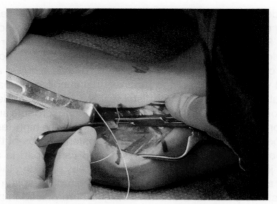

Fig. 6. Repair of the distal portion of the native UCL using the accessory high-tensile suture. One limb of the suture is passed through the anterior and then through the posterior portion of the ligament split, and the other limb is passed through the posterior portion of the ligament split and then through the anterior portion.

CLINICAL RESULTS

In 2018, Dugas and colleagues[18] reported the results of a prospective series of 66 overhead athletes undergoing UCL repair with internal brace augmentation. The

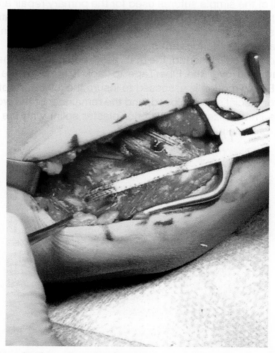

Fig. 7. The FiberTape (Arthrex, Inc., Naples, FL) is passed on top of and superficial to the native ligament, and the isometric point at the medial epicondyle is determined. (*Courtesy of* Arthrex, Inc., Naples, FL)

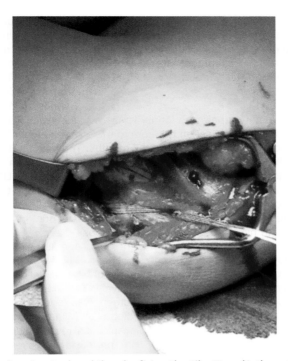

Fig. 8. The second anchor is placed thereby fixing the FiberTape (Arthrex, Inc., Naples, FL.). (*Courtesy of* Arthrex, Inc., Naples, FL.)

minimum follow-up was 1 year. Patients were indicated for repair if they had an avulsion of the proximal or distal UCL with otherwise healthy UCL tissue based on MRI appearance and had a vested interest in shortened rehab. The primary outcome measures at 1 year postop were return to play, time to return to play, and Kerlan-Jobe Orthopedic Clinic (KJOC) scores. Of the 66 overhead athletes who underwent UCL repair, 58 athletes were available for follow-up at 1 year. The average age at the time of surgery was 17.9 years. The athletes were from a variety of sports,

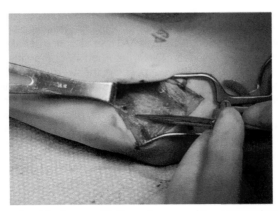

Fig. 9. The final construct is shown with the sutures used to reapproximate the native ligament tied over the InternalBrace. (*Courtesy of* Arthrex, Inc., Naples, FL.)

including 43 baseball pitchers, 8 baseball position players, 4 softball players, 2 football quarterbacks, and 1 javelin thrower. Fifty-four of 56 (93%) of those who desired to return to the same or higher level of competition were able to do so at an average of 6.1 months (range 3.2–12 months) after surgery, with 65% returning in less than 6 months. The average KJOC score was 90.2 at 1-year follow-up. The investigators reported only 1 late failure occurring more than 3 years from the index procedure.

In 2019, Dugas and colleagues[19] reported on a larger series of 111 overhead athletes undergoing primary repair with longer follow-up of 2 years. They reported that 92% (102/111) of those who desired to return to the same or higher level of competition were able to do so at a mean time of 6.7 months. The mean KJOC score at final follow-up was reported as 88.2. They concluded that UCL repair with augmentation is a reasonable option for amateur overhead throwers with selected UCL injuries and that such a surgical technique offered predictable results and a shorter time to return to sports than traditional UCL reconstruction.

Paletta and colleagues (Paletta GA, Milner J. Outcomes of primary repair of the ulanr collateral ligament in high school and college baseball players. Submitted to Am J Sports Med 2020.) have reported on a series of 78 college and high school throwers at a minimum follow-up of 2 years. The average age was 19.9 years (range 15.3–22.7). They reported 74 of 78 (94%) returned to the same or higher level of competition were able at a mean time of 7.5 months postoperatively. The mean KJOC score at final follow-up was reported as 90.4. No revision surgery was required.

Another series by Paletta and colleagues (Paletta GA, Milner, J. Primary repair of ulnar collateral injury in professional baseball players: initial results. Submitted to Orthop J Sports Med 2020.) reported the results in 17 professional players at minimum of 1 year and an average of 27 months postop. In this group, 15 of 17 (88%) were able to return to the same or higher level of play. No advanced performance metrics were used to assess return to the same level of performance. Two athletes required revision surgery with conversion to UCL reconstruction. One athlete had an initial distal injury. Late in his return to throwing program, he suffered reinjury with a tear of the proximal portion of the ligament. The second athlete had continued complaints of pain despite what seemed to be an intact repair. He was ultimately revised to a reconstruction based on an inability to return to throwing due to continued pain. Both athletes returned to the same level of play.

Primary repair has also been used in other groups of athletes including wrestlers and gymnasts. We report here a series of 16 high school and college wrestlers who underwent primary repair of the UCL. These athletes all suffered acute traumatic complete tears of the UCL with extension to the anterior capsule. This injury pattern was more severe than that typically seen in the thrower. All had evidence of valgus laxity or instability of the elbow. Fifteen of sixteen (94%) returned to competitive wrestling at an average of 6.25 months postop. At 1-year post-op, the average KJOC score was 93.1.

Results in gymnasts have been less favorable. The authors report here the results of primary repair in a small series of six level 8 or higher female gymnasts. Interestingly, all 6 had proximal high-grade or complete UCL tears. All underwent standard primary repair. Only 3 of 6 (50%) were able to return to the same level of gymnasts as before injury, and it took an average of 9 months. Thus, in this select group of athletes, the authors now perform reconstruction only rather than primary repair.

SUMMARY

In summary, primary repair of the UCL using InternalBrace augmentation seems to have a predictably high rate of clinical success in properly selected patients. The ideal candidates for primary repair are generally younger athletes with high-grade avulsion type injuries of the proximal or distal portion of the ligament and without evidence of attritional or more diffuse ligament involvement. Continued long-term follow-up is necessary, but short-term results are on par with the results for traditional UCL reconstruction techniques but with shorter return to play times.

REFERENCES

1. Jobe FW, Stark H, Lombardo SJ. Reconstruction of the ulnar collateral ligament in athletes. JBoneJointSurg Am 1986;68(8):1158–63.
2. Norwood LA, Shook JA, Andrews JR. Acute medial elbow ruptures. Am J Sports Med 1981;9(1):16–9.
3. Conway JE, Jobe FW, Glousman RE, et al. Medial instability of the elbow in throwing athletes: treatment by repair or reconstruction of the ulnar collateral ligament. J BoneJointSurg Am 1992;74(1):67–83.
4. Andrews JR, Timmerman LA. Outcome of elbow surgery in professional baseball players. Am J Sports Med 1995;23(4):407–13.
5. Azar FM, Andrews JR, Wilk KE, et al. Operative treatment of ulnar collateral ligament injuries of the elbow in athletes. Am J Sports Med 2000;28(1):16–23.
6. Joyner PW, Bruce J, Hess R, et al. Magnetic resonance imaging-based classification for ulnar collateral ligament injuries of the elbow. J ShoulderElbow Surg 2016;25(10):1710–6.
7. Ford GM, Genuario J, Kinkartz J, et al. Return-to-play outcomes in professional baseball players after medial ulnar collateral ligament injuries: comparison of operative versus nonoperative treatment based on magnetic resonance imaging findings. Am J Sports Med 2016;44(3):723–8.
8. Argo D, Trenhaile SW, Savoie FH, et al. Operative treatment of ulnar collateral ligament insufficiency of the elbow in female athletes. Am J Sports Med 2006;34(3):431–7.
9. Richard MJ, Aldridge JM, Wiesler ER, et al. Traumatic valgus instability of the elbow: pathoanatomy and results of direct repair. J BoneJointSurg Am 2008;90(11):2416–22.
10. Savoie FH, Trenhaile SW, Roberts J, et al. Primary repair of ulnar collateral ligament injuries of the elbow in young athletes: a case series of injuries to the proximal and distal ends of the ligament. Am J Sports Med 2008;36(6):1066–72.
11. Mackay GM, Blyth MJ, Anthony I, et al. A review of ligament augmentation with the InternalBrace™: the surgical principle is described for the lateral ankle ligament and ACL repair in particular, and a comprehensive review of other surgical applications and techniques is presented. SurgTechnol Int 2015;26:239–55.
12. Wilson WT, Hopper GP, Byrne PA, et al. Anterior cruciate ligament repair with internal brace ligament augmentation. SurgTechnol Int 2016;29:273–8.
13. Waldrop NE 3rd, Wijdicks CA, Jansson KS, et al. Anatomic suture anchor versus the Broström technique for anterior talofibular ligament repair: a biomechanical comparison. Am J Sports Med 2012;40(11):2590–6.
14. Clanton TO, Viens NA, Campbell KJ, et al. Anterior talofibular ligament ruptures, part 2: biomechanical comparison of anterior talofibular ligament reconstruction using semitendinosus allografts with the intact ligament. Am J Sports Med 2014;42(2):412–6.
15. Clanton TO, Campbell KJ, Wilson KJ, et al. Qualitative and quantitative anatomical investigation of the lateral ankle ligaments for surgical reconstruction procedures. J BoneJointSurg Am 2014;96(12):e98.

16. Viens NA, Wijdicks CA, Campbell KJ, et al. Anterior talofibular ligament ruptures, Part 1: biomechanical comparison of the augmented Broström repair techniques with the intact anterior talofibular ligament. Am J Sports Med 2014;42(2):405–11.

17. Dugas JR, Walters BL, Beason DP, et al. Biomechanical comparison of ulnar collateral ligament repair with internal bracing versus modified jobe reconstruction. Am J Sports Med 2016;44(3):735–41.

18. Dugas JR, Looze CA, Jones CM, et al. Ulnar collateral ligament repair with internal brace augmentation in amateur overhead throwing athletes. Orthop J Sports Med 2018;6(7 suppl4):1096–102.

19. Dugas JR, Looze CA, Capogna B, et al. Ulnar collateral ligament repair with collagen-dipped fibertape augmentation in overhead-throwing athletes. Am J Sports Med 2019;47(5):1096–102.

Injuries and Conditions Affecting the Elbow Flexor/Pronator Tendons

Rami George Alrabaa, MD*, Nicholas Dantzker, MD,
Christopher S. Ahmad, MD

KEYWORDS

- Elbow • Common flexor pronator tendons • Tendinosis • Medial epicondylitis
- Rupture • Repair

KEY POINTS

- Most patients with medial epicondylitis or flexor-pronator tendon injuries can successfully be treated nonoperatively.
- Operative treatment is reserved for patients with continued symptoms despite adequate nonoperative treatment or in high-level athletes with complete rupture of the common flexor-pronator tendon.
- The physical examination and workup of patients with flexor-pronator tendon injuries should focus on related or concomitant pathologies of the medial elbow, including ulnar collateral ligament injuries, ulnar nerve compression, and the spectrum of injuries associated with valgus extension overload in overhead throwing athletes.
- Surgical treatment of flexor-pronator tendon ruptures or medial epicondylitis includes tendon debridement and reattachment, although alternate techniques have been described in the literature and report favorable functional outcomes.

 Video content accompanies this article at http://www.sportsmed.theclinics.com.

INTRODUCTION
Relevant Anatomy

A thorough understanding of elbow anatomy is critical to an accurate diagnosis in patients presenting with medial elbow pain. The bony, ligamentous, muscular, and nervous structures of the elbow are all potential sources of elbow pain, and concomitant injuries to these structures are common. The bony articulations of the elbow

Department of Orthopedic Surgery, Columbia University Medical Center, 622 West 168th Street, PH-11, New York, NY 10032, USA
* Corresponding author.
E-mail address: ra2830@cumc.columbia.edu

Clin Sports Med 39 (2020) 549–563
https://doi.org/10.1016/j.csm.2020.02.001
0278-5919/20/© 2020 Elsevier Inc. All rights reserved.
sportsmed.theclinics.com

joint include the proximal radioulnar, radiocapitellar, and ulnohumeral joints, which permit a constrained range of motion between −5° and 140° of flexion-extension and 180° of pronosupination.[1,2] The physeal anatomy of the elbow is an important consideration in the adolescent patient, as the medial epicondyle of the humerus does not fuse until late 16 to 18 years of age and is a common source of medial elbow pain in teenage overhead athletes.[3] In the skeletally mature patient, pain over the medial epicondyle is typically indicative of soft tissue injury, as it serves as the proximal origin of the ulnar collateral ligament (UCL) and the common flexor-pronator mass. The ulnar nerve travels posterior to the medial epicondyle and can also be a source of medial elbow pain either in isolation or as a concomitant pathology. Most commonly, the ulnar nerve has no branches in the brachium, giving off its first motor branches the heads of flexor carpi ulnaris (FCU).[1] Protection of the ulnar nerve is paramount during any surgical dissection around the medial elbow. The medial antebrachial cutaneous nerve (MACN), which is a direct branch off of the medial cord of the brachial plexus, is also at risk during the surgical exposure of the medial elbow and should be kept in mind as a potential etiology of medial elbow pain in the thrower.[4,5]

The muscular anatomy of the medial elbow consists of the common flexor-pronator mass, which originates from the medial epicondyle and is the confluence of 5 muscles (**Fig. 1**): pronator teres (PT), flexor carpi radialis (FCR), palmaris longus (PL), flexor digitorum superficialis (FDS), and FCU.[6] There is an additional origin of the FCU from the medial aspect of the coronoid and proximal medial ulna, giving rise to the 2 heads of the FCU. The ulnar nerve travels into the forearm between these 2 heads of the FCU, which is the most common site of ulnar nerve compression and must be addressed during ulnar nerve decompression or transposition. As the common flexor-pronator tendon crosses the ulnohumeral joint, it gives off attachments to the deeper structure of the UCL (**Fig. 2**), which together become confluent with the anteromedial joint capsule.[6] The common flexor tendons and the UCL both originate from the medial epicondyle and project distally, with the flexor tendons being oriented and traveling more anteriorly toward various insertions, while the UCL travels slightly more posteriorly to insert onto the sublime tubercle of the ulna[6]; anatomic distinctions between these 2 medial elbow structures is relevant when assessing for tenderness at specific sites to aid in diagnosis, which will be discussed in subsequent sections. In addition to its motor function in the hand and forearm, the common flexor-pronator mass functions as a dynamic stabilizer to valgus force at the elbow and is susceptible to injury from repetitive tensile stresses such as those seen in overhead throwing.[7,8] It has been suggested that the FDS and FCU are the predominant musculotendinous units responsible for this dynamic stabilization given their position directly over the UCL in elbow flexion, but biomechanical studies have published mixed results regarding this theory.[8–11]

The primary mechanism of injury to the common flexor-pronator tendons results from eccentric loading of the musculotendinous units caused by forearm pronation and wrist flexion combined with a valgus force on the elbow.[12] Pathology of the common flexor-pronator mass includes medial epicondylitis and less commonly flexor-pronator tendon avulsion or rupture. The pathology, epidemiology, clinical evaluation, and management of these tendinous pathologies will be discussed in the following sections.

Elbow Flexor-Pronator Mass Pathology

Medial epicondylitis, often referred to as golfer's elbow, is a common source of elbow pain that typically affects patients in their fourth to sixth decade of life. Although this

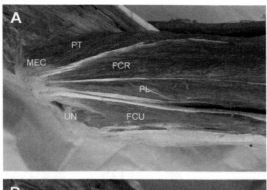

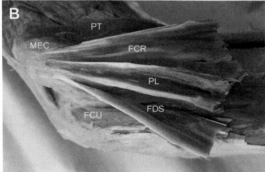

Fig. 1. Photographs A and B of a completed dissection of a cadaveric left elbow showing the ulnar nerve (UN), medial epicondyle (ME), and the muscles of the flexor-pronator mass including the pronator teres (PT), flexor carpi radialis (FCR), palmaris longus (PL), flexor digitorum superficialis (FDS), and flexor carpi ulnaris (FCU). (*From* Springer Nature: Springer Nature, Surg Radiol Anat. Otoshi K, Kikuchi S, Shishido H, Konno S: The proximal origins of the flexor-pronator muscles and their role in the dynamic stabilization of the elbow joint: An anatomic study. 2014;36[3]:289-294; with permission.)

condition is classically associated with occupational settings that require repetitive upper extremity labor, recent studies have reported an increasing incidence of medial epicondylitis among the general population.[12–15] Among athletes, medial epicondylitis is most common in overhead throwers and sports requiring repeated wrist flexion, such as baseball players, javelin throwers, weightlifters, golfers, or bowlers.[16,17] Medial epicondylitis has been reported to be 5 to 20 times less common than lateral epicondylitis.[18] In the occupational setting, medial epicondylitis affects 4% to 5% of individuals, and most these patients (80%) report self-resolving symptoms by 3 years.[19] The etiology of the condition is caused by repetitive stress and eccentric loading of the common flexor tendons, resulting in microtrauma and degeneration. Although most histologic studies focus on lateral epicondylitis, the repeated microtrauma is believed to create damage of the tendon followed by chronic ineffective healing that leads to degeneration and tendinosis.[20] High-level and professional throwing athletes can present with acute strains or ruptures of the flexor pronator mass, and these injuries have been shown to keep athletes away from sport for significant periods of time and found to be a risk factor for subsequent upper extremity injuries including UCL tears.[21] Although overhead throwing athletes may present with an acute injury resulting from avulsion or rupture of the common flexor tendon, most

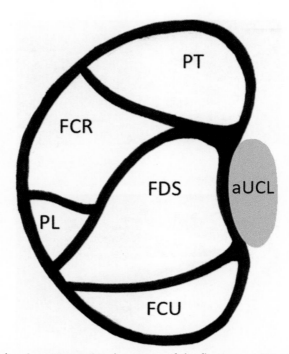

Fig. 2. Diagram showing cross-sectional anatomy of the flexor-pronator mass with the intimately associated anterior bundle of the ulnar collateral ligament (aUCL) just deep to the muscle. (*From* Springer Nature: Springer Nature, Surg Radiol Anat. Otoshi K, Kikuchi S, Shishido H, Konno S: The proximal origins of the flexor-pronator muscles and their role in the dynamic stabilization of the elbow joint: An anatomic study. 2014;36[3]:289-294; with permission.)

cases are degenerative and are characterized by gradual onset and tendinosis.[22] The clinician should keep in mind that common flexor tendon pathology is rare in a skeletally immature patient; thus alternative etiologies involving the medial epicondylar apophysis should be considered.[23] Evaluating the patient or athlete with medial elbow pain can be a diagnostic challenge, and the spectrum of potential etiologies beyond medial epicondylitis should be considered when making a diagnosis.

CLINICAL EVALUATION
History and Differential Diagnosis

When eliciting a patient history, it is important to establish the timing and acuity of symptom onset. The insidious, progressive-onset medial elbow pain without known antecedent trauma is indicative of medial epicondylitis and is typically seen in the general population, whereas the acute onset of pain following a single, distinct injury suggests a common flexor-pronator tendon rupture or avulsion and is more commonly associated with overhead athletes. Symptoms are exacerbated with activity, especially activities requiring wrist flexion and forearm protonation. The pain can radiate distally from the medial epicondyle, and patients may complain of pain with grasping or pulling heavy objects.[24] Symptoms tend to improve with rest and the use of nonsteroidal antiinflammatory drugs (NSAIDs).

Medial elbow pain in the general population or in the athlete can have several different etiologies, and the clinician should be able to differentiate between pathologies based on history, physical examination, and diagnostic imaging. Other than flexor-pronator mass injuries, possible pathologies and associated conditions of medial elbow include ulnar collateral ligament injuries, valgus extension overload, ulnar neuritis or cubital tunnel syndrome, olecranon stress fractures, and medial epicondylar apophysitis or avulsion in skeletally immature throwers. Differentiating between flexor-pronator mass injuries and UCL injuries is critical in overhead athletes, as a UCL injury rarely improves with conservative management may have more serious implications to a player's future. In contrast to patients with UCL injuries, who typically only experience symptoms during sporting activities that exert a valgus force on the elbow, patients with flexor-pronator mass injuries commonly experience symptoms even with low-demand activities and complain of pain with household activities and activities of daily life.[23] The broad differential diagnosis for medial elbow symptoms can be narrowed down further with physical examination and diagnostic imaging.

Physical Examination

Physical examination begins with inspection and assessment of range of motion in flexion-extension and in pronosupination. Mild loss of terminal extension may be present in patients with valgus extension overload and/or in asymptomatic high level throwers.[25] Landmarks about the elbow are palpated. Patients with medial epicondylitis or flexor-pronator mass avulsion injuries will be tender slightly distal (5–10 mm) to the medial epicondyle along a line orthogonal to the anterior aspect of the epicondyle.[12,23] Patients with UCL pathology will be more tender over the ligament itself, which is slightly more posterior along a line extending from the posterior aspect of the epicondyle (**Fig. 3**). The moving valgus stress test should be performed when a UCL injury is suspected and has been reported to have 100% sensitivity with 75% specificity compared with the static valgus stress test.[26] In the authors' practice,

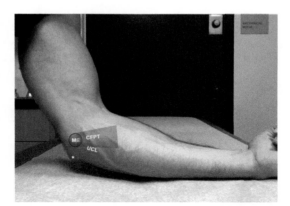

Fig. 3. Photograph of the medial aspect of a patient's left elbow showing the medial epicondyle (ME), and the paths of the common flexor pronator tendon (CFPT) and ulnar collateral ligament (UCL). Although somewhat exaggerated in this schematic, the common flexor-pronator mass tendon is slightly more anterior than the deeper and more posterior UCL. Patients with common flexor mass injuries will be tender more anteriorly, while patients with UCL injuries will be tender more posteriorly over the path of the UCL as it inserts onto the sublime tubercle of the ulna. The olecranon is depicted with the asterisk symbol (*).

the test is performed with the patient supine with the arm in 90° of abduction; a valgus force is applied to the elbow that maximally externally rotates the shoulder, and the examiner ranges the elbow in an arc of flexion-extension (**Fig. 4**). Moreover, patients with flexor-pronator mass injuries or medial epicondylitis will have reproduction of symptoms with resisted forearm protonation and wrist flexion, whereas these maneuvers may only elicit mild symptoms in the athlete with UCL pathology.[23] Patients with symptomatic olecranon osteophytes, valgus extension overload, or olecranon stress fractures will be tender to the posterior olecranon process. As mentioned previously, the throwing athlete may also have a mild flexion contracture associated with such pathology. The thrower may have a positive bounce test in which symptoms are reproduced when the elbow is rapidly brought from flexion to full extension.[27] Patients with ulnar neuritis, cubital tunnel syndrome, or subluxation of the ulnar nerve will complain of paresthesias to the ulnar digits and possibly a snapping sensation over the elbow. The clinician should evaluate for a Tinel sign along the course of the ulnar nerve from midmedial arm to midmedial forearm and assess for a subluxing ulnar nerve or a snapping triceps. As the elbow is brought throughout a range of flexion and extension, a subluxing or dislocating ulnar nerve can be palpated and sometimes visualized as it dislocates anteriorly over the medial epicondyle with flexion and reduces with elbow extension.[28] A provocative maneuver such as the elbow flexion test can be performed to assess for ulnar nerve compression at the cubital tunnel by fully flexing the elbow in combination with wrist extension, which may reproduce symptoms.[29] In advanced cases of ulnar nerve pathology with intrinsic muscle weakness, the patient may demonstrate a positive Froment sign.[30]

In summary, the physical examination for a patient with medial epicondylitis or flexor-pronator mass injury is important to rule out other concomitant pathology, more specifically any ulnar nerve pathology, and in the overhead athlete any UCL injury or pathology associated with valgus extension overload. Localizing precise

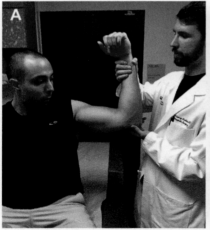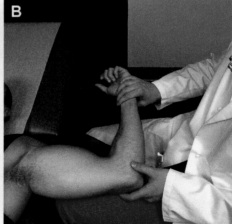

Fig. 4. (*A*) The moving valgus stress test is shown as originally described with the patient upright with the shoulder abducted to 90° and a valgus force applied to the elbow until the shoulder reaches maximal external rotation and the elbow is then extended. The examination is positive when the patient experiences pain with this maneuver. (*B*) The authors prefer to perform the moving valgus stress test with the patient supine as they are able to have more control and stabilization of the humerus as it rests on the examiner's knee.

areas of tenderness, whether over the common flexor-pronator tendons or over the UCL itself, is of great diagnostic value. In addition, examination maneuvers such as the moving valgus stress test and provocative maneuvers for ligament or nerve pathology can help in defining the diagnosis.

Imaging and Diagnostic Examinations

Plain radiographs are obtained for patients complaining of medial elbow pain mostly to rule out any bony pathology. For cases of medial epicondylitis or flexor-pronator mass injuries, standard radiographs are most often unremarkable. Calcification may be present along the medial epicondyle, common flexor tendon, or UCL.[22] Posteromedial olecranon osteophytes or loose bodies can sometimes be identified, especially in high-level throwing athletes and should be further evaluated with computed tomography (CT) scan when present.[31] Plain radiographs are also used to evaluate for olecranon stress fractures, but depending on the chronicity of the injury, the fracture may not be visualized acutely. Advanced imaging such as CT or MRI is obtained when suspecting a stress fracture. The most common olecranon stress fracture pattern observed in adult baseball players has been reported to be oblique fractures running from proximal-medial to distal-lateral.[32]

Ultrasound is a cost-effective imaging modality, but requires experienced ultrasound radiologists and technicians. A dynamic or stress ultrasound is useful to evaluate the soft tissue structures about the elbow, namely the common flexor-pronator tendon and the UCL.[33] A few clinical series have evaluated the use of sonography for the diagnosis of epicondylitis in adults, with sensitivity and specificity values ranging from 75% to over 90%.[34,35]

MRI remains the gold standard for evaluating soft tissues around the elbow and can identify pathology such as medial epicondylitis, common flexor-pronator tendon inflammation or rupture, intra-articular loose bodies, olecranon osteophytes, olecranon stress fractures, and other traumatic causes of elbow pain.[36] An MRI is obtained for overhead throwing athletes with medial elbow pain to differentiate between a flexor-pronator mass and UCL injury (**Fig. 5**). In suspected cases of ulnar nerve pathology, electromyography (EMG) and nerve conduction studies (NCS) are obtained.

MANAGEMENT
Nonoperative

First-line treatment for medial epicondylitis and common flexor-pronator tendon injuries is conservative management with nonoperative treatment, which begins with activity modification and a period of rest, followed by rehabilitation and prevention of future recurrence along with several optional modalities. Activities that require repetitive wrist flexion, forearm protonation, and valgus stress about the elbow should be avoided to alleviate the acute symptoms. Patients who experience exacerbation of acute medial elbow pain may benefit from icing the area and the use of a short course of NSAIDs, thought to reduce the synovitis associated with flexor-pronator tendon degeneration.[12,37] Activity modification and cessation of exacerbating activities such as throwing are continued for 2 to 6 weeks (athletes with concomitant UCL injury are withheld from sport for longer). Range of motion about the wrist and elbow is permitted for activities of daily living to prevent stiffness.

Splints and bracing can be trialed as a nonoperative treatment modality. Nighttime wrist splinting may be used to prevent overt wrist flexion, and elbow extension splints can also be used, especially in patients with concomitant ulnar neuritis or cubital

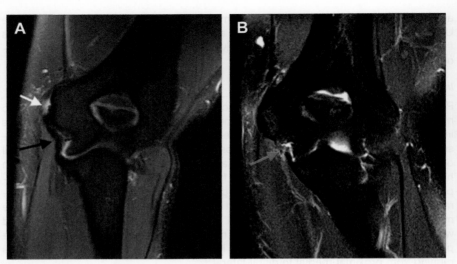

Fig. 5. (A) Coronal T2 MRI of a patient's elbow with medial epicondylitis showing inflammation at the medial epicondyle, the origin of the common flexor tendon (*white arrow*) with an intact UCL (*black arrow*). This is in contrast with the image on the right (*B*), which is a coronal T2 MRI of a patient with a UCL tear that shows a proximal tear of the UCL from its origin on the medial epicondyle (*red arrow*).

tunnel syndrome.[22] Kinesiology taping techniques that act as counterforce bracing have also been described as a treatment method for medial epicondylitis in baseball players.[38] Medial epicondyle injections consisting of corticosteroid, autologous whole blood, or platelet-rich plasma (PRP) injections have been described as well.[39–41] The injection is delivered to the peritendinous and synovial tissues rather than into the tendon itself, with care taken to avoid iatrogenic complications such as subcutaneous atrophy, tendon weakening, or nerve injury.[12] A prospective study of 60 patients with medial epicondylitis treated with corticosteroid injection noted acute improvement in pain within 6 weeks but no difference at 3 months when compared with a control group receiving saline injections.[19] Extracorporeal shock wave therapy (ESWT) has also been described to provide symptomatic relief in patients with tendinopathies, with most of the literature being in regards to the treatment of lateral epicondylitis; studies have mostly been limited to case series and small clinical trials, with mixed results and therefore inconclusive recommendations.[42–47]

After sufficient rest and acute symptoms are alleviated, rehabilitation and physical therapy begin with regaining painless range of motion followed by strengthening exercises and gradual return to sport or activities. Therapy for range of motion consists of wrist and elbow nonweight-bearing exercises and self-directed stretching techniques. Shoulder range-of-motion exercises are also implemented, especially in the throwing athlete to maintain adequate shoulder motion. Eccentric contraction of the flexor-pronator mass is avoided during this stage of rehabilitation to avoid excess stress on the tendon. Once painless range of motion is achieved, strengthening begins with isometric exercises. Increasing resistance and repetitions are implemented until strength is equal to preinjury levels.[24] Shoulder, core, and lower body strengthening exercises are also emphasized in the throwing athlete during rehabilitation.[12] No specific guidelines or protocols exist in terms of return to sport for athletes, although a progressive return to sport has been suggested once the athlete is tolerating eccentric resistance exercises.[22,48]

Operative

Most patients with medial epicondylitis can be successfully treated nonoperatively. Surgical treatment should be reserved for the subset of patients with persistent symptoms for over 6 months despite nonoperative treatment, or athletes with frank rupture of the flexor-pronator tendon. Surgical treatment for rupture of the flexor-pronator tendon is open repair, and that for medial epicondylitis is open debridement and repair of the tendon. The same technique may be applied for both pathologies. Successful arthroscopic debridement has been described for lateral epicondylitis,[49–51] but given the proximity of the ulnar nerve to the medial epicondyle, arthroscopic treatment of medial epicondylitis has been limited.[24,52]

The standard of surgical treatment remains open debridement and repair with or without microfracture of the medial epicondyle, with care taken to protect the medial antebrachial cutaneous nerve (MACN), the ulnar nerve, and the UCL, which is just deep to the common flexor-pronator tendon. Good-to-excellent results have been reported with open debridement and repair in greater than 90% of patients, with most athletes being able to return to sport to their previous level of play.[53,54] Most commonly, repair of the tendon to the medial epicondyle consists of transosseous suture repair. Suture anchor repair of the common flexor-pronator tendon has also been described with excellent functional outcomes in patients with recalcitrant medial epicondylitis.[54,55] Cho and colleagues[56] described a technique for the treatment of medial epicondylitis that involves a small 1.5 cm incision, resection of the common flexor mass, and microfracture of the medial epicondyle to promote healing, without reattachment of the tendon to create an enclosed hematoma for healing. This mini-open technique does not allow for visualization of the ulnar nerve and therefore cannot be performed if concomitant ulnar nerve pathology exists, which would need to be addressed in the form of decompression or transposition. Kwon and colleagues[57] described a fascial elevation and tendon origin resection for the treatment of medial epicondylitis. In their technique, the anterior portion of the tendon origin is excised in order to avoid iatrogenic injury to the UCL, and no tendon reattachment is performed; the authors report 90% patient satisfaction with this technique.

Concomitant medial elbow pathology, namely ulnar nerve compression, should be also addressed at the time of surgery. Preoperative workup including a thorough physical examination and EMG is required for evaluation of ulnar nerve pathology when managing medial epicondylitis or flexor-pronator mass injuries. Surgical treatment of cubital tunnel syndrome with in situ decompression or transposition is performed at the time of surgical debridement and repair of the common flexor tendon. Authors have reported poorer outcomes after surgery in patients with both ulnar neuropathy and medial epicondylitis compared with patients who have medial epicondylitis alone.[58,59] Gong and colleagues[60] described a surgical technique for the treatment of patients who have medial epicondylitis with concomitant ulnar neuritis with excellent outcomes in all patients in their cohort. In this alternative technique, the ulnar nerve is decompressed from proximal to the cubital tunnel up to the 2 heads of the FCU. A Z-lengthening of the flexor-pronator mass is then made so that the proximal flap that contains the FCU remains attached to the medial epicondyle while the distal flap is translated distally and repaired. The ulnar nerve is transposed so that it rests over the brachialis. Overhead throwing athletes can also have UCL injuries in addition to flexor-pronator mass injuries; authors have identified this subset of athletes and noted worse prognosis in these players.[61]

Most commonly, surgical treatment for medial epicondylitis involves open debride-ment and tendon repair. Postoperatively, patients are usually immobilized for a short period of time for wound healing. Rehabilitation begins with range-of-motion exercises at 1 to 2 weeks postoperatively followed by initiation of strengthening exercises at 6 to 8 weeks. Athletes can return to sport-specific exercises and training after 3 months postoperatively.[24]

AUTHORS' PREFERRED SURGICAL TECHNIQUE

The authors prefer their technique of open debridement and tendon repair for the surgical treatment of medial epicondylitis or complete flexor-pronator tendon rup-tures (Video 1). An open technique allows for identification and protection of the ulnar nerve and for concomitant ulnar nerve decompression or transposition if required.

Patient Positioning and Surgical Exposure

The patient is positioned supine with the operative extremity on a hand table. A non-sterile tourniquet is placed on the proximal arm, and the extremity is cleaned and draped in a standard sterile fashion. The medial epicondyle and the proposed skin incision centered just anterior to the medial epicondyle are outlined (**Fig. 6**A). After limb exsanguination with an elastic bandage and tourniquet inflation, an 8 to 10 cm curvilinear incision is made centered over the medial epicondyle. Dissection is carried down the subcutaneous tissue with particular attention to identify the medial antebra-chial cutaneous nerve branches, which are mobilized and protected (**Fig. 6**B). Next, the common flexor tendon is outlined between the flexor carpi ulnaris and the pronator teres (**Fig. 6**C). The tendon is incised along this U-shaped incision and elevated from its origin onto the medial epicondyle while avoiding injury to the UCL. The common

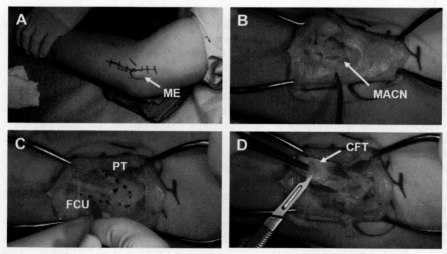

Fig. 6. Patient is positioned supine with the right upper extremity on a hand table. (*A*) The medial epicondyle (ME) and proposed skin incision are outlined. (*B*) The medial antebrachial cutaneous nerve (MACN) is identified and protected during subcutaneous dissection. (*C*) The fascial incision for the common flexor tendon is outlined between the pronator teres (PT) and the flexor carpi ulnaris (FCU). (*D*) The degenerative tissue just deep to the tendon is sharply excised.

flexor tendon is reflected, revealing the degenerative tissue and tendinosis (**Fig. 6D**). The tendinotic tissue is sharply excised.

Bony Preparation and Tendon Repair

Two bone tunnels are then made in the medial epicondyle with a 0.045 mm Kirschner wire (K-wire), while care is taken to protect and avoid the ulnar nerve (**Fig. 7A, B**). The bone tunnels are created with a 5 mm bone bridge, with 1 tunnel more superior and another more posterior in the orientation of the common flexor tendon. A Number 0 nonabsorbable suture is passed from posterior to anterior through each bone tunnel (**Fig. 7C**). A separate suture is then sewn through the substance of each suture limb that was passed through the bone tunnels (**Fig. 7D**). This effectively creates 3 suture limbs available to be shuttled for each tunnel (**Fig. 7E**), yielding a total of 6 suture limbs available for the repair. Small perforations in the bone are then made with a K-wire to create a vascular bed for tendon healing (**Fig. 7F**). All 6 sutures are then passed in simple fashion through the common flexor tendon in order to repair and compress it to its footprint (**Fig. 8A**). The 3 suture limbs from the posterior tunnel are passed more posteriorly through the tendon, and the 3 suture limbs from the anterior tunnel are passed

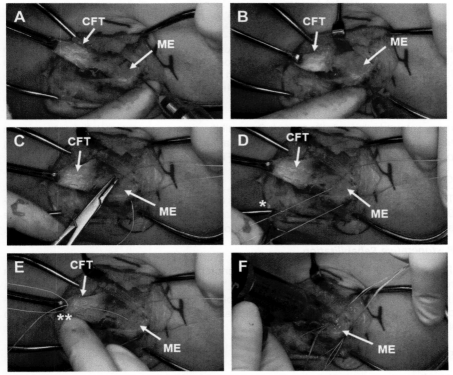

Fig. 7. Two bone tunnels are created through the medial epicondyle (ME) with a 0.045 mm Kirschner wire, 1 more posteriorly (*A*) and the other more anteriorly (*B*). (*C*) A Number 0 nonabsorbable suture is passed from posterior to anterior through each bone tunnel. (*D*) * A new Number 0 nonabsorbable suture is sewn through the substance of each suture that was already passed through the bone tunnel therefore creating 3 suture strands arising from each bone tunnel ** (*E*). (*F*) Small perforations in the medial epicondyle are made with a Kirschner wire to prepare the footprint for healing. CFT, common flexor tendon.

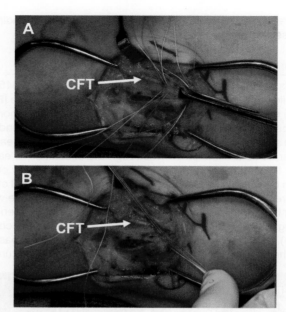

Fig. 8. (*A*) The 3 posterior limbs are passed posteriorly through the common flexor tendon (CFT), and the other 3 limbs are passed anteriorly in simple fashion to restore the tendon to its footprint. (*B*) The limb strands are first tied to themselves, then adjacent limbs in a criss-crossing pattern to compress the tendon to the medial epicondyle.

more anteriorly through the tunnel. Once all the sutures are passed, the sutures from each limb are tied to themselves, then to adjacent suture limbs to create a crossing pattern to compress the tendon to bone (**Fig. 8**B).

Closure and Immobilization

The fascial incision and deep dermal layers are sequentially closed with absorbable 3-0 suture, followed by a running subcuticular layer with 4-0 absorbable suture for the skin. The patient is immobilized in a posterior plaster splint at 70° of flexion for 10 days.

Postoperative Rehabilitation

The patient is initially placed in a posterior plaster splint postoperatively that is removed at the first postoperative visit in 10 to 14 days and then transitioned to a hinged elbow brace that allows for range of motion as tolerated. Strengthening exercises are started at 6 to 8 weeks postoperatively, with return to full activity at 3 to 4 months.

SUPPLEMENTARY DATA

Supplementary data related to this article can be found online at https://doi.org/10.1016/j.csm.2020.02.001.

REFERENCES

1. Morrey B. Anatomy of the elbow joint. In: Morrey B, Sanchez-Sotelo J, editors. The elbow and its disorders. Philadelphia: Saunders Elsevier; 2009. p. 39–63.

2. An K, Zobitz M, Morrey B. Biomechanics of the elbow. In: Morrey B, Sanchez-Sotelo J, editors. The elbow and its disorders. Philadelphia: Saunders Elsevier; 2009. p. 246–67.

3. Smucny M, Kolmodin J, Saluan P. Shoulder and elbow injuries in the adolescent athlete. Sports Med Arthrosc Rev 2016;24(4):188–94.

4. Masear VR, Meyer RD, Pichora DR. Surgical anatomy of the medial antebrachial cutaneous nerve. J Hand Surg Am 1989;14(2 Pt 1):267–71.

5. Cesmebasi A, O'Driscoll SW, Smith J, et al. The snapping medial antebrachial cutaneous nerve. Clin Anat 2015;28(7):872–7.

6. Otoshi K, Kikuchi S, Shishido H, et al. The proximal origins of the flexor-pronator muscles and their role in the dynamic stabilization of the elbow joint: an anatomical study. Surg Radiol Anat 2014;36(3):289–94.

7. Lin F, Kohli N, Perlmutter S, et al. Muscle contribution to elbow joint valgus stability. J Shoulder Elbow Surg 2007;16(6):795–802.

8. Park MC, Ahmad CS. Dynamic contributions of the flexor-pronator mass to elbow valgus stability. J Bone Joint Surg Am 2004;86(10):2268–74.

9. Davidson PA, Pink M, Perry J, et al. Functional anatomy of the flexor pronator muscle group in relation to the medial collateral ligament of the elbow. Am J Sports Med 1995;23(2):245–50.

10. Udall JH, Fitzpatrick MJ, McGarry MH, et al. Effects of flexor-pronator muscle loading on valgus stability of the elbow with an intact, stretched, and resected medial ulnar collateral ligament. J Shoulder Elbow Surg 2009;18(5):773–8.

11. Hamilton CD, Glousman RE, Jobe FW, et al. Dynamic stability of the elbow: electromyographic analysis of the flexor pronator group and the extensor group in pitchers with valgus instability. J Shoulder Elbow Surg 1996;5(5):347–54.

12. Amin NH, Kumar NS, Schickendantz MS. Medial epicondylitis: evaluation and management. J Am Acad Orthop Surg 2015;23(6):348–55.

13. Descatha A, Leclerc A, Chastang JF, et al. Medial epicondylitis in occupational settings: prevalence, incidence and associated risk factors. J Occup Environ Med 2003;45(9):993–1001.

14. Ritz BR. Humeral epicondylitis among gas- and waterworks employees. Scand J Work Environ Health 1995;21(6):478–86.

15. Wiggins AJ, Cancienne JM, Camp CL, et al. Disease burden of medial epicondylitis in the USA is increasing: an analysis of 19,856 patients from 2007 to 2014. HSS J 2018;14(3):233–7.

16. Patel RM, Lynch TS, Amin NH, et al. The thrower's elbow. Orthop Clin North Am 2014;45(3):355–76.

17. Leach RE, Miller JK. Lateral and medial epicondylitis of the elbow. Clin Sports Med 1987;6(2):259–72.

18. Ciccotti MG, Charlton WP. Epicondylitis in the athlete. Clin Sports Med 2001; 20(1):77–93.

19. Stahl S, Kaufman T. The efficacy of an injection of steroids for medial epicondylitis. A prospective study of sixty elbows. J Bone Joint Surg Am 1997;79(11): 1648–52.

20. Regan W, Wold LE, Coonrad R, et al. Microscopic histopathology of chronic refractory lateral epicondylitis. Am J Sports Med 1992;20(6):746–9.

21. Hodgins JL, Trofa DP, Donohue S, et al. Forearm flexor injuries among major league baseball players: epidemiology, performance, and associated injuries. Am J Sports Med 2018;46(9):2154–60.

22. Ciccotti MG, Ramani MN. Medial epicondylitis. Tech Hand Up Extrem Surg 2003; 7(4):190–6.

23. Pearce McCarty L 3rd. Approach to medial elbow pain in the throwing athlete. Curr Rev Musculoskelet Med 2019;12(1):30–40.

24. Petkovic D, Shiu B, Ahmad C. Epicondylitis and baseball players. In: Ahmad C, Romeo A, editors. Baseball sports medicine. Philadelphia: Wolters Kluwer; 2019. p. 66–84.

25. King JW, Brelsford HJ, Tullos HS. Analysis of the pitching arm of the professional baseball pitcher. Clin Orthop Relat Res 1969;67:116–23.

26. O'Driscoll SW, Lawton RL, Smith AM. The "moving valgus stress test" for medial collateral ligament tears of the elbow. Am J Sports Med 2005;33(2):231–9.

27. Wilson FD, Andrews JR, Blackburn TA, et al. Valgus extension overload in the pitching elbow. Am J Sports Med 1983;11(2):83–8.

28. Childress HM. Recurrent ulnar-nerve dislocation at the elbow. Clin Orthop Relat Res 1975;108:168–73.

29. Buehler MJ, Thayer DT. The elbow flexion test. A clinical test for the cubital tunnel syndrome. Clin Orthop Relat Res 1988;233:213–6.

30. Staples JR, Calfee R. Cubital tunnel syndrome: current concepts. J Am Acad Orthop Surg 2017;25(10):e215–24.

31. Ahmad CS, ElAttrache NS. Valgus extension overload syndrome and stress injury of the olecranon. Clin Sports Med 2004;23(4):665–76, x.

32. Paci JM, Dugas JR, Guy JA, et al. Cannulated screw fixation of refractory olecranon stress fractures with and without associated injuries allows a return to baseball. Am J Sports Med 2013;41(2):306–12.

33. Ciccotti MG, Atanda A Jr, Nazarian LN, et al. Stress sonography of the ulnar collateral ligament of the elbow in professional baseball pitchers: a 10-year study. Am J Sports Med 2014;42(3):544–51.

34. Park GY, Lee SM, Lee MY. Diagnostic value of ultrasonography for clinical medial epicondylitis. Arch Phys Med Rehabil 2008;89(4):738–42.

35. Lee MH, Cha JG, Jin W, et al. Utility of sonographic measurement of the common tensor tendon in patients with lateral epicondylitis. AJR Am J Roentgenol 2011; 196(6):1363–7.

36. Kheterpal AB, Bredella MA. Overuse Injuries of the Elbow. Radiol Clin North Am 2019;57(5):931–42.

37. Walz DM, Newman JS, Konin GP, et al. Epicondylitis: pathogenesis, imaging, and treatment. Radiographics 2010;30(1):167–84.

38. Chang HY, Wang CH, Chou KY, et al. Could forearm kinesio taping improve strength, force sense, and pain in baseball pitchers with medial epicondylitis? Clin J Sport Med 2012;22(4):327–33.

39. Hechtman KS, Uribe JW, Botto-vanDemden A, et al. Platelet-rich plasma injection reduces pain in patients with recalcitrant epicondylitis. Orthopedics 2011; 34(2):92.

40. Mishra A, Pavelko T. Treatment of chronic elbow tendinosis with buffered platelet-rich plasma. Am J Sports Med 2006;34(11):1774–8.

41. Suresh SPS, Ali KE, Jones H, et al. Medial epicondylitis: is ultrasound guided autologous blood injection an effective treatment? Br J Sports Med 2006; 40(11):935–9.

42. Lee SS, Kang S, Park NK, et al. Effectiveness of initial extracorporeal shock wave therapy on the newly diagnosed lateral or medial epicondylitis. Ann Rehabil Med 2012;36(5):681–7.

43. Sems A, Dimeff R, Iannotti JP. Extracorporeal shock wave therapy in the treatment of chronic tendinopathies. J Am Acad Orthop Surg 2006;14(4):195–204.

44. Guler NS, Sargin S, Sahin N. Efficacy of extracorporeal shockwave therapy in patients with lateral epicondylitis: A randomized, placebo-controlled, double-blind clinical trial. North Clin Istanb 2018;5(4):314–8.

45. Aydin A, Atic R. Comparison of extracorporeal shock-wave therapy and wrist-extensor splint application in the treatment of lateral epicondylitis: a prospective randomized controlled study. J Pain Res 2018;11:1459–67.

46. Stasinopoulos D. Can extracorporeal shock-wave therapy be used for the management of lateral elbow tendinopathy? World J Methodol 2018;8(3):37–9.

47. Krischek O, Hopf C, Nafe B, et al. Shock-wave therapy for tennis and golfer's elbow–1 year follow-up. Arch Orthop Trauma Surg 1999;119(1–2):62–6.

48. Hoogvliet P, Randsdorp MS, Dingemanse R, et al. Does effectiveness of exercise therapy and mobilisation techniques offer guidance for the treatment of lateral and medial epicondylitis? A systematic review. Br J Sports Med 2013;47(17):1112–9.

49. Stiefel EC, Field LD. Arthroscopic lateral epicondylitis release using the "bayonet" technique. Arthrosc Tech 2014;3(1):e135–9.

50. Byram IR, Kim HM, Levine WN, et al. Elbow arthroscopic surgery update for sports medicine conditions. Am J Sports Med 2013;41(9):2191–202.

51. Moradi A, Pasdar P, Mehrad-Majd H, et al. Clinical outcomes of open versus arthroscopic surgery for lateral epicondylitis, evidence from a systematic review. Arch Bone Jt Surg 2019;7(2):91–104.

52. do Nascimento AT, Claudio GK. Arthroscopic surgical treatment of medial epicondylitis. J Shoulder Elbow Surg 2017;26(12):2232–5.

53. Vangsness CT Jr, Jobe FW. Surgical treatment of medial epicondylitis. Results in 35 elbows. J Bone Joint Surg Br 1991;73(3):409–11.

54. Vinod AV, Ross G. An effective approach to diagnosis and surgical repair of refractory medial epicondylitis. J Shoulder Elbow Surg 2015;24(8):1172–7.

55. Grawe BM, Fabricant PD, Chin CS, et al. Clinical outcomes after suture anchor repair of recalcitrant medial epicondylitis. Orthopedics 2016;39(1):e104–7.

56. Cho BK, Kim YM, Kim DS, et al. Mini-open muscle resection procedure under local anesthesia for lateral and medial epicondylitis. Clin Orthop Surg 2009;1(3):123–7.

57. Kwon BC, Kwon YS, Bae KJ. The fascial elevation and tendon origin resection technique for the treatment of chronic recalcitrant medial epicondylitis. Am J Sports Med 2014;42(7):1731–7.

58. Gabel GT, Morrey BF. Operative treatment of medial epicondylitis - influence of concomitant ulnar neuropathy at the elbow. J Bone Joint Surg Am 1995;77a(7):1065–9.

59. Kurvers H, Verhaar J. The results of operative treatment of medial epicondylitis. J Bone Joint Surg Am 1995;77(9):1374–9.

60. Gong HS, Chung MS, Kang ES, et al. Musculofascial lengthening for the treatment of patients with medial epicondylitis and coexistent ulnar neuropathy. J Bone Joint Surg Br 2010;92(6):823–7.

61. Osbahr DC, Swaminathan SS, Allen AA, et al. Combined flexor-pronator mass and ulnar collateral ligament injuries in the elbows of older baseball players. Am J Sports Med 2010;38(4):733–9.

Sprains, Strains, and Partial Tears of the Medial Ulnar Collateral Ligament of the Elbow

Felix H. Savoie III, MD*, Michael O'Brien, MD

KEYWORDS

- Shoulder • Ligament • UCL • Sprain • Partial tear

KEY POINTS

- Strains and partial tears are more common injuries than complete tears in non- professional athletes.
- These lower grade injuries are best managed more conservatively than immediate surgery in young athletes.
- If surgery is required, repair with or without an internal brace is a much better option in non-professional athletes.

INTRODUCTION

The anterior bundle of the ulnar collateral ligament (UCL) complex is the primary stabilizer of the elbow to valgus stress from 20° to 120° of flexion,[1–8] the primary arc of motion used in overhead throwing. Isolated UCL deficiency was first identified in javelin throwers by Waris[9] in 1946, and was once thought to be a career-ending injury. The initial operative intervention for the condition involved repair of the native ligament, which was supported by Barnes and Tullos,[10] who noted that athletes with UCL injury had better clinical outcomes after repair in comparison with nonoperative treatment. Much of the current operative management of UCL deficiency is focused on symptomatic valgus instability in the high-level throwing athlete and usually requires some variation of the reconstructive procedure pioneered by Jobe in 1974 for return to play.[11–15] However, there has been a substantial increase in the number of patients sustaining a more acute form of this injury at younger ages,[16,17] for which a reconstruction may not be warranted. In contrast to elite athletes who have sustained repetitive microtrauma over years of high-level competition with resultant ligament damage through its length and secondary

Department of Orthopaedic Surgery, Tulane University. 1430 Tulane Avenue, SL-32, New Orleans, LA 70112, USA
* Corresponding author.
E-mail address: fsavoie@tulane.edu

Clin Sports Med 39 (2020) 565–574
https://doi.org/10.1016/j.csm.2020.02.007
0278-5919/20/Published by Elsevier Inc.
sportsmed.theclinics.com

pathologic changes in the elbow from chronic valgus extension overload syndrome,[11,13] the younger or acutely injured athlete can be expected to have a ligament of better quality, with isolated damage to one area, and a more biomechanically stable joint.[18–23] In these patients the injury is more likely to be a sprain or partial tear. If the tear is complete, it only involves a single area of injury at the proximal or distal end of the ligament. In these young patients nonoperative treatment can be very successful, and in most cases if surgery is needed primary repair of the UCL has proved to be a viable option, with reliable results and a quicker return to sports than the standard reconstruction.[24]

EXAMINATION AND IMAGING

In many young overhead athletes, medial elbow pain signifies an injury to the anterior band of the medial ulnar collateral ligament (MUCL). The patient may report a slow onset of pain with repetitive use of the arm or may have a history of a single "pop" followed by an inability to throw accurately or with velocity.

Examination of the athlete starts from the ground up. The patient's stance, body habitus, and resting posture are noted. A single leg squat can test hip and core strength. Hip internal and external rotation on both the plant leg and lead leg should be measured and recorded. The shoulder is evaluated with Whipple, O'Brien, and Dynamic Label Shear tests both without and then with scapular assist.

The elbow is then evaluated for alignment and motion. Tender areas are noted. It is crucial to palpate the proximal and distal ends of the MUCL, the ulnar nerve, the capitellum, and plica during the examination. Valgus and varus testing at 30°, 70°, and 90° of flexion can be compared with the opposite side. Valgus extension overload testing and moving valgus stress test may confirm the diagnosis. As described by O'Driscoll and colleagues,[25] the moving valgus stress test is performed on a patient in the upright position with the shoulder abducted to 90°, in maximal external rotation with the elbow fully flexed. The examiner then extends the elbow while applying a constant valgus load. A positive test will reproduce medial elbow pain that the patient experiences with provocative activities and should be maximal between the positions of 120° and 70° of elbow extension, correlating with the late cocking and early acceleration phases of throwing. Other physical examination findings that are usually positive include the Milk test and the valgus extension overload test.

Imaging should include standard radiographs to evaluate for bony changes, loose bodies, and osteochondritis dissecans. Standard radiographic evaluation of the elbow begins with anteroposterior, lateral, and oblique views. A true lateral view of the hyperflexed elbow or an axial olecranon view in 110° of flexion may identify posteromedial osteophytes, suggestive of a chronic valgus extension overload syndrome. Comparative stress radiographs may help identify ligamentous laxity, and a greater than 5-mm side-to-side difference may be sufficient as a diagnostic study. In younger patients, contralateral comparison views may be helpful to identify growth disturbances and variant ossification centers.

Advanced imaging is usually needed, and the authors prefer magnetic resonance arthrograms in these patients. The advanced imaging will show strains, partial tears, or complete tears and also allow an accurate assessment of the quality of the noninjured ligament.[26]

Ultrasonography can also provide an excellent image of the ligament, delineating both the area of injury and evaluating the body's response to the injury with Doppler assessment of the vascular response. Dynamic ultrasonography, performing the examination while doing a moving valgus stress test, has been shown to be an effective tool in evaluating injuries of the MUCL.

NONOPERATIVE MANAGEMENT
Sprains

In many young overhead athletes, the MUCL may only have interstitial damage (sprain) or have a small partial tear. In the first group (sprains) an aggressive form of nonoperative treatment has been reasonably successful in the authors' patients. The patient is placed in a hinged elbow brace set to allow a pain-free range of motion, usually 30° to 90° on the first visit. The patient is referred to physical therapy for leg, hip, core, scapula, and shoulder rehabilitation, maintaining the brace at all times. Once the entire body is balanced, the elbow is added to the rehabilitation. A full, pain-free range of motion must be achieved before the patient is allowed to start a return to hit and throw program in the brace, usually 3 to 4 weeks. As this progresses and the instability examination normalizes negative, the brace is discontinued and the patient is allowed to return to full sports. The entire recovery time from a sprain is usually 6 to 8 weeks.

Partial Tears

Partial MUCL tears can also be managed nonoperatively with a program similar to that for MUCL sprains. In these cases, supplementation with biologics is also discussed. The authors have previously published results on the use of leukocyte-rich platelet-

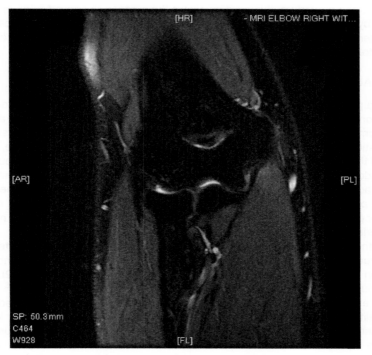

Fig. 1. MRI of post-PRP UCL showing complete reconstitution.

rich plasma (PRP) (Harvest; Terumo BCT, Lakewood, CO), which produced excellent healing in both proximal and distal partial tears (**Fig. 1**).[27]

In these cases, the history and imaging confirm a partial tear and its location. PRP injections are offered as an option to add to the nonoperative treatment. A series of 2 injections 2 weeks apart are administered while continuing the physical therapy and bracing program described for sprains. A "study" MRI of a few coronal cuts is performed 2 to 4 weeks after the second PRP and thereafter, dynamic ultrasonography is used to monitor the status of the ligament. The brace is continued for a minimum of 6 weeks and the usual return to play without the brace is 12 weeks. The program has allowed successful return to play in 85% of injured athletes with partial MUCL tears.

INDICATIONS AND CONTRAINDICATIONS FOR SURGICAL REPAIR

Indication for surgery is the presence of a significant proximal or distal tear in an older (age >15 years) athlete. Contraindications include ligaments with midsubstance injuries, evidence of damage over an extended length of the ligament, and a ligament of general poor quality with calcifications or defects noted on MRI or ultrasonography. In these cases, a standard graft reconstruction procedure is required.

PATIENT POSITIONING IN SURGERY

For the authors' UCL repair protocol, preference is to place the patient in the standard prone arthroscopy position with the shoulder abducted to 90° and the elbow flexed to 90° over a block. This position eliminates the need for traction, allows for easier intraoperative manipulation of the elbow, permits access to the posterior aspect of the joint, and affords a more stable position to the elbow.[28] Following the arthroscopic portion of the procedure, this position allows the surgeon to convert to an open procedure by internally rotating the shoulder and placing the hand on an arm board near the patient's hip, exposing the medial side of the elbow while providing a constant varus stress for the repair.

SURGICAL TECHNIQUE

With the patient in the prone arthroscopy position already described, a thorough examination under anesthesia is performed to evaluate the elbow for instability and motion, comparing the injured elbow with the opposite, uninjured side. A standard diagnostic arthroscopy is then performed to evaluate the articular cartilage, specifically of the capitellum and the posterolateral plica. Although rare in these young athletes, additional pathologic features including loose bodies and ulnohumeral spurs can be addressed if present. The arthroscopic stress test of Field and Altchek[29] can also be performed at this time, which produced positive findings of medial opening 3 mm or greater in all of the authors' 60 patients investigated in a previously reported case series on MUCL repair.[24]

With the arthroscopic portion of the case complete, the surgery is converted to an open procedure with the arm positioning change already described. A skin incision is made on the tip of the medial epicondyle and extended distally 5 cm (**Fig. 2**). A pronator muscle-splitting approach as described by Smith and colleagues[15] is then used to expose the UCL (**Fig. 3**A–C). The outer surface of the UCL is evaluated for tissue quality and the location of the tear (see **Fig. 3**A). Depending on the tear location and extent, a longitudinal incision is then made along either the anterior border (for a simple repair) or in the middle (for a repair + internal brace [Arthrex, Naples, FL]) of the MUCL and the remainder of the ligament inspected (see **Fig. 3**B).

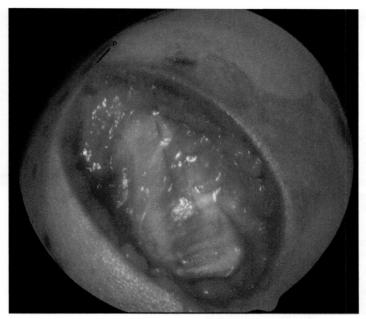

Fig. 2. Initial approach to the MUCL showing the flexor pronator fascia.

If a simple partial humeral avulsion is encountered, the bone in the area of the origin of the UCL from the distal, lateral aspect of the medial epicondyle and adjacent trochlea is lightly debrided and rasped. Angling toward the olecranon fossa, a double-loaded suture anchor is then placed at the apex of the "V" formed by the junction of the trochlea and medial epicondyle. The sutures are passed in horizontal mattress configuration through the most proximal area of the undamaged ligament: one set at the proximal end of the normal ligamentous tissue and one set 5 mm distal to the first mattress stitch (see **Fig. 3C**). Each set of mattress sutures is placed at the anterior and posterior aspect of the ligament (**Fig. 4**, completed MUCL repair). One should be aware of the position of the ulnar nerve adjacent to the posterior edge of the MUCL. In most cases, it is safe to expose the nerve and retract it at the level of the suture passage to prevent inadvertent injury. Alternatively, direct suture repair without anchors can be accomplished proximally by placing convergent drill holes from the medial tip of the epicondyle and the origin site of the UCL. The drill holes are then connected with a curved Keith needle, and the suture is shuttled from the origin site through the medial hole. Care must be taken not to tether the ulnar nerve along the posterior aspect of the ligament with sutures.

In the more complex injuries (usually the ones requiring surgery), the authors have adopted a more solid repair based on the work of Dugas's group.[30] In these cases, once the ligament is exposed and the proximal injury is evaluated, a longitudinal incision is made in the middle of the MUCL to evaluate the rest of the ligament. If the ligament is of good quality, the first anchor of the internal brace is inserted into the anatomic origin of the MUCL on the medial epicondyle. The drill hole for the second anchor, placed 1 to 2 mm distal to the insertion site on the sublime tubercle, is also made at this time because the joint is exposed and intra-articular placement can be avoided. The suture attached to the first anchor is then passed through the ligament distal to the tear and the injury repaired. Two plication stitches are used to close the

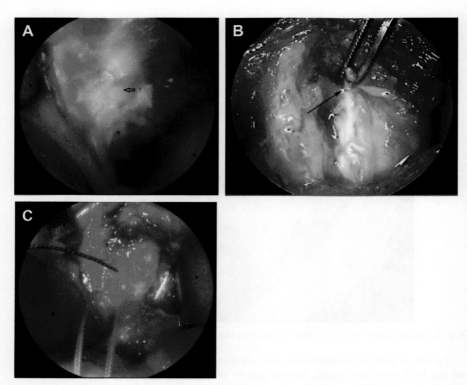

Fig. 3. (*A*) On initial exposure of the medial ulnar collateral ligament (MUCL), a visual in-spection of the ligament may reveal the tear, here in the proximal ligament (T). The flexor pronator muscles are split, held apart by the 2 army-navy retractors (R). The distal part of the ligament is normal (N). (*B*) The view of the MUCL after a longitudinal split to further assess the amount of damage to the ligament. The forceps are holding a small fragment of the bone of the origin site that was avulsed as part of the injury. (*C*) The MUCL with initial su-tures used in the repair (T, tear; R, retractor) passing through the edge of the tear (*green stitch*) and through the normal ligament (*purple stitch*).

split in the ligament. The second anchor for the internal brace is then placed with 15.5 to 16 mm of "extra" tape to accommodate the depth of the tunnel and prevent over-tensioning into the distal drill hole. One extra absorbable suture is used to stabilize the midportion of the fibertape (**Fig. 5**).

In the case of distal avulsions, the first anchor of the internal brace is placed directly into the sublime tubercle or 1 to 2 mm distal to it and angled away from the joint to avoid violating the ulnohumeral joint. The sutures are passed through the most distal aspect of the undamaged ligament in a way similar to that used for the proximal su-tures, with the same precautions regarding the ulnar nerve.

The ligament is then tensioned and tied. The elbow is taken through a complete range of motion to evaluate the isometrics of the repair.[24]

POSTOPERATIVE PROTOCOL

The elbow is immobilized in a posterior slab splint at 90° of flexion for 1 week. Active range of motion is started at 1 week in a hinged brace set at 30° to 90° and increased 10° in each direction until full motion is achieved. Physical therapy focused on the hip,

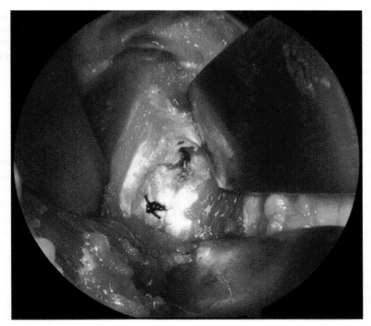

Fig. 4. Completed UCL repair with all sutures in place.

core, and scapula is started at this time. At 3 to 4 weeks, strengthening exercises for the wrist, forearm, and rotator cuff are added to the core program while maintaining the brace on the elbow at all times. Patients are started on an activity-specific program at 6 weeks. At this time, plyometrics are incorporated along with sport-specific activity

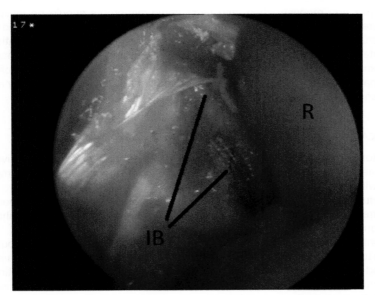

Fig. 5. The internal brace has been added to complete the repair of the MUCL: IB, internal brace; R, retractor.

in the brace. Throwing and hitting are initiated at between 8 and 12 weeks in the brace depending on shoulder posture, scapular position, and core strength, and progressed as tolerated provided there is no pain over the repaired UCL. The sport-specific rehabilitation is continued without the brace beginning at 12 weeks and continued until full activity is achieved, usually by 16 to 24 weeks.[24]

RESULTS

Historically, surgical repair of the UCL after failed nonoperative management has produced varied results. However, in the appropriately selected patient, repair of the ligament in the absence of secondary pathologic changes can produce a reliable result and allow a more rapid return to sports in comparison with standard reconstruction. In a recent case series, 60 patients younger than 22 years with symptomatic valgus instability of the elbow underwent MUCL repair after failing nonoperative management. Overall, 93% of the patients achieved good to excellent results according to the Andrews-Carson elbow outcome score, and 56 (93%) of the 60 patients returned to sports within 6 months at the same or higher level of competition. Four patients were considered to have failures based on their functional results and Andrews-Carson rating scale.[24] A similar study by Richard and colleagues[31] reported comparable success.

Recently, the authors reviewed their first series of UCL repairs with added internal bracing. Forty-nine of 50 (98%) patients returned to the same or higher level of play by 18 weeks after surgery. Only one did not return to play (Savoie and colleagues, unpublished data).

POTENTIAL COMPLICATIONS

Ulnar nerve neuropraxia has been shown to be a common complication following both UCL repair and reconstruction, and ulnar nerve symptoms should be evaluated if discovered preoperatively. Most often, the symptoms are transient and related to sensory disturbances in the distribution of the ulnar nerve. Rarely this complication may necessitate a neurolysis or transposition procedure, and postoperative ulnar nerve symptoms are not likely to affect the outcome.[13,24,32] Postoperative arthrofibrosis, which may require prolonged therapy and/or additional arthroscopic capsular release, has been shown to occur.[24]

TECHNICAL PEARLS

1. Do not operate too soon: These patients may respond well to conservative management of bracing, rest, periscapular and core strengthening, and improved throwing mechanics.
2. Carefully examine the ligament on preoperative imaging and on direct inspection to ensure that it is adequate for repair. If there is any doubt, a reconstruction should be performed.
3. The internal brace has been a wonderful addition to the repair, enabling young athletes to return to sport more rapidly than with reconstruction. If the results are maintained for 5 to 10 years, this may well prove to be superior to reconstruction.
4. Careful attention must be paid to the location of the ulnar nerve to avoid vigorous retraction or tethering with sutures. In patients with a preoperative Tinel sign or ulnar nerve subluxation, many authors recommend a transposition.

DISCLOSURE

The authors have nothing to disclose.

REFERENCES

1. An K, Morrey BF, Chao EYS. The effect of partial removal of proximal ulna on elbow constraint. Clin Orthop Relat Res 1986;209:270–9.
2. Andrews JR, Heggland EJ, Fleisig GS, et al. Relationship of ulnar collateral ligament strain to amount of medial olecranon osteotomy. Am J Sports Med 2001;29: 716–21.
3. Morrey BF, An KN. Articular and ligamentous contributions to the stability of the elbow. Am J Sports Med 1983;11:315–9.
4. Morrey BF, An KN. Functional anatomy of the ligaments of the elbow. Clin Orthop Relat Res 1985;201:84–90.
5. Morrey BF, Tanaka S, An K. Valgus stability of the elbow: a definition of primary and secondary constraints. Clin Orthop Relat Res 1991;265:187–95.
6. Regan WD, Korinek SL, Morrey BF, et al. Biomechanical study of ligaments around the elbow joint. Clin Orthop Relat Res 1991;271:170–9.
7. Schwab GH, Bennett JB, Woods GW, et al. Biomechanics of elbow instability: the role of the medial collateral ligament. Clin Orthop Relat Res 1980;146:42–52.
8. Sojbjerg JO, Ovesen J, Nielsen S. Experimental elbow instability after transaction of the medial collateral ligament. Clin Orthop Relat Res 1987;218:186–90.
9. Waris W. Elbow injuries of javelin-throwers. Acta Chir Scand 1946;93(6):563–75.
10. Barnes DA, Tullos HS. An analysis of 100 symptomatic baseball players. Am J Sports Med 1978;6:62–7.
11. Jobe FW, Stark H, Lombardo SJ. Reconstruction of the ulnar collateral ligament in athletes. J Bone Joint Surg Am 1986;68:1158–63.
12. Azar FM, Andrews JR, Wilk KE, et al. Operative treatment of ulnar collateral ligament injuries of the elbow in athletes. Am J Sports Med 2000;28:16–23.
13. Conway JE, Jobe FW, Glousman RE, et al. Medial instability of the elbow in throwing athletes: treatment by repair or reconstruction of the ulnar collateral ligament. J Bone Joint Surg Am 1992;74:67–83.
14. Thompson WH, Jobe FW, Yocum LA, et al. Ulnar collateral ligament reconstruction in athletes: muscle-splitting approach without transposition of the ulnar nerve. J Shoulder Elbow Surg 2001;10:152–7.
15. Smith GR, Altchek DW, Pegnani MJ, et al. A muscle-splitting approach to the ulnar collateral ligament of the elbow. Am J Sports Med 1996;24:575–80.
16. Petty DH, Andrews JR, Fleisig GS, et al. Ulnar collateral ligament reconstruction in high school baseball players: clinical results and injury risk factors. Am J Sports Med 2004;32(5):1158–64.
17. Olsen SJ, Fleisig GS, Dun S, et al. Risk factors for shoulder and elbow injuries in adolescent baseball pitchers. Am J Sports Med 2006;34:905–12.
18. Fleisig GS, Barrentine SW. Biomechanical aspects of the elbow in sports. Sports Med Arthrosc Rev 1995;3:149–59.
19. Fleisig GS, Andrews JR, Dillman CJ, et al. Kinetics of baseball pitching with implications about injury mechanisms. Am J Sports Med 1995;23:233–9.
20. Gainor BJ, Piotrowski G, Puhl J, et al. The throw: biomechanics and acute injury. Am J Sports Med 1980;8:114–8.
21. Kenter K, Behr CT, Warren RF, et al. Acute elbow injuries in the National Football League. J Shoulder Elbow Surg 2000;9:1–5.

22. Mirabello SC, Loeb PE, Andrews JR. The wrist: field evaluation and treatment. Clin Sports Med 1992;11:1–25.
23. Norwood LA, Shook JA, Andrews JR. Acute medial elbow ruptures. Am J Sports Med 1981;9:16–9.
24. Savoie FH 3rd, Trenhaile SW, Roberts J, et al. Primary repair of ulnar collateral ligament injuries of the elbow in young athletes: a case series of injuries to the proximal and distal ends of the ligament. Am J Sports Med 2008;36:1066–72.
25. O'Driscoll SW, Lawton RL, Smith AM. The "moving valgus stress test" for medial collateral ligament tears of the elbow. Am J Sports Med 2005;33:231–9.
26. Glajchen N, Schwartz ML, Andrews JR, et al. Avulsion fracture of the sublime tubercle of the ulna: a newly recognized injury in the throwing athlete. AJR Am J Roentgenol 1998;170:627–8.
27. Deal JB, Smith E, Heard W, et al. Platelet-rich plasma for primary treatment of partial ulnar collateral ligament tears: MRI correlation with results. Orthop J Sports Med 2017;5(11). 2325967117738238.
28. Poehling GG, Whipple TL, Sisco L, et al. Elbow arthroscopy: a new technique. Arthroscopy 1989;5:222–4.
29. Field LD, Altchek DW. Evaluation of the arthroscopic valgus instability test of the elbow. Am J Sports Med 1996;24:177–81.
30. Wilk KE, Arrigo CA, Bagwell MS, et al. Repair of the ulnar collateral ligament of the elbow: rehabilitation following internal brace surgery. J Orthop Sports Phys Ther 2019;49(4):253–61.
31. Richard MJ, Aldridge JM 3rd, Wiesler ER, et al. Traumatic valgus instability of the elbow: pathoanatomy and results of direct repair. Surgical technique. J Bone Joint Surg Am 2009;91(Suppl 2):191–9.
32. Cain EL Jr, Andrews JR, Dugas JR, et al. Outcome of ulnar collateral ligament reconstruction of the elbow in 1281 athletes: results in 743 athletes with minimum 2-year follow-up. Am J Sports Med 2010;38(12):2426–34.

Olecranon Stress Fracture

Dylan N. Greif, BA*, Christopher P. Emerson, MS, Paul Allegra, MD,
Brandon J. Shallop, MD, Lee D. Kaplan, MD

KEYWORDS

- Elbow • Olecranon • Stress fracture • Overuse injury • Throwing injuries • MRI

KEY POINTS

- Olecranon stress fracture is an elbow injury that primarily affects athletes involved with throwing sports or other activities that emphasize repetitive motion of the elbow.
- Tenderness over the olecranon after or during throwing, especially the medial side, is a key physical examination finding suggestive of olecranon stress fracture.
- MRI has been reported as the gold standard for detecting stress fractures.
- Nonoperative treatment has been successful in the few reports of stress reactions in the literature. However, operative management is the mainstay treatment option.
- The return to sport rate after olecranon stress fracture is very high, with both nonoperative or operative management.

INTRODUCTION

Olecranon stress fracture (OSF) is an overuse elbow injury that primarily affects athletes who perform repetitive throwing motions. The first reported description of the injury was linked to a javelin thrower in 1946. Currently, baseball players are the most susceptible to this injury.[1] The incidence of OSF in other sports such as wrestling, diving, gymnastics, and archery is also increasing.[2–4] OSF can be a challenge to manage, because there is limited literature describing the disease process, diagnosis, and treatment of this condition. This article describes the epidemiology, anatomy, and pathophysiology of OSF and summarizes the current literature regarding diagnosis, management, and prognostic outcome of this condition.

EPIDEMIOLOGY

Stress fractures are rare injuries. Only 0.8% of fractures in high school athletes are stress related, and only 2.8% of those injuries involve the upper extremity.[5] The olecranon has an incidence of 58% of stress fractures in baseball players. Pitchers are the most predominant position at risk of injury.[6] OSF is increasing in prevalence in

University of Miami Sports Medicine Institute, 5555 Ponce De Leon Boulevard, Coral Gables, FL 33146, USA
* Corresponding author.
E-mail address: d.greif@med.miami.edu

pediatric patients owing to the recent increased number of children participating in competitive sports (currently 45 million children in the United States play in organized youth sports).[7,8] This factor is of particular significance given that 31% of pediatric athletes experience elbow pain over the course of 1 year, with 5% of young baseball pitchers sustaining a serious throwing injury necessitating surgical repair or extended cessation of sport within 10 years.[9–11]

ANATOMY

The osseous anatomy of the elbow joint is complex, consisting of 3 functionally separate articulations: the proximal radioulnar, radiocapitellar, and ulnohumeral articulations. These articulations allow for a range of motion in extension and flexion from −5° to 140°, as well as forearm rotational motion from 90° pronation to 90° of supination.[12] The olecranon's importance lies in its role in articulating with the humeral trochlea (**Fig. 1**). The humeral trochlea articulates with the proximal ulna via the sigmoid notch, and the olecranon is the most proximal aspect of this notch, with the coronoid process the most distal. Hence, the olecranon assists in creating a hinge motion in the elbow owing to its cupping of the lower end of the humerus.

Resistance to valgus stress is provided by the anterior band of the ulnar collateral ligament (UCL) and the radial head, whereas varus stress is countered by the lateral collateral ligament complex.[13,14] The triceps brachii and the anconeus insert onto the posterior third of the olecranon and proximal ulna, making the olecranon process periosteum and triceps tendon closely associated. Finally, the brachialis inserts onto the coronoid process of the ulna, which helps to distribute the compressive forces across the elbow joint during contraction.

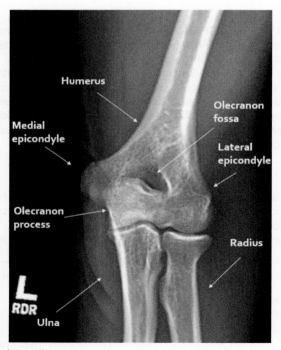

Fig. 1. Anatomy of the elbow.

PATHOPHYSIOLOGY

Stress fractures occur owing to 2 mechanisms, the first being owing to an increased amount of cyclical repetitions occurring at a lower intensity than maximum bone strength on nonpathologic bone tissue.[15] Although the intensity is not enough to cause an acute fracture at onset, the continued stress on the bone prevents it from appropriately remodeling.[16] This abnormal remodeling process is the result of osteoblasts laying down bone at a rate slower than osteoclasts resorbing bone.[17] Because remodeling and strengthening of bone is lagging behind resorption of damaged bone, microdamage accumulates over time.[18] From this repetitive microdamage, a fracture can develop during normal sustainable loads.

Stress fractures may also occur owing to trabecular bone having insufficient density. Such bone has reduced mechanical properties at onset, therefore, even normal intensity loads are at higher risk of stress fractures over time.[16] The most common example of this presentation is in female softball players when combined with poor diet, such as diminished calcium intake, or menstrual disturbances related to exercise.[19] Although women are at increased risk for stress fractures owing to this specific mechanism, among athletes, the overall difference in incidence between men and women is minimal.[15]

For baseball players in particular, OSF has been attributed to rapid and repetitive valgus extension. The UCL is the main ligamentous stabilizer for the medioposterior part of the elbow, and absorbs approximately 50% of the valgus stress (around 64 Nm) placed on the elbow.[20] As rapid elbow extension occurs, the tip of the olecranon is forced into the olecranon fossa and, with increased laxity of the UCL comes a compensatory increase in compression on the medial aspect of the olecranon–olecranon fossa articulation during extension.[21] Excessive tensile forces of the triceps on the olecranon during the acceleration phase of throwing also exacerbate this process.[22] Aguinaldo and Chambers[23] reported that there are several mechanical factors in the throwing motion that predispose the elbow to additional excessive valgus loads, including late trunk rotation, reduced shoulder external rotation, increased elbow flexion, and sidearm motions.

Additionally, recurrent UCL injuries, ranging from strains or minimal tears to multiple reconstructive procedures, increase the laxity and subsequent contact pressure in the posteromedial aspect of the elbow during extension. This process is also associated with medial epicondylar apophysitis and avulsion fractures (**Fig. 2**) owing to repetitive stress placed on the medial elbow. This structure is vital for valgus stability because dynamic and static stabilizers attach here.[12]

PEDIATRIC POPULATION

Unlike the adult elbow, the pediatric elbow contains 6 active ossification centers that occur predictably depending on age: capitellum at 1 year, radial head and medial epicondyle at 5 to 6 years, trochlea and olecranon at 8 to 10 years, and lateral epicondyle at 10 years, with the sequence the same in both boys and girls, although boys tend to lag behind up to 2 years on average.[24] The significance of open physes is that they present weak biomechanical points and are therefore more susceptible to failure when faced with increased or recurrent force.[25] Open physes are weaker and less elastic and, unlike adults who have a high incidence of soft tissue failures, because the soft tissue tend to absorb the majority of biomechanical stresses, in pediatric athletes the physes absorb these biomechanical stresses.[7]

During growth spurts, the growth plate is also at an increased risk for fracture owing to decreased physeal strength during this period, where bone mineralization lags

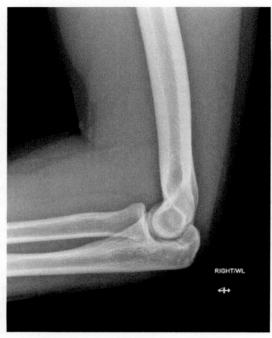

RIGHT/WL

Fig. 2. Avulsion fracture.

behind linear bone growth, creating porous bone.[26] Repetitive loading at this time can lead to altered metaphyseal perfusion, interfering with the mineralization of bone. Therefore, ischemic conditions and osseous necrosis with deformity of the developing ossification center may develop.[27] Asymmetric or complete cessation of growth can also occur, decreasing the olecranon's ability to handle repetitive stress.

Common risk factors seen in adolescent patients with OSF include average of 12 years of onset, playing a pitcher or catcher role in a throwing sport, playing more than 100 games a year, or throwing a breaking ball (a type of pitch that increases rotational and angular forces on the elbow), which has been recommended not be thrown before the age of 14 to 16 years, and increased velocity.[28,29]

CLINICAL HISTORY

When assessing elbow pathology, the patient history is of utmost importance. Certain activities and distributions of discomfort can help to rule OSF in or out of the differential diagnosis. When dealing with a thrower, it is imperative to ask at what point in the throwing motion symptoms occur, because pitchers with pain medially at the onset of arm acceleration tend to have UCL pathology, whereas patients with posterior or posteromedial elbow pain at ball release (when the elbow nears terminal extension) should be evaluated further for OSF.[30] Posterolateral pain may also be reported. Patients will also note loss of terminal elbow extension, hence an inability to complete their pitch, maintain control, or a sense of reduced velocity on the pitch.[31]

Patients also most likely emphasize pain with repetitive motion, which may improve with rest, anti-inflammatory medication, icing, or compression. Extension of the elbow causes the most significant amount of pain, but patients also tend to report pain during pronation and supination of the forearm. Any discomfort will most likely be reported as increasing in intensity over time, as the bone becomes weaker to the point of failure.

PHYSICAL EXAMINATION

The examiner should proceed with a complete elbow examination: inspection, palpation, range of motion, strength testing, stability testing, and a neurovascular examination. Inspect and palpate for any swelling at or near the olecranon and localize any tenderness over the region. Point tenderness to palpation over the olecranon, especially on the medial side, is a key physical examination finding suggestive of OSF, although posterolateral pain may also be elicited.[32] Palpation of the ulnar nerve, UCL, distal medial triceps, and flexor–pronator group should also be performed to ensure that these nearby structures are not involved.[30]

During range of motion testing, assess for pain that is reproducible with resisted elbow extension. Beforehand, it is important for the examiner to recognize that throwers tend to have some loss of elbow extension in their throwing elbow at baseline compared with their nonthrowing arm, and therefore, a minor comparable deficit of extension should not be a major concern. There are 2 focused examination maneuvers that often reproducibly elicit pain in patients with an OSF. The snapping extension test and the arm bar test. The snapping extension test, demonstrated in **Fig. 3**, involves placing continuous valgus stress on the elbow followed by extension from 30° flexion to full extension. The examiner repeats the examination without valgus stress while palpating the posteromedial olecranon for tenderness. The arm bar examination, demonstrated in **Fig. 4**, involves having the examiner place the fully pronated and extended elbow on his or her shoulder and applies downward pressure on the proximal forearm and midhumerus.[33]

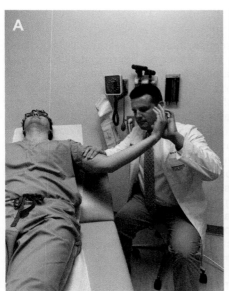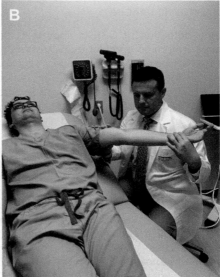

Fig. 3. (*A*, *B*): Posterior elbow impingement examination. (*A*), the examiner attempts to recreate symptoms by grasping the wrist at 20 to 30° of flexion, then forcibly extending the elbow while applying a valgus stress as seen in Figure B.

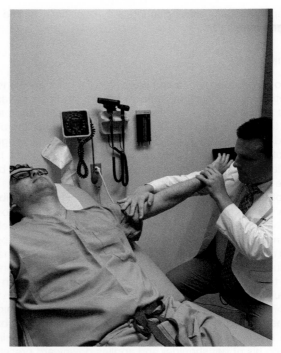

Fig. 4. Arm bar examination. The examiner places the fully pronated and extended elbow on his/her shoulder, applying downward pressure on the proximal forearm and midhumerus.

DIAGNOSTIC IMAGING

Early detection of OSF is important, because there is a statistically significant earlier return to sport or activity when a stress injury is appropriately diagnosed within 3 weeks of symptom onset compared with later than 3 weeks (return time of 10.4 weeks vs 18.4 weeks, respectively).[34] Patients with OSF may or may not have radiologic findings. Plain radiographs of the elbow should be taken owing to their cost effectiveness and readily available access. Standard anteroposterior, lateral, and axial views should always be ordered; however, although not required, 2 oblique views may also be obtained to assist with better visualization of the posteromedial olecranon.[30] Typical findings, as seen in **Fig. 5**, include osteophyte formation in the posteromedial olecranon fossa, loose bodies from fragmentation of the capitellum, possible calcium deposits on the medial ulnar collateral ligament, and hypertrophy of the humerus resulting from decreased spacing for articulation of the olecranon process within the fossa. It is important to note that stress fractures may not appear on a typical radiograph if not significant enough in size. Therefore, if a stress fracture is suspected based on the physical examination and/or clinical judgment, but not confirmed via radiograph, additional imaging may be required.

Multidetector computed tomography (CT) imaging has been described as a useful imaging modality when it comes to detecting early stress injuries owing to its ability to identify cortical abnormalities.[35,36] Cortical abnormalities are very early signs of fatigue damage to the cortical bone and tend to not be seen on typical radiographs

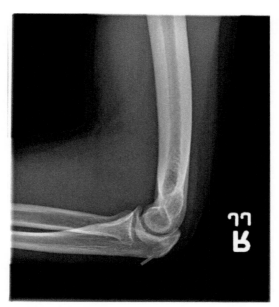

Fig. 5. Radiograph of OSF (*arrow*).

owing to the lack of sensitivity to minute osseous pathology when patients are presenting with pain with only a few weeks onset. CT scans can also detect increased resorption activity via increased hypoattenuation, bone marrow edema via attenuation of yellow marrow, and periosteal edema, which would present as a soft tissue mass adjacent to the periosteal surface of the bone.[36] Late bony changes such as increased medullary density, endosteal sclerosis, sclerotic lines in trabecular bone, and periosteal thickening are also easily detected by a CT scan.[37] However, for OSF specifically, there are other imaging modalities that are more sensitive and specific compared with CT imaging.

Bone scintigraphy is a traditional variant of nuclear medicine that is very sensitive to stress fractures. Scintigraphy examination allows for very early detection of bony changes, necessitating only 3 to 5 days after symptom onset compared with 1 to 2 weeks for a CT scan (**Fig. 6**).[38] This is because radiopharmaceutical tracers become concentrated in affected regions where there is increased bone remodeling, microfractures of the trabecular bone, bone calluses, and any other periosteal reactions.[39] That being said, although scintigraphy is highly sensitive to stress fractures, it lacks specificity because it cannot differentiate a stress fracture from a physiologic stress reaction, thus limiting their diagnostic usefulness. Furthermore, this imaging modality is not as cost appropriate as its counterparts, is time consuming, and exposes the patient to a significant amount of radiation. Therefore, it is only recommended when CT scanning or MRI is not available.[40]

MRI has been reported as the gold standard for detecting stress fractures as determined by the American College of Radiology.[16] Although the specificity of both a CT and MRI is very high, the sensitivity for detection via MRI is higher.[41] Compared with bone scintigraphy, both modalities have similar sensitivity, but MRI has more significant specificity.[42] Abnormalities caused by the fracture can be identified within 2 days from onset of symptoms, along with early detection of edema in the bone tissue

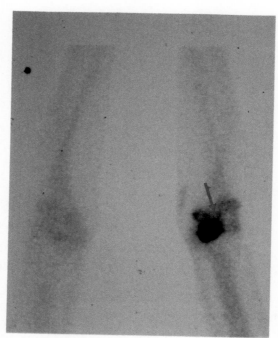

Fig. 6. Bone scan of the olecranon (*arrow*).

and adjacent areas (**Fig. 7**). Therefore, it is possible to differentiate medullary damage from cortical, endosteal, and periosteal damage, allowing gradation of the lesions regarding their severity and prognosis. Because intramedullary endosteal edema is one of the first signs of bone remodeling, its detection is of utmost importance, particularly for smaller lesions. MRI is also the gold standard for detecting ligamentous lesions, which is important owing to the relationship between OSF and UCL damage.[40]

Owing to the rarity of OSF, there have been limited attempts to classify OSF into different subtypes, which may improve diagnosis and clarify the mechanism of onset. Furushima and colleagues[43] classified OSF baseball players by identifying fractures via radiographs, CT scans, and MRI. This comparison was made by comparing the throwing arm with the nonthrowing arm of each patient, with particular emphasis on assessing the epiphyseal plate if patients had pediatric imaging. A total of five types of fracture lines were deduced based on the origin and direction of the fracture plane: physeal (mean age of onset [MAOO], 14.1 years), classic (MAOO, 18.6 years), transitional (MAOO, 16.9 years), sclerotic (MAOO, 18 years), and distal (MAOO, 19.6 years). According to Furushima and colleagues, the physeal type fracture is the most common pediatric OSF while the classic type is the most common adult OSF presentation. Classic OSF originates from the olecranon articular surface and runs in the dorsal–proximal direction. Physeal OSF occurs when delayed closure or nonunion is found along the line of epiphyseal plate and is staged depending on severity: stages 1 and 2 have delayed epiphyseal plate closure compared with the nonthrowing arm, whereas stage 3 involves minor epiphyseal plate dehiscence. Stage 4 involves complete dehiscence of the epiphyseal plate. This study also concluded that all OSF types were complicated with medial elbow disorders, most commonly UCL injury or avulsion fracture.

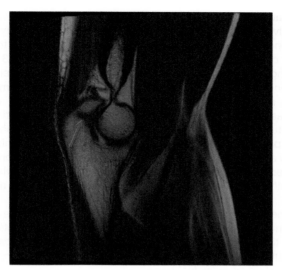

Fig. 7. MRI of an OSF (*arrow*).

NONSURGICAL MANAGEMENT

Nonsurgical management is typically indicated for sclerotic stress fractures, but may also be attempted for physeal, classical, transitional, or distal fracture patterns and is attempted for a 3-month period.[43] Patients begin management with active rest via cessation of throwing and other inciting activities. This period is followed by rehabilitation exercises that focus on increasing rotator cuff and flexor–pronator strength. Rehabilitation culminates by addressing the biomechanics behind the inciting injury.[30] Any continued throwing or propagation of any form of valgus stress, even if at a reduced level, may delay healing or worsen the fracture. Nonsteroidal anti-inflammatory drugs may also be used. Administration of a single intraarticular dose of soluble corticosteroids has not been found to be useful, nor harmful in OSF management.[30]

In a case series of 7 professional throwing athletes, Schickendantz and colleagues[44] placed patients in a customized hinged elbow orthosis set between full flexion and 20° short of full extension. At 2 weeks, light forearm and progressive resistance exercises were allowed. At 4 weeks, the orthosis was discontinued, and a full range of motion with light resistance training was initiated. Six of the athletes successfully return to competitive sports without need of surgical intervention. Other authors agree that a progressive throwing program should can be initiated 2 to 3 months after the diagnosis of OSF.[45,46] After this period, patients were allowed to return to sport.

A systematic review by Smith and colleagues[47] involving 14 studies with 52 patients found that return to sport and resolution of symptoms is acceptable with nonoperative management and comparable with operative management with the main advantage being no surgical complications. In fact, all those treated nonoperatively returned to sport except for one patient lost to follow-up. Typically, nonoperative candidates had symptoms for a mean duration of 2.8 months, much shorter than the 6.7 months of their operative counterparts, which may be related to less severe symptoms and less significant radiographic findings, allowing for a decreased time to return to play.

However, the authors also found that 33% of the operative cases were due to prior failed nonoperative management. This finding may be related to delayed radiographic union seen in nonoperative management, where radiographic union took nearly twice as long to occur compared with operative management (29.6 vs 14.3 weeks, respectively). This finding correlates with the fact that stress fractures heal slower than complete fractures and, in some cases, can take up to 6 months for complete resolution when managed nonoperatively.[22] However, according to Smith and colleagues, despite a decreased time to symptomatic and radiographic resolution for operative management, return to sport was longer in the operative group compared with nonoperatively treated patients (16.0 weeks vs 25.7 weeks, respectively). This finding may be attributed to only a handful of studies reporting a time to return to sport, return to sport in operative patients being delayed by complications or need for revision, and added caution from athletes to restart participation in sports soon after a surgical procedure.[47]

Overall, nonoperative management has been shown to be successful in allowing athletes to return to sport with minimal or no symptomatic or functional difficulties. However, given the time restrictions of competitive athletes who cannot afford the possibility of failure of nonoperative management, the decision to operate is subsequently considered on an individual basis.

SURGICAL MANAGEMENT

The persistence of symptoms and/or the inability to return to sport after nonoperative management are indicative of surgical intervention. According to the literature, up to 77% of patients do opt for a surgical procedure.[47] It has been suggested that the presence of a fracture line on plain radiographs indicates a low chance of spontaneous healing in the overhead throwing athlete.[31] Using their classification system, Furushima and colleagues[43] stated that surgery is indicated for stage 3 and 4 physeal OSF, as well as classic, transitional, and distal OSF after approximately 3 months of nonoperative management. It was noted that sclerotic OSF was not an indication for operative management. Overall, despite the class of OSF, debridement of the injury site and excision of any osteophytes or loose bodies are performed if indicated.

The most common and successful technique described in literature is open reduction internal fixation, although cannulated screws may be used if warranted.[35,48–50] If a cannulated screw must be placed, a guide pin is placed under fluoroscopic control, with orientation perpendicular to the fracture plane. The guide pin is then overreamed for the appropriately sized cannulated screw, followed by a single cannulated screw being placed. The results are shown in **Fig. 8**. Paci and colleagues[48] reported that 17 of 18 athletes treated with cannulated screw fixation after failed nonoperative management of OSF returned to sports at an average of 29 weeks after surgery and on average played an additional 3.2 years of baseball. However, 6 athletes requires a subsequent surgery for hardware removal.

Less common techniques that have been described are the use of bone grafting owing to nonunion and excision of the olecranon tip. For bone grafting, an autogenous bone graft was inlaid across the defect. Histologic examination demonstrated new bone formation, and radiographic imaging 3 months later showed union across the defect.[51,52] Although rarer, if a stress fracture extends to the tip of the olecranon, it is possible to simply excise the fractured tip via arthroscopy. When Hulkko and colleagues[53] opted to simply remove the tip of the olecranon in a throwing athlete, they reported optimal healing within 2 months with the patient throwing normally after that.

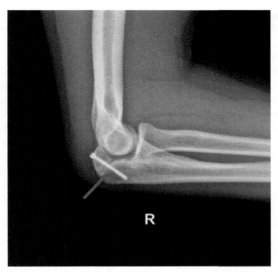

Fig. 8. Open reduction, internal fixation of OSF with cannulated screw (*arrow*).

According to Smith and colleagues, symptomatic resolution occurred in 97.5% of patients with less time to symptom resolution compared with nonoperative management. They also found that 72.5% of patients returned to preinjury competition level and 22.5% returning to competition above their preinjury level. However, 9 reported complications were documented, resulting in an overall complication rate of 17.3%, though only 3 of complications required an additional surgery for revisional purposes; all patients returned to sports with no additional complications. Rettig and colleagues[49] reported patients having symptoms related to hardware leading to removal of 3 screws, but symptoms resolved in all patients after hardware removal. Despite increased complication risk, surgical intervention nonetheless remains the mainstay of OSF treatment.

PROGNOSTIC OUTCOME

The return to sport rate after OSF is very high, irrespective of treatment modality. Almost all the patients in Smith and colleagues' systematic review (96.2%) returned at minimum to their preinjury level of sport, with almost one-fourth of those returning to a higher level of performance thereafter. Complications are typically only seen with surgical management of OSF, but the current literature suggests that these typically resolve.

Nonunion in OSF is rare given that athletes tend to have a healthy overall bone density and do not have underlying health problems that slow healing. It is also possible for patients to experience loss of motion even after treatment, although this would only manifest as a loss of a few degrees of extension.

SUMMARY

OSFs are a rare overuse injury associated with competitive athletes in throwing sports such as baseball and can affect both adult and pediatric patients. They can be challenging to manage. Stress fracture treatment involves either active rest or surgery, which take time away from training and competition. Operative management remains the gold standard intervention, because nonoperative management requires more time for symptom resolution and radiographic union while carrying the risk of failure, necessitating operative management in the future.

There are still few studies in the literature on this topic, with limited patient numbers. There is no clear classification of injury or standardization of management and return to play in this population, and as a result, larger prospective studies are required to further study this pathology. Despite continued lack of literature, the prognosis of this fracture depends on optimal patient management, whether it be through operative or nonoperative management. Patients who are diagnosed appropriately and follow appropriate treatment rehabilitation instructions will have a better prognosis, which based on current literature includes the vast majority.

DISCLOSURE

The authors have nothing to disclose.

REFERENCES

1. Waris W. Elbow injuries of javelin-throwers. Acta Chir Scand 1946;93(6):563–75.
2. Hetling T, Bourban P, Gojanovic B. Stress fracture and nonunion of coronoid process in a gymnast. Case Rep Orthop 2016;2016:9172483.
3. Clark RR, McKinley TO. Bilateral olecranon epiphyseal fracture non-union in a competitive athlete. Iowa Orthop J 2010;30:179–81.
4. Yavuz U, Sokucu S, Demir B, et al. An unusual stress fracture in an archer with hypophosphatasia. Case Rep Orthop 2013;2013:350236.
5. Changstrom BG, Brou L, Khodaee M, et al. Epidemiology of stress fracture injuries among US high school athletes, 2005-2006 through 2012-2013. Am J Sports Med 2015;43(1):26–33.
6. Iwamoto J, Takeda T. Stress fractures in athletes: review of 196 cases. J Orthop Sci 2003;8(3):273–8.
7. Caine D, DiFiori J, Maffulli N. Physeal injuries in children's and youth sports: reasons for concern? Br J Sports Med 2006;40(9):749–60.
8. Merkel DL. Youth sport: positive and negative impact on young athletes. Open Access J Sports Med 2013;4:151–60.
9. Matsuura T, Suzue N, Kashiwaguchi S, et al. Elbow injuries in youth baseball players without prior elbow pain: a 1-year prospective study. Orthop J Sports Med 2013;1(5). 2325967113509948.
10. Fleisig GS, Andrews JR, Cutter GR, et al. Risk of serious injury for young baseball pitchers: a 10-year prospective study. Am J Sports Med 2011;39(2):253–7.
11. Makhni EC, Morrow ZS, Luchetti TJ, et al. Arm pain in youth baseball players: a survey of healthy players. Am J Sports Med 2015;43(1):41–6.
12. Pearce McCarty L 3rd. Approach to medial elbow pain in the throwing athlete. Curr Rev Musculoskelet Med 2019;12(1):30–40.
13. Duclos ME, Roualdes O, Cararo R, et al. Significance of the serum CTX-II level in an osteoarthritis animal model: a 5-month longitudinal study. Osteoarthritis Cartilage 2010;18(11):1467–76.
14. Newman SD, Mauffrey C, Krikler S. Olecranon fractures. Injury 2009;40(6): 575–81.
15. Astur DC, Zanatta F, Arliani GG, et al. Stress fractures: definition, diagnosis and treatment. Rev Bras Ortop 2016;51(1):3–10.

16. Carmont MR, Mei-Dan O, Bennell KL. Stress fracture management: current classification and new healing modalities. Oper Techn Sport Med 2009;17(2):81–9.
17. Knapp TP, Garrett WE. Stress fractures: general concepts. Clin Sports Med 1997; 16(2):339–56.
18. Kaeding CC, Spindler KP, Amendola A. Management of troublesome stress fractures. Instr Course Lect 2004;53:455–69.
19. Myburgh KH, Hutchins J, Fataar AB, et al. Low bone density is an etiologic factor for stress fractures in athletes. Ann Intern Med 1990;113(10):754–9.
20. Fleisig GS, Andrews JR, Dillman CJ, et al. Kinetics of baseball pitching with implications about injury mechanisms. Am J Sports Med 1995;23(2):233–9.
21. Mauro CS, Hammoud S, Altchek DW. Ulnar collateral ligament tear and olecranon stress fracture nonunion in a collegiate pitcher. J Shoulder Elbow Surg 2011; 20(7):e9–13.
22. Ahmad CS, ElAttrache NS. Valgus extension overload syndrome and stress injury of the olecranon. Clin Sports Med 2004;23(4):665–76, x.
23. Aguinaldo AL, Chambers H. Correlation of throwing mechanics with elbow valgus load in adult baseball pitchers. Am J Sports Med 2009;37(10):2043–8.
24. Iyer RS, Thapa MM, Khanna PC, et al. Pediatric bone imaging: imaging elbow trauma in children–a review of acute and chronic injuries. AJR Am J Roentgenol 2012;198(5):1053–68.
25. Rudzki JR, Paletta GA Jr. Juvenile and adolescent elbow injuries in sports. Clin Sports Med 2004;23(4):581–608, ix.
26. Morscher E. Strength and morphology of growth cartilage under hormonal influence of puberty. Animal experiments and clinical study on the etiology of local growth disorders during puberty. Reconstr Surg Traumatol 1968;10:3–104.
27. Leveau BF. Skeletal Injury in the Child - Ogden,Ja. Phys Ther 1984;64(8):1297–8.
28. Benjamin HJ, Briner WW Jr. Little league elbow. Clin J Sport Med 2005;15(1): 37–40.
29. Lyman S, Fleisig GS, Andrews JR, et al. Effect of pitch type, pitch count, and pitching mechanics on risk of elbow and shoulder pain in youth baseball pitchers. Am J Sports Med 2002;30(4):463–8.
30. Dugas JR. Valgus extension overload: diagnosis and treatment. Clin Sports Med 2010;29(4):645–54.
31. Cain EL, Moroski NM. Elbow surgery in athletes. Sports Med Arthrosc Rev 2018; 26(4):181–4.
32. Greiwe RM, Saifi C, Ahmad CS. Pediatric sports elbow injuries. Clin Sports Med 2010;29(4):677–703.
33. Zwerus EL, Somford MP, Maissan F, et al. Physical examination of the elbow, what is the evidence? A systematic literature review. Br J Sports Med 2018;52(19): 1253–60.
34. Ohta-Fukushima M, Mutoh Y, Takasugi S, et al. Characteristics of stress fractures in young athletes under 20 years. J Sports Med Phys Fitness 2002;42(2): 198–206.
35. Fujioka H, Tsunemi K, Takagi Y, et al. Treatment of stress fracture of the olecranon in throwing athletes with internal fixation through a small incision. Sports Med Arthrosc Rehabil Ther Technol 2012;4(1):49.
36. Gaeta M, Minutoli F, Scribano E, et al. CT and MR imaging findings in athletes with early tibial stress injuries: comparison with bone scintigraphy findings and emphasis on cortical abnormalities. Radiology 2005;235(2):553–61.
37. Blake SP, Connors AM. Sacral insufficiency fracture. Br J Radiol 2004;77(922): 891–6.

38. Sofka CM. Imaging of stress fractures. Clin Sports Med 2006;25(1):53–62, viii.
39. Schneiders AG, Sullivan SJ, Hendrick PA, et al. The ability of clinical tests to diagnose stress fractures: a systematic review and meta-analysis. J Orthop Sports Phys Ther 2012;42(9):760–71.
40. Jarraya M, Hayashi D, Roemer FW, et al. Radiographically occult and subtle fractures: a pictorial review. Radiol Res Pract 2013;2013:370169.
41. Fredericson M, Jennings F, Beaulieu C, et al. Stress fractures in athletes. Top Magn Reson Imaging 2006;17(5):309–25.
42. Ishibashi Y, Okamura Y, Otsuka H, et al. Comparison of scintigraphy and magnetic resonance imaging for stress injuries of bone. Clin J Sport Med 2002; 12(2):79–84.
43. Furushima K, Itoh Y, Iwabu S, et al. Classification of olecranon stress fractures in baseball players. Am J Sports Med 2014;42(6):1343–51.
44. Schickendantz MS, Ho CP, Koh J. Stress injury of the proximal ulna in professional baseball players. Am J Sports Med 2002;30(5):737–41.
45. Nuber GW, Diment MT. Olecranon stress fractures in throwers. A report of two cases and a review of the literature. Clin Orthop Relat Res 1992;278:58–61.
46. Mamanee P, Neira C, Martire JR, et al. Stress lesion of the proximal medial ulna in a throwing athlete. A case report. Am J Sports Med 2000;28(2):261–3.
47. Smith SR, Patel NK, White AE, et al. Stress fractures of the elbow in the throwing athlete: a systematic review. Orthop J Sports Med 2018;6(10). 2325967118799262.
48. Paci JM, Dugas JR, Guy JA, et al. Cannulated screw fixation of refractory olecranon stress fractures with and without associated injuries allows a return to baseball. Am J Sports Med 2013;41(2):306–12.
49. Rettig AC, Wurth TR, Mieling P. Nonunion of olecranon stress fractures in adolescent baseball pitchers: a case series of 5 athletes. Am J Sports Med 2006;34(4): 653–6.
50. Suzuki K, Minami A, Suenaga N, et al. Oblique stress fracture of the olecranon in baseball pitchers. J Shoulder Elbow Surg 1997;6(5):491–4.
51. Pavlov H, Torg JS, Jacobs B, et al. Nonunion of olecranon epiphysis: two cases in adolescent baseball pitchers. AJR Am J Roentgenol 1981;136(4):819–20.
52. Torg JS, Moyer RA. Non-union of a stress fracture through the olecranon epiphyseal plate observed in an adolescent baseball pitcher. A case report. J Bone Joint Surg Am 1977;59(2):264–5.
53. Hulkko A, Orava S, Nikula P. Stress fractures of the olecranon in javelin throwers. Int J Sports Med 1986;7(4):210–3.

The Lacertus Syndrome of the Elbow in Throwing Athletes

Steve E. Jordan, MD

KEYWORDS

- Medial elbow pain • Differential diagnosis • Lacertus syndrome

KEY POINTS

- It is important to take a complete history and perform a careful examination in order to avoid confirmation bias when evaluating throwers with medial elbow pain. Lacertus syndrome is a postexertional compartment syndrome, and the history can help elucidate this.
- The Lacertus syndrome is more common than pronator syndrome, which involves the median nerve, and can be distinguished with a careful workup. Other more common pathologies should be ruled out with a routine workup.
- Include inspection of the flexor pronator muscle group and consider evaluating after throwing when examining a thrower with postexertional elbow pain.

HISTORY OF THE TECHNIQUE

In 1959, George Bennett summarized his experiences caring for throwing athletes. The following paragraph is excerpted in its entirety from that article.[1]

"There is a lesion which produces a different syndrome. A pitcher in throwing a curveball is compelled to supinate his wrist with a snap at the end of his delivery. On examination, one will note distinct fullness over the pronator radii teres. These are covered by a strong fascial band, a portion of which is the attachment of the biceps, which runs obliquely across the pronator muscle. A pitcher may be able to pitch for two or three innings but then the pain and swelling become so great that he has to retire. A simple linear and transverse division of the fascia covering the muscles has relieved tension on many occasions and rehabilitated these men so that they were able to return to the game."

This is the first known reference to a condition that has undoubtedly disabled many players and possibly ended careers of an untold number of throwing athletes. Although Bennett did not fully understand the causes or even the mechanics involved (ie, he thought the pitcher supinates instead of pronates on release of the baseball), he did describe a simple operative treatment that has allowed us to

The Andrews Institute, The Andrews Research and Education Foundation, 1040 Gulf Breeze Parkway, Suite 203, Gulf Breeze, FL 32561, USA
E-mail address: jordan.se@gmail.com

Clin Sports Med 39 (2020) 589–596
https://doi.org/10.1016/j.csm.2020.03.004
0278-5919/20/© 2020 Elsevier Inc. All rights reserved.

prolong the careers of throwing athletes. To help distinguish this condition from pronator teres syndrome that involves compression of the median nerve, we have named it the lacertus syndrome.

HISTORY AND PHYSICAL EXAMINATION

Athletes with the lacertus syndrome usually present with a vague history of slowly increasing discomfort in the flexor-pronator muscles after throwing. The discomfort is described as an achy painful tightness of the medial elbow, which develops in the first few hours after activity. Specifically there are not any distal neurologic symptoms or findings, and a Tinel's sign over the anteromedial elbow is not present. This would suggest pronator teres syndrome and involvement of the median nerve.

Pronator teres syndrome is an uncommon but distinct condition in which the median nerve is compressed and irritated as it courses across the elbow region.[2] Possible areas of compression classically include between the 2 heads of the pronator muscle, beneath the lacertus fibrosus, proximal to the elbow at the ligament of Struthers, beneath the fibrous arch of the flexor digitorum superficialis, and more rarely as it crosses under the flexor palmaris longus or Gantzer muscle (**Fig. 1**). Pertinent findings and complaints include symptoms similar to carpal tunnel syndrome and the presence of a Tinel sign at the area of the lacertus fascia and convergence of the 2 heads of the pronator teres muscle anterior and 3 to 5 cm distal to the medial epicondyle. Symptoms of pronator syndrome can also be elicited with resisted protonation and extension in symptomatic patients. One should be thorough and open minded when evaluating any athlete with elbow discomfort in an effort to avoid confirmation bias and perhaps miss the diagnosis of an uncommon condition.

In players with lacertus syndrome the symptoms early on may be minor and are often ignored. A few hours rest leads to complete relief. As the condition progresses, the symptoms may develop earlier during throwing and become more severe. Symptoms may also require longer periods of rest to resolve—days instead of hours. Just as Dr Bennett described, these symptoms may progress to the point that the player

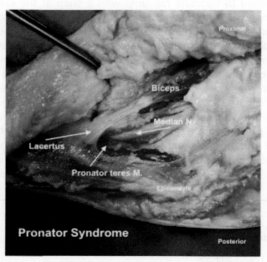

Fig. 1. Dissection of right medial elbow—distal is to left. Note median nerve entering the forearm between the 2 heads of the pronator teres muscle and below the lacertus fascia.

cannot continue throwing. For position players in baseball, this problem is often not debilitating; however, for pitchers it may be. Football quarterbacks complain most often during the repetition of practice but rarely after or during games. It is at the point when the symptoms have progressed to a degree that they interfere with competition that a player usually presents to the athletic trainer or doctor.

The duration of symptoms may vary markedly. In the authors' experience with 60 patients, the duration of acute symptoms ranged from 8 hours to 4 days before resolving, only to begin again when the athlete returned to throwing. Duration of recurrent symptoms ranged from 6 months to 3 years. In all patients the symptoms were disabling if the throwing activity resumed before the acute symptoms had resolved.

The key feature of the history in patients with the lacertus syndrome is the delayed onset of symptoms, which is like that seen in exertional compartment syndromes of the leg in runners. This, together with the history of no neurologic impairment and that a period of rest allows the athlete to resume throwing without discomfort, is diagnostic. Trauma to the elbow is usually not a factor in the etiology of the lacertus syndrome. The physician should take a careful history and perform a thorough physical examination of the elbow to help rule out more common abnormalities such as medial epicondylitis, ulnar collateral ligament injuries, and cubital tunnel syndrome or ulnar neuritis. Other conditions that can cause medial elbow pain and discomfort in throwers are bicipital tendinitis and stress fractures and rarely musculocutaneous nerve entrapment. Pronator teres syndrome or intraarticular pathologies should also be considered and ruled out.

In patients who have a history of postexertional medial elbow pain and tightness and who have the lacertus syndrome as part of their differential diagnosis, it is essential to examine the player after a workout. The examination should begin with a careful inspection of the arm, looking for exaggerated contours of the medial musculature just distal to the medial epicondyle. In players with severe or advanced cases, the proximal portions of the flexor pronator muscles seem grossly swollen, and the distinct oblique band of the lacertus fibrosus is readily visible (**Fig. 2**). The patient should be asked to flex and pronate the wrist, which may demonstrate more clearly

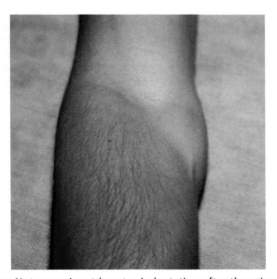

Fig. 2. Right elbow. Note prominent lacertus indentation after throwing.

any abnormality in the area of the lacertus fascia. Palpation of this area will likely reveal tenderness in the muscle directly beneath and just distal to the crossing fascial band. Any tenderness should be distinguished from a Tinel's sign over the median nerve.

Radiographs and MRI examinations are performed to help exclude other more common diagnoses. There are no findings on these studies to confirm the diagnosis of lacertus syndrome, but the tests are obviously helpful in ruling out other conditions. The diagnosis of lacertus syndrome can usually be made with a careful history and physical examination alone. Ancillary studies are done to rule out associated pathologies.

High-speed video of the pitching motion of course has revealed that pitches are released with a terminal pronation of the hand and forearm.[3] Although Bennett was incorrect in his assertion that curveball pitchers supinate on release, he was correct in his belief that curveball pitchers are more prone to develop the lacertus syndrome. Seventy percent of the pitchers in our series listed the breaking ball as their prominent pitch. The curveball is held during the acceleration phase of pitching with greater supination of the hand, putting more stretch on the pronator teres than seen in a fastball or change-up, both of which are normally held in a forearm neutral position during acceleration.[4] This may lead to more work for the pronator muscles in the release of a breaking ball and thus account for the greater propensity of breaking ball pitchers to develop the condition. Repetitive pronation of the forearm is the mechanism that leads to the symptoms.

The pathophysiology of the lacertus syndrome is somewhat similar to that of exertional compartment syndrome in the legs of runners in that the symptoms develop after a period of exertion.[5] The success of a fasciotomy in cases of lacertus syndrome supports this observation. The 2 syndromes are similar in their presentation. Both are conditions brought on by exertion and relieved by rest. The symptoms in both conditions usually peak 1 to 2 hours after exertion.

However, the lacertus syndrome does differ from compartment syndromes of the leg due to the peculiar anatomy of the lacertus fascia. The lacertus fibrosus fascia is not the primary muscle fascia for the flexor pronator group of muscles. It is a fascial continuation of the distal biceps muscle that separates from the distal tendon and courses medially to blend into the fascia of the medial flexor pronator muscles (**Fig. 3**). It does not define an entire compartment; it merely invests and covers a portion of the muscle compartment and may thus act as an extrinsic constrictor preventing normal tissue expansion during and after exercise. Postexercise compartmental pressure measurements taken in symptomatic patients revealed pressures 15 to 22 mm Hg greater under the area of the lacertus fascia than in the same muscles proximal to the crossing lacertus fascia. Therefore, the pathophysiology of the lacertus syndrome is that of a partial compartment syndrome. Only the tissue below the crossing fascia has elevated pressures, and it is here that the symptoms are generated. It is also here that surgical attention should be directed.

NONOPERATIVE TREATMENT

The first priority of nonoperative treatment again is to rule out more common causes of elbow pain in throwers and to make a definitive diagnosis. Once the diagnosis is made, patient education, activity modification, and treatment can be implemented. For example, players may be able to manage the condition after gaining a better understanding of the cause. Some players may elect to avoid surgery when nearing the end of their competitive careers, choosing to finish up without taking time off to recover from an "elective" procedure. Others may simply learn to manage the symptoms by avoiding overuse when possible. With the support of the coaching staff,

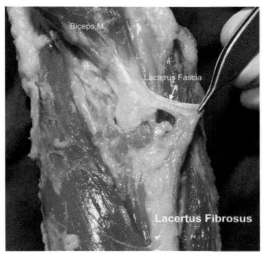

Fig. 3. Cadaver dissection of right elbow. Note lacertus fascia extending medially from biceps tendon.

position players and situational relief pitchers can avoid surgery by limiting any unnecessary throwing and pronator muscle overuse. Resting the arm and avoiding repetitive protonation are the essentials of nonoperative treatment in the lacertus syndrome.

SURGICAL INDICATIONS AND TECHNIQUE

The lacertus fibrosus fascia has been known by several names through the years. These include the more formal aponeurosis musculus bicipitis brachii and the simpler bicipital fascia or aponeurosis.[6] Henry described it as a "sort of retinaculum" arising from the biceps muscle and tendon and extending over the median nerve and the distal end of the brachial artery, attaching or investing into the fascia of the medial muscles of the forearm.[7] In the days of the barber surgeons this aponeurosis was called the "grace a Dieu" fascia (praise to God fascia), because it protected the artery and nerve during phlebotomy.[8] The fascia arises from the medial border of the bicipital tendon and the lower medial portion of the muscle; it has a thickened proximal edge, which, in some patients can be seen and palpated. It passes distally and medially to fuse with the deep fascia of the flexor pronator muscles in the upper forearm until it ultimately reaches the ulna posteromedially.[9] During surgery the fibers of the lacertus fibrosus can be distinguished from the investing muscle fascia by the oblique orientation of its fibers wrapping down and around the musculature (**Fig. 4**).

The basilic vein and the anterior and ulnar branches of the medial antebrachial cutaneous nerve are the only structures of immediate significance when exposing the lacertus fibrosus (see **Fig. 4**). Each usually crosses the elbow anterior to the medial epicondyle. Typically, the dissection is well anterior to the cubital tunnel, and the ulnar nerve is not at risk when releasing the fascia. However, one must be aware of the branches of the ulnar nerve, especially the first motor branch, which supplies the humeral head of the flexor carpi ulnaris. This branch can have a higher than normal origin within the cubital tunnel and it may encroach on the field of surgery at the most medial aspect.[10]

The indication for surgery is failure of nonoperative treatment to allow the athlete to participate in sports. After ruling out other possible causes for the patient's pathology

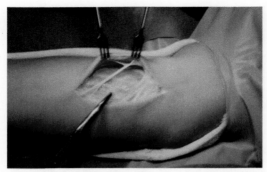

Fig. 4. Surgical dissection of medial elbow. Note fascial band of lacertus (scissors) and medial antebrachial cutaneous nerve branches crossing the field.

and exhausting conservative treatments measures, the patient is prepared for surgery. Patients are asked to throw 30 to 50 times the day before or the morning of surgery when possible. This makes the area of compression under the lacertus fascia more distinct.

The patient is positioned supine with the arm extended on a hand table. A tourniquet is used about the upper arm to control bleeding and improve visualization. A 4- to 6-cm longitudinal incision is made centered over the lacertus indentation in the flexor-pronator muscle group. The skin and subcutaneous tissue are carefully dissected away from the underlying muscle and fascial layers. Care is taken to protect the branches of the medial antebrachial cutaneous nerve.

Once the muscles are visualized, the lacertus fibers are identified. The proximal edge is usually the easiest to see, and it is typically the area of the most prominent indentation of the muscles. One or two simple fasciotomies are made from proximal to distal, always under direct visualization.

These releases should restore the contour to the muscles and eliminate the indentation caused by the crossing lacertus fibrosus (**Fig. 5**). The distinctness and width (proximal to distal) of the lacertus fibrosus varies from patient to patient. In some patients the proximal fibers are thick and the area of compression is narrow. In others the fibers are less distinct and the fibers extend 3 to 4 cm from proximal to distal. The surgeon should feel that a releasing fasciotomy has been done over the proximal flexor

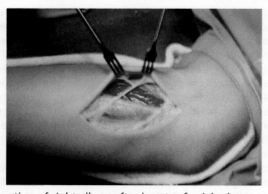

Fig. 5. Surgical dissection of right elbow after lacertus fascial release.

pronator muscle group, restoring the normal muscle contour, before closing. There have been no complications due to overreleasing the fascia, whereas there may be recurrence if it is underreleased. Irrigation and a simple wound closure complete the case.

POSTOPERATIVE CARE

The patients are placed in a soft dressing and given a sling to wear for 2 weeks. Routine postoperative wound checks are performed. Gentle range of motion is begun as tolerated or needed for daily personal care. Players are encouraged to refrain from vigorous exercise with the affected arm for the first month and then they are released to progress as tolerated. Return to throwing is individualized, and the decision is based on the patient's examination. If the player is pain free and the wounds are completely healed, there is no contraindication to begin tossing with advancement to throwing as tolerated. Players are told this usually begins at 4 weeks, and return to full-effort throwing is normally expected at about 6 weeks. Postoperative complications are rare. Persistence of symptoms indicates either inadequate fascial release or the presence of unrecognized pathology such as median nerve involvement.

SUMMARY

The lacertus syndrome is a postexertional or overuse syndrome affecting the medial elbow of throwing athletes. The pathology and presentation are identical to that of a compartment syndrome caused by the constriction of active muscles by an overlying fascia. The lacertus fibrosus fascia constricts the flexor pronator muscles in predisposed athletes, causing pain and discomfort that can lead to an inability to throw regularly. The diagnosis can be made with a careful history and physical examination. The treatment is a simple release of the tight lacertus fibrosus.

ACKNOWLEDGMENTS

The author wishes to thank Rick Williams, ATC and Isabel Holland for their invaluable assistance throughout the course of this project.

DISCLOSURE

The author has nothing to disclose.

REFERENCES

1. Bennett GE. Elbow and shoulder lesions of baseball players. Am J Surg 1959; 98:484.
2. Johnson R, Spinner M, Shrewsbury M. Median nerve entrapment syndrome in the proximal forearm. J Hand Surg Am 1979;4(1):48–51.
3. Jobe FW, Nuber G. Throwing injuries of the elbow. Clin Sports Med 1986; 5(4):621.
4. Barrentine SW, Matsuo T, Escamilla RF, Fleisig GS. Kinematic analysis of the wrist and forearm during baseball pitching. J Appl Biomech 1998;14:24–39.
5. Black KP, Schultz TK, Cheung NL. Compartment syndrome in athletes. Clin Sports Med 1990;9:471.
6. Goss CM. Gray's Anatomy. 29th edition. Philadelphia: Lea and Feiberger; 1973.

7. Henry A. Extensile Exposure. 2nd edition. Edinburgh: Churchill Livingstone; 1973.
8. Ellis H. Clinical Anatomy. London: Blackwell Scientific Publications; 1977.
9. Hollingshead WH. Textbook of Anatomy. 2nd edition. Hagerstown: Harper Row; 1967.
10. Jordan SE. Surgical anatomy of the elbow, operative techniques in upper extremity sports injuries. St Louis (MO): Mosby; 1996.

Conditions and Injuries Affecting the Nerves Around the Elbow

Mark S. Schickendantz, MD*, Sercan Yalcin, MD

KEYWORDS

- Peripheral nerve • Elbow • Sports injury

KEY POINTS

- Peripheral nerve injuries account for less than 0.5% of all sports-related injuries.
- Sports-related peripheral neuropathies account for 6% of all peripheral neuropathies and most commonly involve the upper extremity.
- The majority of these conditions respond well to nonsurgical care. Accurate and timely diagnosis are the keys to good outcomes.

 Video content accompanies this article at http://www.sportsmed.theclinics.com.

MECHANISMS OF ATHLETIC NERVE INJURY

Peripheral nerve injuries account for less than 0.5% of all sports-related injuries. Sports-related peripheral neuropathies account for 6% of all peripheral neuropathies and most commonly involve the upper extremity.[1] Sunderland[2] described the route of the median, radial, and ulnar nerves in 1945 (**Fig. 1**). They are positioned in arrangements of pulleys and sheaths to glide smoothly around the elbow. However, this anatomic relationship exposes each nerve to a risk for compression.[3]

The underlying mechanisms of the athletic nerve injury are compression, ischemia, traction, and friction.[4] Chronic athletic nerve compression may cause damage with moderate or low pressure for long or intermittent periods of time (eg, ulnar nerve injury from long distance bicycling riding), and is the primary factor.[5–7]

Cleveland Clinic Sports Health Center, 5555 Transportation Boulevard, Garfield Heights, Ohio 44125, USA
* Corresponding author.
E-mail address: schickm@ccf.org

Clin Sports Med 39 (2020) 597–621
https://doi.org/10.1016/j.csm.2020.02.006
0278-5919/20/© 2020 Elsevier Inc. All rights reserved.

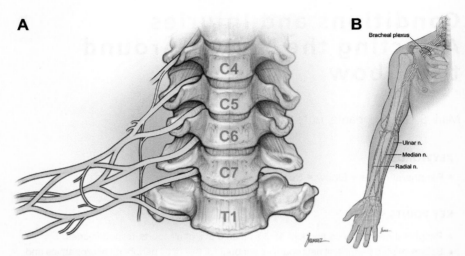

Fig. 1. Brachial plexus (*A*) and major nerves of the upper extremity (*B*). (*Reprinted* with permission, Cleveland Clinic Center for Medical Art & Photography © 2020. All Rights Reserved.)

ULNAR NERVE

The ulnar nerve is most commonly injured nerve around the elbow.[8] Acute injury usually occurs by a direct impact to the posterior elbow during a collision or a fall.[9] However, overuse injuries are much more common in sports. The underlying mechanisms are traction and/or compressive forces and excessive valgus stress at the elbow during overhead athletic activity.[1,10] In weightlifters, the hypertrophy of the medial head of the triceps muscle may cause compression.[11,12] During the acceleration phase of the throwing motion, the ulnar nerve is exposed to longitudinal traction.[13] Recurrent subluxation of the nerve may also occur.[14] During elbow flexion the ulnar nerve subluxes anteriorly, comes in contact with the epitrochlear head of the flexor carpi ulnaris (FCU) and anterior part of the tight Osborne's arcade. This causes compression in overhead athletes.[12,15] Throwing may increase angular velocity around the elbow up to 7000°/s, and is suggested to be responsible for the ulnar nerve involvement in athletes.[16] Elbow flexion coupled with wrist extension was shown to increase the pressure on the ulnar nerve inside the cubital tunnel up to 3 times and the late cocking position while throwing increases up to 6 times.[17] It was also reported that the ulnar nerve elongates about 4.7 mm with elbow flexion, which increases the tension during throwing motion.[18]

Anatomy

The ulnar nerve derives from C8 and T1 nerve roots and is the largest terminal branch of the medial cord of the brachial plexus[3,11,19] (**Fig. 2**). About 6 to 8 cm above the medial epicondyle, it pierces the medial intermuscular septum and descends with the ulnar artery on the anterior surface of the medial head of the triceps.

At the level of the elbow, the ulnar nerve enters the cubital tunnel (see **Fig. 4**). The roof of the cubital tunnel is formed by the FCU fascia and the arcuate ligament of Osbourne, which runs transversely from the medial epicondyle to the olecranon and is about 4 mm wide.[20] The ulnar nerve leaves the cubital tunnel and passes between the humeral and ulnar heads of the FCU.

In the first part of the cubital tunnel, the ulnar nerve provides an articular branch. The ulnar nerve innervates the FCU, the flexor digitorum profundus (FDP) of the fourth and

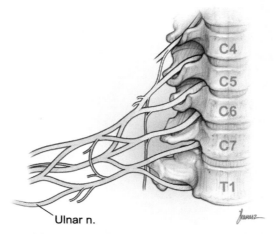

Fig. 2. The formation of the ulnar nerve from C8 and T1 nerve roots in the brachial plexus. (*Reprinted* with permission, Cleveland Clinic Center for Medical Art & Photography © 2020. All Rights Reserved.)

fifth digits in the forearm, and hypothenar muscles, medial lumbrical muscles, dorsal interossei, palmar interossei, adductor pollicis, deep head of the flexor pollicis brevis, and palmaris brevis in hand. The ulnar nerve also provides sensory innervation to the palmar aspect of the fifth digit, the ulnar half of the fourth digit, and the palmar/medial aspect of the hand.[9]

Ulnar Neuritis

Ulnar neuritis occurs in athletes owing to the ulnar nerve's anatomic position along the medial elbow, which exposes the nerve to compression, traction, and inflammation by the neighboring structures, particularly during the acceleration phase of throwing.[13,21] It has been reported to be present in more than 40% of athletes with valgus instability. Approximately 60% of athletes with medial epicondylitis develop ulnar nerve symptoms.[22,23] Repetitive tensile force on the ulnar nerve has been implicated as a cause of ulnar neuritis.[14]

Athletes typically present with gradually increasing pain in the medial forearm and sensory disturbance on ulnar side of the hand, as well as the fourth and fifth fingers. Motor findings may present as loss of ball control and difficulty with performance of complex tasks.[21]

The nerve should be examined for subluxation or dislocation with palpation and during flexion and extension. Tinel's sign and elbow flexion tests may be positive.[24]

Electromyography (EMG) and nerve conduction velocity may be obtained as part of the diagnostic workup. Positive results are usually seen in advanced nerve entrapment. In cases with dynamic compression, tests may result negative. Therefore, results should be interpreted with caution.[21,25,26] On MRI, the ulnar nerve is typically enlarged and demonstrates bright fascicles with varying sizes[27] (**Fig. 3**).

The initial treatment includes cessation of provocative activities, rest, ice, and nonsteroidal anti-inflammatory drugs (NSAIDs). After the symptoms resolve, stretching of the elbow, forearm, and wrist are allowed, followed by progressive isometric strengthening program and gradual return to sports.[21,26]

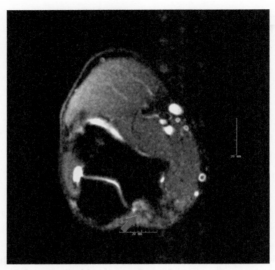

Fig. 3. An axial T2-wegihted MRI showing an enlarged ulnar nerve (*red arrow*).

Surgery is indicated for refractory symptoms or athletes with advanced symptoms such as motor weakness or muscle wasting. Surgical options include in situ decompression, medial epicondylectomy, and subcutaneous or submuscular anterior transposition of the ulnar nerve. The peer reviewed literature supports anterior transposition over in situ decompression in athletes with ulnar neuritis owing to its proposed advantage of protecting the nerve better compared with decompression. Decompression alone may not adequately decrease the compressive and tensile forces across the cubital tunnel that occur with repetitive elbow flexion activities such as throwing.[14,26,28–30]

Cubital Tunnel Syndrome

Ulnar nerve compression is the second most common nerve entrapment syndrome of the upper extremity following carpal tunnel syndrome.[1,19,31–34] Its incidence is 0.75 per 1.000 person per year.[35] Baseball is the most commonly reported sports, but recreational skiing, weightlifting, and racquet sports are also reported.[36]

In athletes, the ulnar nerve is potentially compressed at 5 sites around the elbow. The cubital tunnel is the most common site in baseball catchers, bicycle riders, and paraplegic wheelchair athletes.[37–39] Osborne's ligament is the dominant compression site in the cubital tunnel[40] (**Fig. 4**). During elbow flexion, this ligament tightens, narrows the tunnel, and increases the pressure within the tunnel up to 7 times.[18] The concomitant contraction of the FCU further increases the pressure to more than 20 times.[41] Other potential entrapment sites include the arcade of Struthers, the medial epicondyle, the medial intermuscular septum, and most distally between the 2 heads of the FCU[42,43] (**Fig. 5**). Throwing athletes using repetitive elbow flexion are at risk. Weight lifting and racquet sports are also reported to cause ulnar nerve injury.[14]

Athletes usually present with pain over the medial joint line, paresthesia and numbness of the fourth and fifth fingers, loss of grip strength, and hypothenar muscle atrophy.[35,44] Throwing athletes complain of the loss of ball control or coordination.[40] Chronic cases may also present with a claw hand.[45] Masse's sign, defined as the

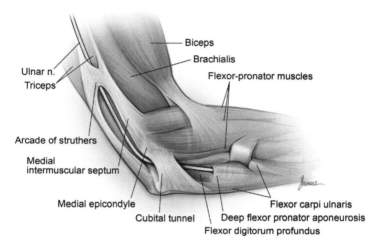

Fig. 4. Possible sites of ulnar nerve entrapment at the elbow: the arcade of Struthers, the medial intermuscular septum, the medial epicondyle, the cubital tunnel, and the deep flexor–pronator aponeurosis. (*Reprinted* with permission, Cleveland Clinic Center for Medical Art & Photography © 2020. All Rights Reserved.)

flattening of the metacarpal arch from atrophy of the opponens digiti quinti and interossei, may be positive.[46] Sensory deficiency usually precedes motor deficiency.

Physical examination reveals impaired sensation in the ulnar nerve distribution and ulnar intrinsic muscle weakness. The presence of hypothenar skin wrinkling indicates a significant ulnar neuropathy. The most common and classical finding is positive elbow flexion test in which pain is elicited with supination of the forearm, extension of the wrist, and flexion of the elbow past 90° for 3 minutes.[34]

The Froment and the Wartenberg signs also indicate ulnar neuropathy.[47–49] Tinel's sign and the pressure provocation test, in which a firm pressure is applied on the ulnar nerve just proximal to the cubital tunnel with the elbow in 20° flexion and maintained for 60 seconds, may also be used as provocative tests.[1] The sensitivity and specificity of the Tinel's sign are 70% and 54%, respectively. However, the negative predictive value of the Tinel's sign was reported to be 98%.[40,50] The sensitivity and specificity of the pressure provocation test are 75% and 46%, respectively. However, if combined with elbow flexion and applied over 60 seconds, the sensitivity increases to 98%.[51] The carrying angle with abnormally valgus angulation may also predispose to traction injury of the ulnar nerve.[40]

Although a clinical diagnosis of the ulnar neuropathy is usually possible, diagnostic studies are often used. Nerve conduction studies and EMG can localize the site of ulnar nerve entrapment. However, changes may not be seen until disease has advanced, and a negative electrodiagnostic test does not rule out compression.[40,52] The cubital tunnel syndrome is considered positive if the ulnar nerve motor conduction velocity is less than 50 m/s, and if there is a 10 m/s difference in velocity or a 20% decrease in the amplitude compared with the contralateral elbow.[53] Ultrasound examination may also be used to demonstrate compression.[9] Radiographs of the elbow joint help in identifying the potential bony sources of compression. MRI can be useful to evaluate soft tissue masses causing nerve compression and to assess for concomitant pathology.[19,54,55]

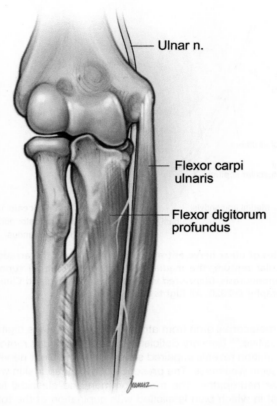

Fig. 5. The ulnar nerve may potentially be compressed between the 2 heads of the FCU. (*Reprinted* with permission, Cleveland Clinic Center for Medical Art & Photography © 2020. All Rights Reserved.)

Initial conservative treatment in the early phase includes rest, NSAIDs, and functional rehabilitation, which addresses sports specific biomechanics. Usually, symptoms resolve with rest.[1] Nocturnal splinting in semiextension or elbow pads could be considered.[40] The use of the localized corticosteroid injection is controversial.[1,9,40] In overhead athletes, throwing is not allowed for 6 weeks, followed by the implementation of a return to throwing program. Athletes with associated valgus instability secondary to ulnar collateral ligament insufficiency have higher risks of recurrence of symptoms.[1]

Surgery to treat cubital tunnel syndrome is indicated for refractory neuritis symptoms, neuropathy with motor changes, and tension neuropraxia. Surgical options include in situ decompression of the cubital tunnel, medial humeral epicondylectomy with ulnar nerve decompression, anterior transposition of the ulnar nerve (subcutaneous or submuscular), and endoscopic decompression.[1,56–58] In athletes, anterior transposition of the ulnar nerve using a subcutaneous technique is the preferred surgical treatment (Video 1).[59–61]

Ulnar Nerve Instability

Blattmann[62] first described the ulnar nerve instability in 1851. It is a chronic condition in which the ulnar nerve repetitively subluxes and relocates at the elbow.[1,62,63] As the elbow joint is flexed, the ulnar nerve leaves its sulcus on distal humerus and is compressed by the medial humeral epicondyle. In well-developed athletes, the ulnar nerve is further pushed out of the sulcus by the hypertrophied medial head of the triceps.[64]

On examination, the ulnar nerve can be palpated subluxing anterior out of the ulnar groove during elbow flexion and is usually accompanied by a palpable click as it snaps across the medial epicondyle.[65]

Mild, intermittent, or positional symptoms are managed with conservative treatment, including NSAIDs and avoidance of activities that involve repetitive elbow flexion and extension. In some sports such as bodybuilding, judo, and gymnastics, the atypical development of muscle groups is held responsible for the low response to conservative treatment.[35]

Surgery is indicated for refractory symptoms. Subcutaneous anterior transposition of the ulnar nerve is usually preferred by the majority of surgeons because of its simplicity and early return to activity. However, submuscular anterior transposition might be a better option in select cases.[66] The medial head of the triceps should be examined preoperatively and intraoperatively for snapping during flexion and extension, because failure in recognizing its snapping may cause persistent discomfort and symptomatic snapping despite surgery.[67,68]

Anconeus Epitrochlearis

The anconeus epitrochlearis, also known as the accessory anconeus muscle, is an accessory muscle that originates from the medial border of the olecranon and inserts to the medial epicondyle (**Fig. 6**). It should not be confused with the anconeus muscle, which is present at the lateral aspect of the elbow.[69] It is believed to protect the ulnar nerve and assist the triceps in preventing subluxation.[70] It is the most common anomalous muscle in the upper extremity and has been reported to be present in up to 34%.[40,71] When present, it may cause ulnar nerve compression during elbow flexion. The anconeus epitrochlearis is a known cause of cubital tunnel syndrome and has been postulated as a source of medial elbow pain in overhead athletes.[70] Its incidence in patients with cubital tunnel syndrome was reported to be as high as 25%.[71]

On MRI, it is best viewed on axial images[72] (**Fig. 7**: Axial MRI image).

In athletes who have persistent pain despite a trial of conservative management, surgical treatment options include excision of the muscle alone, or excision combined with anterior transposition of the ulnar nerve.[21,71,73]

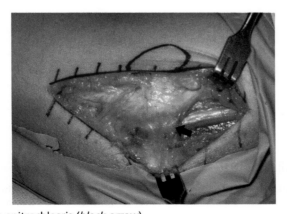

Fig. 6. Anconeus epitrochlearis (*black arrow*).

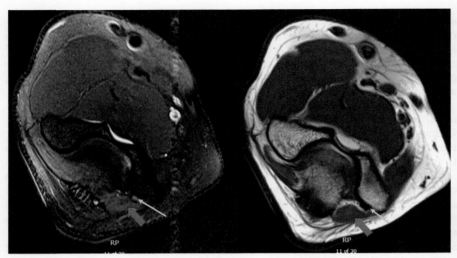

Fig. 7. Anconeus epitrochlearis on axial MRI, both on T1- and T2-weighted images (*red arrows*). *Yellow arrows* correspond to N. Ulnaris on both images.

MEDIAN NERVE
Anatomy

The median nerve arises from the medial and lateral cords of the brachial plexus. It contains nerve fibers from the C6 to T1 roots[11,19,31,74] (**Fig. 8**). It descends on the

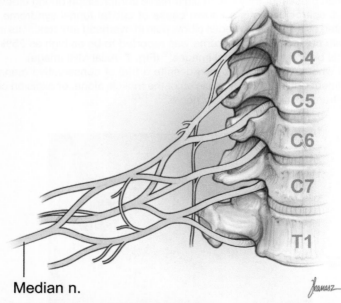

Fig. 8. The formation of the median nerve from the C6 to the T1 roots in the brachial plexus. (*Reprinted* with permission, Cleveland Clinic Center for Medical Art & Photography © 2020. All Rights Reserved.)

median side of the arm, lateral to the median artery, between the brachialis and biceps. Above the antecubital fossa, it passes under the ligament of Struthers, runs between the brachialis muscle and the medial intermuscular septum distally. Then, it passes through the antecubital fossa, deep to the lacertus fibrosus, and descends between the 2 heads of the pronator teres (PT) into the forearm between the flexor digitorum superficialis (FDS) and FDP. The anterior interosseous nerve (AIN) originates close to the deep head of PT and the arch of FDS.[9,75,76]

The median nerve innervates all the flexor muscles in the forearm except the FCU and the medial 2 digits of FDP. In the hand, it innervates the first and second lumbricals, opponens pollicis, abductor pollicis brevis, and flexor pollicis brevis. The median nerve provides sensory innervation to the palmar/lateral aspect of the hand, including the first 3 and one-half digits.[77]

In athletes, median nerve compression is usually the result of excessive and repetitive movements in the elbow and forearm. Common sites of median nerve compression in athletes are the PT (resulting in PT syndrome), the ligament of Struthers and the FDS (leading to AIN syndrome), and the lacertus fibrosis (resulting in lacertus syndrome). Athletes present with proximal forearm pain and numbness in the hand except for isolated AIN injury, which is a pure motor nerve.[9] The AIN anatomically serves as the division point between high and low median nerve injuries.[77] AIN syndrome and pronator syndrome are clinical entities of proximal median neuropathy in the forearm that have similar, but uniquely different, presentations and etiologies.

Pronator Teres Syndrome

First described by Seyffarth in 1951, the pronator syndrome results from overuse in athletes.[78,79] The most common site of entrapment is between the 2 heads of the PT (**Fig. 9**). Other sites include the overlying bicipital aponeurosis (lacertus fibrosus) and the FDS (sublimis bridge).

Pronator syndrome is common in athletes performing repeated pronation and gripping, such as tennis, baseball, archery and weight lifting.[9,11,16,79] Athletes usually present with pain and numbness along the median nerve distribution and may note pain while throwing and swinging a racquet.[31,34,80–83]

Symptoms may be elicited either by manual compression of the median nerve over the PT or with resisted wrist flexion and pronation of the forearm.[80,82,84] Alternatively, applying a direct pressure over the PT while the arm is supinated may elicit paresthesia in the median nerve distribution within 1 minute.[47] Interestingly, weakness may be present in all muscles innervated by the median nerve except for the PT, because it receives its innervation proximal to the most common site of compression.[19]

Initial treatment consists of rest, NSAIDs, an elbow splint, and physical therapy, which focuses on functional restoration and proper sports specific mechanics.[9] After symptoms subside, the athlete may be allowed to start simple hand exercises (ball squeeze), followed by light wrist flexion–extension, and pronation–supination exercises.[34] There are no randomized controlled studies investigating the treatment outcomes in pronator syndrome and no evidence to guide the duration of conservative management.

Surgery is indicated for refractory symptoms.[19,31,85] Different approaches have been described to expose the proximal median nerve including oblique, transverse, and lazy S-shaped incisions.[86–88] Basically, the nerve is explored, and fibrous bands are released and excised until the nerve passes freely in the pronator tunnel.[19,84] Minimally invasive and endoscopic median nerve release have also been described more recently.[89,90] The athlete is allowed to return to play once pain is resolved and the cause of compression is addressed.[34]

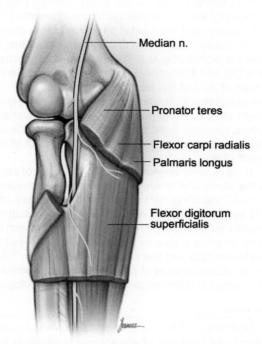

Median n.

Pronator teres

Flexor carpi radialis
Palmaris longus

Flexor digitorum
superficialis

Fig. 9. The median nerve may be compressed between 2 heads of the PT. (*Reprinted* with permission, Cleveland Clinic Center for Medical Art & Photography © 2020. All Rights Reserved.)

Lacertus Syndrome

The lacertus fibrosus is a broad, flattened, fibrous band arising from the lower medial border of the biceps tendon[91](**Fig. 10**). The median nerve passes through a tunnel at the level of lacertus fibrosus, where the bottom of the tunnel is medial trochlea, the lateral wall is the brachialis muscle, the medial wall is pronator muscles, and the roof of the tunnel is the lacertus fibrosus.[92] It may be thickened and cause compression of the median nerve as the nerve passes deep to it. Although it is traditionally considered a component of the pronator syndrome, Hagert[92] suggested lacertus syndrome to be distinguished from other levels of nerve entrapment.

The characteristic clinical triad includes (1) weakness of muscles innervated by the median nerve distal to the lacertus fibrosus, especially the FPL, FDP II, and flexor carpi radialis, (2) pain with external pressure over the median nerve at the level of lacertus fibrosus, and (3) a positive scratch collapse test over the median nerve at the level of the lacertus fibrosus.[50,92] Flexion–supination of the elbow against resistance demonstrates the presence or absence of entrapment of the nerve by the lacertus fibrosus.[84,92] Seitz and colleagues[93] reported 7 cases of acute compression of the median nerve by the lacertus fibrosus. The mechanism of the acute compression in their case series was a sudden severe elbow flexion against a severe counterforce.

Athletes commonly complain of loss of key and tip pinch strength and fine motor skills, sense of clumsiness, and rarely, transient paresthesia in the median nerve innervated region of the hand.[94] The may also have burning and numbness in the palmar cutaneous branch of the median nerve distribution.[95]

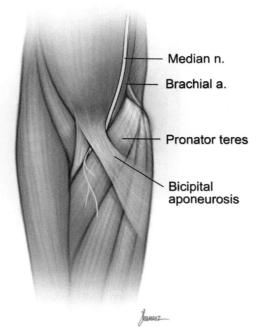

Median n.

Brachial a.

Pronator teres

Bicipital
aponeurosis

Fig. 10. Lacertus fibrosus. (*Reprinted* with permission, Cleveland Clinic Center for Medical Art & Photography © 2020. All Rights Reserved.)

The lacertus fibrosus can be surgically released either through an S-shaped incision or minimally invasive technique using wide awake anesthesia.[92]

Ligament of Struthers

The ligament of Struthers is a fibrous band extending from a supracondylar spur on the distal humerus to the medial epicondyle[31] (**Fig. 11**). It is reported to be present in 0.7% to 2.7% of the population.[96,97]

Athletes usually present with pain in the wrist or medial forearm and numbness along the thumb and index finger. Pain is worsened with supination of the forearm. Palpation may not always be possible because of body habitus.[77] Internal oblique elbow radiographs may reveal the spur.[98] EMG may be helpful in making a diagnosis. However, it has been shown that only 5% of symptomatic patients will have a positive test.[99] Treatment consists of surgical removal of the bony process and excision of the ligament.[100,101]

Anterior Interosseous Nerve Syndrome (Kiloh-Nevin Syndrome)

The AIN is a pure motor nerve. It innervates pronator quadratus, lateral 2 heads of the FDP, and the FPL.[9,34] It can be compressed by the fibrous edge of the FDS, the deep head of PT, or the forearm musculature in athletes.[11]

Symptoms include vague pain in the proximal forearm and weakness in the nerve's distribution.[34] Athletes usually complain of a dull and aching pain as well as difficulty using the thumb and index finger.

Physical examination reveals weakness of flexion of the thumb, index and middle fingers, and difficulty performing OK sign.[102–106] Symptoms could be elicited by

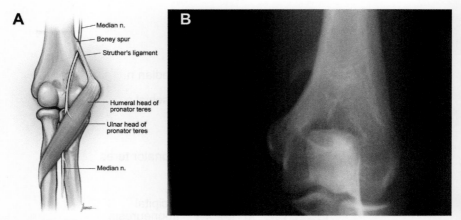

Fig. 11. Pronator syndrome (*A*) and ligament of Struthers (*red arrows*) (*A, B*). ([A] *Reprinted with permission, Cleveland Clinic Center for Medical Art & Photography © 2020. All Rights Reserved.*)

resisted elbow flexion, pronation, and index and middle finger flexion.[47] Because the AIN is a pure motor branch, sensory findings are not present.

The diagnosis may be established using EMG, which reveals fibrillations, sharp waves, abnormal latency, and abnormal compound motor action potentials.[107]

Many authors reported spontaneous recovery with conservative management.[19,108–110] However, there is no consensus on the time to allow for spontaneous resolution. A minimum of 12 months of conservative treatment is suggested before offering a surgical intervention.[103]

Surgery is indicated for refractory symptoms. The proximal median nerve is exposed using the lazy S-shaped incision over the volar forearm, and is released in a proximal to distal fashion. The AIN is identified and released from the overlying tissue, as it courses into the distal forearm.[19] Some authors suggested that hourglass-like constrictions exist around the AIN owing to multifocal nerve compressions, and a combination of neurolysis with or without resection of the hourglass constriction and direct coaptation or interpositional nerve graft have been suggested to have satisfactory outcomes.[111–113] Minimally invasive endoscopic decompression is also reported for AIN syndrome.[114]

RADIAL NERVE

The radial nerve is rarely injured in athletes.[11] It may be entrapped in multiple anatomic locations proximally along the humerus or distally along the forearm and can affect the posterior interosseous nerve (PIN), a motor branch of the radial nerve.[31] In athletes, it most commonly occurs as a result of excessive and repetitive elbow extension such as in racket sports.

Anatomy

The radial nerve derives from the posterior cord of the brachial plexus. It contains nerve fibers from the C5 to T1 roots and is the largest branch of the brachial plexus[11,19] (**Fig. 12**). Distal to its groove on the humerus, the radial nerve moves laterally, pierces the intermuscular septum and runs in the anterior compartment between the biceps and brachialis muscles.[115] At the radiohumeral joint, approximately 3 to 4 cm proximal

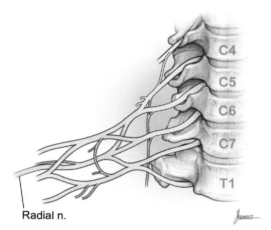

Radial n.

Fig. 12. The formation of the radial nerve from the C5 to T1 roots in the brachial plexus. (*Reprinted* with permission, Cleveland Clinic Center for Medical Art & Photography © 2020. All Rights Reserved.)

to the superior border of the supinator muscle, the radial nerve bifurcates into the PIN and superficial radial nerve.[75]

The PIN passes adjacent to the joint capsule at the level of the radial head, courses obliquely through the supinator muscle, and enters into the extensor compartment of the forearm. The PIN is a predominantly motor branch that travels between the 2 heads of the supinator muscle and continues down between the superficial and deep extensor muscles of the forearm.

The superficial radial nerve arises at the level of the radiohumeral joint, continues distally in the forearm lateral to the radial artery and in the deep surface of the BR, pierces the fascia on the ulnar side of this tendon about 7 cm about the wrist.[76] It provides sensory innervation to the lateral forearm.

Posterior Interosseous Entrapment (Supinator Syndrome)

PIN entrapment is usually seen in athletes who have an overgrowth of muscles, such as bodybuilders, mixed marital arts fighters, rope skippers, and wrestlers, as well as in athletes who undergo repetitive supination and pronation such as swimmers and tennis players.[19,116]

The PIN may be entrapped while it courses under the supinator muscle at the entrance of the arcade of Frohse, which is a tendinous thickening of the proximal edge of the supinator muscle and is one of the most common locations for radial nerve compression[117](**Fig. 13**). The arcade of Frohse is present in 30% to 50% of the population.[118] It is tightened during pronation and may cause nerve compression.[119] Other sites of PIN entrapment include the fibrous bands of tissue between brachialis and brachioradialis (BR), the medial proximal edge of extensor carpi radialis brevis, the recurrent radial blood vessels at the radial neck, known as the leash of Henry, and the distal margin of the superficial part of supinator.[11,120,121]

Athletes usually present with burning or pain along the lateral forearm, which worsens with supination resistance with the elbow at 90°. Physical examination may reveal weakness of the extensor muscles of wrist and gradual loss of digit and thumb extension. The function of the BR and extensor carpi radialis longus is preserved. No sensory loss occurs with the PIN lesion.[19] Pain may be elicited by applying pressure over the supinator

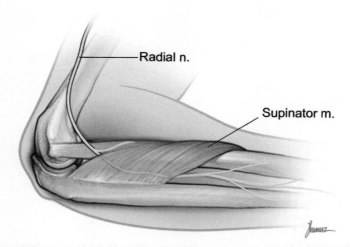

—Radial n.

Supinator m.

Fig. 13. The PIN may be entrapped while it courses under the supinator muscle. (*Reprinted with permission, Cleveland Clinic Center for Medical Art & Photography © 2020. All Rights Reserved.*)

canal.[119] Roles' sign, defined as pain with resisted extension of the third finger, may be positive. However, it is also usually positive in lateral epicondylitis.[119]

EMG is the preferred diagnostic study and is characterized by abnormalities in spontaneous or voluntary activity of PIN-innervated muscles. The BR and the extensor carpi radialis longus are preserved.[31,122] Imaging studies are not routinely used; however, MRI may be useful to demonstrate mass lesions including ganglia, fibromas, lipomas, hemangiomas, and tumors, all of which have been described as causative factors.[19,123]

Treatment includes rest and functional physical therapy, with a focus on the kinetic chain and proper mechanics. Surgical release is indicated for refractory symptoms.[9] Surgical approaches include both the posterior and the anterior approaches. In the posterior approach, the extensor carpi radialis brevis and the extensor digitorum communis are identified superficial to the supinator muscle, followed by the identification and release of the PIN proximal to the arcade of the Frohse. In the anterior approach, the radial nerve is identified between the BR and the biceps, followed distally as it bifurcates as PIN and superficial radial nerve. The arcade of Frohse is then released, and the entire length of the supinator is visualized and completely released.[124]

IATROGENIC AND SURGICAL INJURIES

Iatrogenic peripheral nerve injuries during sports-related surgeries are rare. However, complications related to these injuries may have a substantial effect on the athlete's career and life. Orthopedic surgery has been reported to be the most common cause of iatrogenic peripheral nerve injury requiring treatment, with the median nerve being the most commonly injured nerve in the upper extremity.[125,126]

The nerve may be directly injured during dissection or with surgical instruments and implants such as plates, drill bits, K-wires, and minimally invasive techniques.[127] Indirect mechanisms of injury include stretching and thermal damage.[125] Most iatrogenic injuries could be prevented with an adequate knowledge of surgical anatomy and an awareness of the types of procedures in which peripheral nerves are particularly vulnerable.[128]

Iatrogenic Injuries to the Ulnar Nerve

Ulnar collateral ligament reconstruction

Jobe performed the first ulnar collateral ligament reconstruction in 1974.[129] Relatively high ulnar nerve–related complication rates associated with his original technique (which involves complete detachment of the common flexor origin) led to the development of alternative approaches that use a muscle splitting approach.[98,126,130–139]

In a recent systematic review including 1368 patients, Watson and colleagues[129] compared complication rates of different ulnar collateral ligament reconstruction techniques. They reported the overall prevalence of the ulnar nerve injury to be 12.9%. They suggested that modifications to the Jobe technique decreased complication rates from 51.4% to 6.0% (*P*<.05).

In a recent meta-analysis investigating the outcomes of different ulnar collateral ligament reconstruction techniques, Somerson and colleagues[130] reported the overall prevalence of the ulnar nerve injury to be 6.7%. They showed that the docking technique had lower ulnar nerve complication rates and higher rates of excellent Conway scores. They attributed the high rates of complications with the earlier techniques to the transposition of the ulnar nerve.

Elbow arthroscopy

The prevalence of nerve complications after elbow arthroscopy is reported to be between 0% and 14%. Most of these complications are transient.[131,132]

Underlying injury mechanisms were proposed to include compression or direct injury from instruments, excessive joint distension, aggressive manipulation, or postoperative continuous passive motion device.[131,133] Some authors have suggested that local anesthetics and regional nerve blocks do not allow evaluation of the nerve and discouraged the use of local anesthetic immediately after surgery.[131,133–135]

The ulnar nerve may be iatrogenically injured as portals are blindly created in athletes with prior subcutaneous ulnar nerve transposition.[136] Therefore, a history of prior anterior transposition should be obtained before the surgery.[133] In cases with prior transposition and palpable ulnar nerve, a 1-cm incision and blunt dissection to the capsule without identification is possible. However, if the nerve is not palpable, then it is advised to identify and protect the ulnar nerve first.[137] The ulnar nerve may also be injured if the anteromedial portals are placed over 2 cm proximal to the medial epicondyle.[138] The ulnar nerve is also at risk while debriding the medial gutter during posterior compartment arthroscopy.[133]

Kelly and colleagues[131] suggested that underlying rheumatoid arthritis and contracture are the most significant risk factors for ulnar nerve injury during elbow arthroscopy. Blonna and O'Driscoll[139] suggested that simultaneous ulnar nerve transposition and retractor use could reduce complications. Ulnar neuropathy has the worst prognosis for returning of motor function, and intrinsic hand weakness may be permanent.[140]

Iatrogenic Injuries to the Median Nerve

The median nerve could may iatrogenically injured in a variety of procedures; it is reported to have the highest iatrogenic injury rate among the upper limb nerves.[125]

Palmaris graft harvest

The palmaris longus (PL) originates from the common flexor tendon on the medial epicondyle of the humerus. It is generally the only tendon superficial to the antebrachial fascia of the forearm, and is one of the most variable muscles, with the most common variation being its absence.[141,142]

The PL is a commonly used donor tendon for transfer and grafting. At the level of the wrist, it lies immediately superficial to the median nerve.[143,144] This anatomic relationship exposes the median nerve to risk during tendon harvesting procedures. In athletes with an absent PL tendon, misidentification of the median nerve as the PL tendon causes it to be harvested as a graft unintentionally.[145–149]

There are a few ways to distinguish the median nerve from the PL tendon. First, the median nerve has tubular shape, whereas the PL tendon is flat and broad. Second, it has a larger diameter than the PL tendon. In addition, it has vasa nervorum running along its volar aspect.[144] Choo and colleagues[144] suggested the following strategies to prevent median nerve injury during PL harvesting:

1. Preoperative: Examine the presence of PL by asking the athlete to flex wrist while opposing thumb to small finger.
2. Intraoperative
   a. Assess for tenting of skin and cupping of palm when applying upward traction on tendon.
   b. Assess for a flattened shape of the tendon in contrast with the tubular shape of a nerve.
   c. Assess for the absence of the vasa nervorum.
   d. Extend the incision proximally and/or distally until the PL is unequivocally identified.

Distal biceps repair

The treatment choice for the acute rupture of the distal biceps tendon in athletes is surgical reattachment. The reported postoperative complication rate of the distal biceps tendon repair is between 16% and 40%.[150,151] The prevalence of the median nerve injury during distal biceps tendon repair is reported to be 4%.

Initially, a single anterior incision via the Henry approach was used to anatomically reattach the distal biceps to the radial tuberosity. Boyd and Anderson developed a 2-incision technique owing to the high rates of nerve injury with Henry approach. Failla later modified the 2-incision technique.[152] Current biceps tendon fixation techniques include suture anchors, bio-interference screws, and cortical buttons. This has led to a trend back to the single incision approach being more commonly used.[152]

Injury may result from aberrant dissection and/or aggressive retraction medially on the neurovascular bundle.[153]

The identification of anatomic landmarks and avoidance of aggressive medial retraction are important to prevent median nerve injury during distal tendon repair. Wide retractors increase access to the repair site, dissipate the force over a large area, and are recommended to be used. Dissection should be directed lateral to the brachial artery and medial dissection should be avoided.[153]

In cases of median nerve deficit after distal biceps tendon reattachment, the initial treatment is observation of the symptoms and function. Surgery is indicated for cases with no improvement in functions and nerve studies. Nerve repair is preferred in acute neurotmesis, whereas chronic cases are generally treated with tendon transfers to recover thumb opposition, finger flexion, and wrist flexion.[153]

Iatrogenic Injuries to the Radial Nerve

The radial nerve and its branches have been reported to be iatrogenically injured during distal bicep tendon repair. Fortunately, most of these injuries cause transient and recovery mostly occurs within 6 months, although it may take longer owing to the long course of the nerve.

A PIN injury was reported in about 1% to 5% of distal biceps repairs using a single anterior incision and it is considered the most severe complication of this surgery.[154–156] The PIN may be injured during both the 1-incision and 2-incision approaches, and may occur via mechanical nerve compression (such as during retraction while exposing the radial tuberosity), by direct injury such as errant drill bit placement, entrapment under a cortical button, or dissection along the proximal radius.[153,157] The most dangerous drill bit orientation is distal and radially directed drilling at the level of the radial tuberosity.[153] Placing the forearm in full supination during deep dissection to the radial tuberosity helps to avoid PIN injury.

Clinically, patients with PIN deficits present with weakness with finger and thumb extension and radial deviation with attempted wrist extension. Fortunately, most PIN injuries are neuropraxia and ultimately recover. Cohen[158] suggested the presence of motor unit action potentials in the muscles of the dorsal forearm to be a positive prognostic sign.

In a cadaver study, Lo and colleagues[159] investigated the effect of drill trajectory on proximity to the PIN during cortical button distal biceps repair. They recommended drilling across the radius at 90° to its longitudinal axis, and aiming for 0° to 30° ulnarly, with the athlete's forearm in full supination to provide an increased margin of safety and thereby prevent injury to the PIN.

If a PIN injury is detected intraoperatively, standard nerve repair techniques should be applied.[153] The investigators reported different recovery time after the injury.[157] Cohen reported that stretch injuries recover in less than 8 weeks and recommended the use of a dynamic digital extension splint. If nerve functions do not return in 8 weeks, electrical studies could be obtained. Surgical exploration could be considered in the absence of recovery at 3 months after injury.[158,160]

Superficial radial nerve

The superficial radial nerve provides sensation to the dorsoradial aspect of the hand and thumb. Injury to the nerve is encountered in 5% to 10% of distal biceps repairs. It is generally a neuropraxia caused by aggressive lateral traction.

Some authors recommended the use of skin hooks instead of lateral retractors to prevent injury to the superficial radial nerve.[153]

Initial treatment is usually observation of the symptoms because the numbness improves in most cases. Permanent damage and neuromas may also develop, but symptomatic treatment is generally recommended.[153]

DISCLOSURE

The authors have nothing to disclose.

SUPPLEMENTARY DATA

Supplementary data related to this article can be found online at https://doi.org/10.1016/j.csm.2020.02.006.

REFERENCES

1. Güner MD, Demirtaş AM. Ulnar nerve problems in sportsmen. In: Elbow and sport. Switzerland: Springer; 2016. p. 209–17.

2. Sunderland S. The intraneural topography of the radial, median and ulnar nerves. Brain 1945;68(4):243–98.

3. Kumar SD, Bourke G. Nerve compression syndromes at the elbow. Orthop Trauma 2016;30(4):355–62.
4. Akuthota V, Maslowski E. Causes of numbness and tingling in athletes. In: Nerve and vascular injuries in sports medicine. Switzerland: Springer; 2009. p. 3–15.
5. Dyck PJTP. Peripheral neuropathy. 4th edition. Philadelphia: Elsevier Saunders; 2005.
6. Lundborg G, Rydevik B. Effects of stretching the tibial nerve of the rabbit. A preliminary study of the intraneural circulation and the barrier function of the perineurium. J Bone Joint Surg Br 1973;55(2):390–401.
7. Ochoa J, Danta G, Fowler TJ, et al. Nature of the nerve lesion caused by a pneumatic tourniquet. Nature 1971;233(5317):265–6.
8. Weinstein S, Herring S. Nerve problems and compartment syndromes in the hand, wrist, and forearm. Clin Sports Med 1992;11(1):161–88.
9. Hainline BW. Peripheral nerve injury in sports. Continuum (Minneap Minn) 2014; 20(6):1605–28.
10. Hang Y-S. Tardy ulnar neuritis in a little league baseball player. Am J Sports Med 1981;9(4):244–6.
11. Feinberg JH, Nadler SF, Krivickas LS. Peripheral nerve injuries in the athlete. Sports Med 1997;24(6):385–408.
12. Dangles CJ, Bilos ZJ. Ulnar nerve neuritis in a world champion weightlifter: a case report. Am J Sports Med 1980;8(6):443–5.
13. Schickendantz MS. Diagnosis and treatment of elbow disorders in the overhead athlete. Hand Clin 2002;18(1):65–75.
14. Glousman R. Ulnar nerve problems in the athlete's elbow. Clin Sports Med 1990; 9(2):365–77.
15. Barnes DA, Tullos HS. An analysis of 100 symptomatic baseball players. Am J Sports Med 1978;6(2):62–7.
16. Sicuranza M. Compressive neuropathies in the upper extremity of athletes. Hand Clin 1992;8(2):263–73.
17. Pechan J, Juliš I. The pressure measurement in the ulnar nerve. A contribution to the pathophysiology of the cubital tunnel syndrome. J Biomech 1975;8(1):75–9.
18. Apfelberg DB, Larson SJ. Dynamic anatomy of the ulnar nerve at the elbow. Plast Reconstr Surg 1973;51(1):76–81.
19. Ali ZS, Heuer GG, Zager EL. Nerve compression/entrapment sites of the upper limb. In: Nerves and nerve injuries. Netherlands: Elsevier; 2015. p. 725–53.
20. Pecina M, Markiewitz A. Tunnel syndrome in athletes in tunnel syndromes: peripheral nerve compression syndrome. New York: Taylor & Francis; 2001.
21. Warrell CS, Osbahr DC, Andrews JR. Thrower's elbow 25. In: Volpi P, editor. Arthroscopy and sport injuries: applications in high-level athletes. Switzerland: Springer; 2016. p. 185.
22. Conway J, Jobe FW, Glousman R, et al. Medial instability of the elbow in throwing athletes. Treatment by repair or reconstruction of the ulnar collateral ligament. J Bone Joint Surg Am 1992;74(1):67–83.
23. Gabel GT, Morrey B. Operative treatment of medial epicondylitis. J Bone Joint Surg Am 1995;77(7):1065–9.
24. Buehler MJ, Thayer DT. The elbow flexion test. A clinical test for the cubital tunnel syndrome. Clin Orthop Relat Res 1988;(233):213–6.
25. Del Pizzo W, Jobe FW, Norwood L. Ulnar nerve entrapment syndrome in baseball players. Am J Sports Med 1977;5(5):182–5.
26. Hariri S, Safran MR. Ulnar collateral ligament injury in the overhead athlete. Clin Sports Med 2010;29(4):619–44.

27. Anderson MW, Alford BA. Overhead throwing injuries of the shoulder and elbow. Radiol Clin 2010;48(6):1137–54.
28. Boatright J, D'Alessandro D. Nerve entrapment syndromes at the elbow. In: Jobe FW, editor. Operative techniques in upper extremity sports injuries. St Louis (MO): Mosby-Year Book; 1996. p. 518–37.
29. Childress HM. Recurrent ulnar-nerve dislocation at the elbow. Clin orthopaedics Relat Res 1975;108:168–73.
30. Jobe FW, Stark H, Lombardo S. Reconstruction of the ulnar collateral ligament in athletes. J Bone Joint Surg Am 1986;68(8):1158–63.
31. Yang AJ, Akuthota V. Nerve injuries in sports. In: Nerves and nerve injuries. Netherlands: Elsevier; 2015. p. 655–63.
32. Filippou G, Mondelli M, Greco G, et al. Ulnar neuropathy at the elbow: how frequent is the idiopathic form? An ultrasonographic study in a cohort of patients. Clin Exp Rheumatol 2010;28(1):63.
33. Norkus S, Meyers MC. Ulnar neuropathy of the elbow. Sports Med 1994;17(3): 189–99.
34. Ibrahim V, Weiss E. Elbow and forearm injuries. In: Essential sports medicine. Switzerland: Springer; 2008. p. 61–76.
35. Adamczyk G. Nerve entrapment of upper extremities in sports. In: Doral MN, Karlsson J, editors. Sports injuries: prevention, diagnosis, treatment and rehabilitation. Berlin: Springer Berlin Heidelberg; 2015. p. 603–13.
36. Fulkerson JP. Transient ulnar neuropathy from Nordic skiing. Clin orthopaedics Relat Res 1980;(153):230–1.
37. Jobe F, Nuber G. Throwing injuries of the elbow. Clin Sports Med 1986;5(4): 621–36.
38. Eckman PB, Perlstein G, Altrocchi PH. Ulnar neuropathy in bicycle riders. Arch Neurol 1975;32(2):130–1.
39. Dozono K, Hachisuka K, Hatada K, et al. Peripheral neuropathies in the upper extremities of paraplegic wheelchair marathon racers. Spinal Cord 1995; 33(4):208.
40. Pellegrini A, Calderazzi F, Lunini E, et al. The throwing elbow. In: The elbow. Switzerland: Springer; 2018. p. 447–65.
41. Werner C-O, Ohlin P, Elmqvist D. Pressures recorded in ulnar neuropathy. Acta Orthop Scand 1985;56(5):404–6.
42. Gellman H. Compression of the ulnar nerve at the elbow: cubital tunnel syndrome. Instr Course Lect 2008;57:187–97.
43. Elhassan B, Steinmann SP. Entrapment neuropathy of the ulnar nerve. J Am Acad Orthop Surg 2007;15(11):672–81.
44. Eygendaal D, Safran M. Postero-medial elbow problems in the adult athlete. Br J Sports Med 2006;40(5):430–4.
45. Duchenne G-B. Physiology of motion demonstrated by means of electrical stimulation and clinical observation and applied to the study of paralysis and deformities. Philadelphia: WB Saunders; 1959.
46. Earle AS, Vlastou C. Crossed fingers and other tests of ulnar nerve motor function. J Hand Surg 1980;5(6):560–5.
47. Popinchalk SP, Schaffer AA. Physical examination of upper extremity compressive neuropathies. Orthop Clin North Am 2012;43(4):417–30.
48. Wartenberg R. A sign of ulnar palsy. J Am Med Assoc 1939;112(17):1688.
49. Mackinnon SE. Surgery of the peripheral nerve. In: Mackinnon SE, Dellon AL, editors. Carpal Tunnel Syndrome. New York: Thieme; 1988. p. 146–69.

50. Cheng CJ, Mackinnon-Patterson B, Beck JL, et al. Scratch collapse test for evaluation of carpal and cubital tunnel syndrome. J Hand Surg 2008;33(9):1518–24.

51. Palmer BA, Hughes TB. Cubital tunnel syndrome. J Hand Surg 2010;35(1):153–63.

52. Posner MA. Compressive ulnar neuropathies at the elbow: I. Etiology and diagnosis. J Am Acad Orthop Surg 1998;6(5):282–8.

53. Medicine AAoE. AAEM practice topics in electrodiagnostic medicine. Practice parameter for electrodiagnostic studies in ulnar neuropathy at the elbow: summary statement. Muscle Nerve 1999;22:408–11.

54. Dellon A. Patient evaluation and management considerations in nerve compression. Hand Clin 1992;8(2):229.

55. Beekman R, Schoemaker MC, van der Plas JPL, et al. Diagnostic value of high-resolution sonography in ulnar neuropathy at the elbow. Neurology 2004;62(5):767–73.

56. Hahn SB, Choi YR, Kang HJ, et al. Decompression of the ulnar nerve and minimal medial epicondylectomy with a small incision for cubital tunnel syndrome: comparison with anterior subcutaneous transposition of the nerve. J Plast Reconstr Aesthet Surg 2010;63(7):1150–5.

57. Tsai TM, Bonczar M, Tsuruta T, et al. A new operative technique: cubital tunnel decompression with endoscopic assistance. Hand Clin 1995;11(1):71–80.

58. Amadio P, Gabel G. Treatment and complications of failed decompression of the ulnar nerve at the elbow. In: Gelberman, editor. Oper nerve repair reconstructionvol. 2. Philadelphia: Lippincitt Williams and Wilkins; 1991. p. 1107–19.

59. Charles YP, Coulet B, Rouzaud J-C, et al. Comparative clinical outcomes of submuscular and subcutaneous transposition of the ulnar nerve for cubital tunnel syndrome. J Hand Surg 2009;34(5):866–74.

60. Chung KC. Treatment of ulnar nerve compression at the elbow. J Hand Surg 2008;33(9):1625–7.

61. Mackinnon SE. Comparative clinical outcomes of submuscular and subcutaneous transposition of the ulnar nerve for cubital tunnel syndrome. J Hand Surg 2009;34(8):1574–5.

62. Blattmann A. Beobachtung einer Dislokation des N. ulnaris. Dtsch Klin 1851;435–7.

63. Bednar M, Blair S, Light T. Complications of the treatment of cubital tunnel syndrome. Hand Clin 1994;10(1):83–92.

64. Molnar SL, Lang P, Skapinyecz J, et al. Dislocation of the ulnar nerve at the elbow in an elite wrestler. BMJ Case Rep 2011;2011. bcr0220113806.

65. Peck E, Strakowski JA. Ultrasound evaluation of focal neuropathies in athletes: a clinically-focused review. Br J Sports Med 2015;49(3):166–75.

66. Xarchas K, Psillakis I, Koukou O, et al. Ulnar nerve dislocation at the elbow: review of the literature and report of three cases. Open Orthop J 2007;1:1.

67. Haws M, Brown RE. Bilateral snapping triceps tendon after bilateral ulnar nerve transposition for ulnar nerve subluxation. Ann Plast Surg 1995;34(5):550–1.

68. Spinner RJ, Goldner RD. Snapping of the medial head of the triceps and recurrent dislocation of the ulnar nerve. Anatomical and dynamic factors. J Bone Joint Surg Am 1998;80(2):239–47.

69. Deng F, Jindani I. Anconeus epitrochlearis. Available at: https://radiopaedia.org/articles/anconeus-epitrochlearis?lang=us.

70. Li X, Dines JS, Gorman M, et al. Anconeus epitrochlearis as a source of medial elbow pain in baseball pitchers. Orthopedics 2012;35(7):e1129–32.

71. Masear VR, Hill JJ Jr, Cohen SM. Ulnar compression neuropathy secondary to the anconeus epitrochlearis muscle. J Hand Surg 1988;13(5):720–4.
72. Byun S-D, Kim C-H, Jeon I-H. Ulnar neuropathy caused by an anconeus epitrochlearis: clinical and electrophysiological findings. J Hand Surg Eur Vol 2011; 36(7):607–8.
73. Chalmers J. Unusual causes of peripheral nerve compression. Hand 1978;(2): 167–75.
74. Rigoard P. Atlas of anatomy of the peripheral nerves: the nerves of the limbs–student edition. Springer; 2017.
75. Crosio A, Mattei L, Blonna D, et al. Anatomy and specimens. In: The elbow. Switzerland: Springer; 2018. p. 19–28.
76. Celli A. Anatomy and biomechanics of the elbow. In: Treatment of elbow lesions. Switzerland: Springer; 2008. p. 1–11.
77. Neal SL, Fields KB. Peripheral nerve entrapment and injury in the upper extremity. Am Fam Physician 2010;81(2):147–55.
78. Seyffarth H. Primary myoses in the M. pronator teres as cause of lesion of the N. medianus (the pronator syndrome). Acta Psychiatr Neurol Scand Suppl 1951; 74:251.
79. Radić B, Radić P, Duraković D. Peripheral nerve injury in sports. Acta Clin Croat 2018;57(3):561–9.
80. Hartz CR, Linscheid R, Gramse R, et al. The pronator teres syndrome: compressive neuropathy of the median nerve. J Bone Joint Surg Am 1981;63(6):885–90.
81. Arendt EA. Stress fractures. In: Mellion MB, editor. Sports medicine secrets. 2nd edition. Philadelphia: Hanley & Belfus; 1999. p. 331–7.
82. Morris HH, Peters BH. Pronator syndrome: clinical and electrophysiological features in seven cases. J Neurol Neurosurg Psychiatry 1976;39(5):461–4.
83. Solnitzky O. Pronator syndrome: compression neuropathy of the median nerve at level of pronator teres muscle. Georgetown Med Bull 1960;13:232–8.
84. Johnson RK, Spinner M, Shrewsbury MM. Median nerve entrapment syndrome in the proximal forearm. J Hand Surg 1979;4(1):48–51.
85. Eversmann W. Proximal median nerve compression. Hand Clin 1992;8(2): 307–15.
86. Olehnik WK, Manske PR, Szerzinski J. Median nerve compression in the proximal forearm. J Hand Surg 1994;19(1):121–6.
87. Mackinnon S, Dellon A, Hudson A, et al. Chronic human nerve compression–a histological assessment. Neuropathol Appl Neurobiol 1986;12(6):547–65.
88. Koo JT, Szabo RM. Compression neuropathies of the median nerve. J Am Soc Surg Hand 2004;4(3):156–75.
89. Lee AK, Khorsandi M, Nurbhai N, et al. Endoscopically assisted decompression for pronator syndrome. J Hand Surg 2012;37(6):1173–9.
90. Zancolli ER III, Zancolli EP IV, Perrotto CJ. New mini-invasive decompression for pronator teres syndrome. J Hand Surg 2012;37(8):1706–10.
91. Swiggett R, Ruby LK. Median nerve compression neuropathy by the lacertus fibrosus: report of three cases. J Hand Surg 1986;11(5):700–3.
92. Hagert E. Clinical diagnosis and wide-awake surgical treatment of proximal median nerve entrapment at the elbow: a prospective study. Hand 2013;8(1):41–6.
93. Seitz WH Jr, Matsuoka H, McAdoo J, et al. Acute compression of the median nerve at the elbow by the lacertus fibrosus. J Shoulder Elbow Surg 2007; 16(1):91–4.

94. Paletta GA, Wright RW. The modified docking procedure for elbow ulnar collateral ligament reconstruction: 2-year follow-up in elite throwers. Am J Sports Med 2006;34(10):1594–8.

95. Lalonde D. Lacertus syndrome: a commonly missed and misdiagnosed median nerve entrapment syndrome. BMC Proceedings. Switzerland: Springer; 2015.

96. Miller TT, Reinus WR. Nerve entrapment syndromes of the elbow, forearm, and wrist. Am J Roentgenol 2010;195(3):585–94.

97. Hrdlička A. Incidence of the supracondyloid process in whites and other races. Am J Phys Anthropol 1923;6(4):405–12.

98. Lordan J, Rauh P, Spinner RJ. The clinical anatomy of the supracondylar spur and the ligament of Struthers. Clin Anat 2005;18(7):548–51.

99. Lee MJ, LaStayo PC. Pronator syndrome and other nerve compressions that mimic carpal tunnel syndrome. J Orthop Sports Phys Ther 2004;34(10):601–9.

100. Suranyi L. Median nerve compression by Struthers ligament. J Neurol Neurosurg Psychiatry 1983;46(11):1047–9.

101. Bilge T, Yalaman O, Bilge S, et al. Entrapment neuropathy of the median nerve at the level of the ligament of Struthers. Neurosurgery 1990;27(5):787–9.

102. Stern MB. The anterior interosseous nerve syndrome (the Kiloh-Nevin syndrome). Report and follow-up study of three cases. Clin orthopaedics Relat Res 1984;(187):223–7.

103. Rodner CM, Tinsley BA, O'Malley MP. Pronator syndrome and anterior interosseous nerve syndrome. J Am Acad Orthop Surg 2013;21(5):268–75.

104. Kiloh LG, Nevin S. Isolated neuritis of the anterior interosseous nerve. Br Med J 1952;1(4763):850.

105. Plancher KD, Peterson RK, Steichen JB. Compressive neuropathies and tendinopathies in the athletic elbow and wrist. Clin Sports Med 1996;15(2):331–71.

106. Spinner M. The functional attitude of the hand afflicted with an anterior interosseous nerve paralysis. Bull Hosp Joint Dis 1969;30(1):21–2.

107. Seror P. Posterior interosseous nerve conduction: a new method of evaluation. Am J Phys Med Rehabil 1996;75(1):35–9.

108. Miller-Breslow A, Terrono A, Millender LH. Nonoperative treatment of anterior interosseous nerve paralysis. J Hand Surg 1990;15(3):493–6.

109. Seki M, Nakamura H, Kono H. Neurolysis is not required for young patients with a spontaneous palsy of the anterior interosseous nerve: retrospective analysis of cases managed non-operatively. J Bone Joint Surg Br 2006;88(12):1606–9.

110. Ulrich D, Piatkowski A, Pallua N. Anterior interosseous nerve syndrome: retrospective analysis of 14 patients. Arch Orthop Trauma Surg 2011;131(11):1561.

111. Haussmann P, Patel MR. Intraepineurial constriction of nerve fascicles in pronator syndrome and anterior interosseous nerve syndrome. Orthop Clin North Am 1996;27(2):339–44.

112. Kotani H, Miki T, Senzoku F, et al. Posterior interosseous nerve paralysis with multiple constrictions. J Hand Surg 1995;20(1):15–7.

113. Pan Y-w, Wang S, Tian G, et al. Typical brachial neuritis (parsonage-turner syndrome) with hourglass-like constrictions in the affected nerves. J Hand Surg 2011;36(7):1197–203.

114. Damert H-G, Hoffmann R, Kraus A, et al. Minimally invasive endoscopic decompression for anterior interosseous nerve syndrome: technical notes. J Hand Surg 2013;38(10):2016–24.

115. Hazani R, Engineer NJ, Mowlavi A, et al. Anatomic landmarks for the radial tunnel. Eplasty 2008;8.

116. Chien AJ, Jamadar DA, Jacobson JA, et al. Sonography and MR imaging of posterior interosseous nerve syndrome with surgical correlation. Am J Roentgenol 2003;181(1):219–21.
117. Clavert P, Lutz J, Adam P, et al. Frohse's arcade is not the exclusive compression site of the radial nerve in its tunnel. Orthop Traumatol Surg Res 2009; 95(2):114–8.
118. Andreisek G, Crook DW, Burg D, et al. Peripheral neuropathies of the median, radial, and ulnar nerves: MR imaging features. Radiographics 2006;26(5): 1267–87.
119. Rovesta C, Marongiu MC, Corradini A, et al. Different treatment modalities in the nerve entrapments of upper extremity. In: Sports injuries: prevention, diagnosis, treatment and rehabilitation. 2015. p. 513–26.
120. Dang AC, Rodner CM. Unusual compression neuropathies of the forearm, part I: radial nerve. J Hand Surg 2009;34(10):1906–14.
121. Lorei MP, Hershman EB. Peripheral nerve injuries in athletes. Sports Med 1993; 16(2):130–47.
122. De Araujo MP. Electrodiagnosis in compression neuropathies of the upper extremities. Orthop Clin North Am 1996;27(2):237–44.
123. Terrono AL, Millender LH. Management of work-related upper-extremity nerve entrapments. Orthop Clin North Am 1996;27(4):783–93.
124. Naam NH, Nemani S. Radial Tunnel Syndrome. Orthop Clin North Am 2012; 43(4):529–36.
125. Pulos N, Shin EH, Spinner RJ, et al. Management of iatrogenic nerve injuries. J Am Acad Orthop Surg 2019;27(18):e838–48.
126. Smith GR, Altchek DW, Pagnani MJ, et al. A muscle-splitting approach to the ulnar collateral ligament of the elbow: neuroanatomy and operative technique. Am J Sports Med 1996;24(5):575–80.
127. Zhang Q, Sun N, Huang Q, et al. Minimally invasive plating osteosynthesis in the treatment of humeral shaft fractures: a meta-analysis. J Invest Surg 2017;30(2): 133–42.
128. Zhang J, Moore AE, Stringer MD. Iatrogenic upper limb nerve injuries: a systematic review. ANZ J Surg 2011;81(4):227–36.
129. Watson JN, McQueen P, Hutchinson MR. A systematic review of ulnar collateral ligament reconstruction techniques. Am J Sports Med 2014;42(10):2510–6.
130. Somerson JS, Petersen JP, Neradilek MB, et al. Complications and outcomes after medial ulnar collateral ligament reconstruction: a meta-regression and systematic review. JBJS Rev 2018;6(5):e4.
131. Kelly EW, Morrey BF, O'Driscoll SW. Complications of elbow arthroscopy. J Bone Joint Surg Am 2001;83(1):25.
132. Lattermann C, Romeo AA, Anbari A, et al. Arthroscopic debridement of the extensor carpi radialis brevis for recalcitrant lateral epicondylitis. J Shoulder Elbow Surg 2010;19(5):651–6.
133. King GJ. Elbow arthroscopy complications. In: Elbow arthroscopy. Switzerland: Springer; 2013. p. 103–12.
134. Andrews JR, Carson WG. Arthroscopy of the elbow. Arthroscopy 1985;1(2): 97–107.
135. O'Driscoll SW, Morrey B. Arthroscopy of the elbow. Diagnostic and therapeutic benefits and hazards. J Bone Joint Surg Am 1992;74(1):84–94.
136. Gay DM, Raphael BS, Weiland AJ. Revision arthroscopic contracture release in the elbow resulting in an ulnar nerve transection: a case report. J Bone Joint Surg Am 2010;92(5):1246–9.

137. Sahajpal DT, Blonna D, O'Driscoll SW. Anteromedial elbow arthroscopy portals in patients with prior ulnar nerve transposition or subluxation. Arthroscopy 2010; 26(8):1045–52.

138. Dumonski ML, Arciero RA, Mazzocca AD. Ulnar nerve palsy after elbow arthroscopy. Arthroscopy 2006;22(5):577.e1-3.

139. Blonna D, O'Driscoll SW. Delayed-onset ulnar neuritis after release of elbow contracture: preventive strategies derived from a study of 563 cases. Arthroscopy 2014;30(8):947–56.

140. Maak TG, Osei D, Delos D, et al. Peripheral nerve injuries in sports-related surgery: presentation, evaluation, and management: AAOS exhibit selection. J Bone Joint Surg Am 2012;94(16):e121.

141. Drake RL, Vogl A, Mitchell A, et al. Gray's atlas of anatomy, vol. 30. Philadelphia: Churchill Livingstone, Elsevier; 2008. p. 1672–5.

142. Thompson N, Mockford B, Cran G. Absence of the palmaris longus muscle: a population study. Ulster Med J 2001;70(1):22.

143. Tountas CP, Bergman RA. Anatomic variations of the upper extremity. New York: Churchill Livingstone; 1993.

144. Choo J, Wilhelmi BJ, Kasdan ML. Iatrogenic injury to the median nerve during palmaris longus harvest: an overview of safe harvesting techniques. Hand 2017;12(1):NP6–9.

145. Geldmacher J. Median nerve as free tendon graft. Hand 1972;4(1):56.

146. Kovacsy A. Removal of the median nerve instead of the palmaris longus tendon. Magy Traumatol Orthop Helyreallito Seb 1980;23(2):156.

147. Toros T, Vatansever A, Ada S. Accidental use of the median nerve as an interposition material in first carpometacarpal joint arthroplasty. J Hand Surg 2006; 31(5):574–5.

148. Vastamäki M. Median nerve as free tendon graft. J Hand Surg Br 1987;12(2): 187–8.

149. Weber RV, Mackinnon SE. Median nerve mistaken for palmaris longus tendon: restoration of function with sensory nerve transfers. Hand 2007;2(1):1–4.

150. Bisson L, Moyer M, Lanighan K, et al. Complications associated with repair of a distal biceps rupture using the modified two-incision technique. J Shoulder Elbow Surg 2008;17(1):S67–71.

151. Chavan PR, Duquin TR, Bisson LJ. Repair of the ruptured distal biceps tendon: a systematic review. Am J Sports Med 2008;36(8):1618–24.

152. Fajardo MR, Rosenberg Z, Christoforou D, et al. Multiple nerve injuries following repair of a distal biceps tendon rupture: case report and review of the literature. Bull Hosp Jt Dis (2013) 2013;71(2):166.

153. Garon MT, Greenberg JA. Complications of distal biceps repair. Orthop Clin North Am 2016;47(2):435–44.

154. Gallinet D, Dietsch E, Barbier-Brion B, et al. Suture anchor reinsertion of distal biceps rupture: clinical results and radiological assessment of tendon healing. Orthop Traumatol Surg Res 2011;97(3):252–9.

155. Kelly EW, Morrey BF, O'Driscoll SW. Complications of repair of the distal biceps tendon with the modified two-incision technique. J Bone Joint Surg Am 2000; 82(11):1575.

156. Boyd H, Anderson L. A method for reinsertion of the distal biceps brachii tendon. J Bone Joint Surg Am 1961;43(7):1041–3.

157. Reichert P, Królikowska A, Witkowski J, et al. Surgical management of distal biceps tendon anatomical reinsertion complications: iatrogenic posterior interosseous nerve palsy. Med Sci Monit 2018;24:782.

158. Cohen MS. Complications of distal biceps tendon repairs. Sports Med Arthrosc Rev 2008;16(3):148–53.

159. Lo EY, Li C-S, Van den Bogaerde JM. The effect of drill trajectory on proximity to the posterior interosseous nerve during cortical button distal biceps repair. Arthroscopy 2011;27(8):1048–54.

160. Miyamoto RG, Elser F, Millett PJ. Distal biceps tendon injuries. J Bone Joint Surg Am 2010;92(11):2128–38.

Elbow Fractures

Kaare S. Midtgaard, MD[a,b,c], Joseph J. Ruzbarsky, MD[a],
Thomas R. Hackett, MD[a], Randall W. Viola, MD[a,*]

KEYWORDS

- Elbow fracture • Elbow dislocation • Terrible triad • Olecranon fracture
- Radial head fracture • Open reduction and internal fixation • Olecranon osteotomy

KEY POINTS

- Most fractures about the elbow are treated with open reduction and internal fixation and aggressive postoperative mobilization.
- Extra-articular distal humerus fractures can be treated by a variety of approaches. Complex intra-articular distal humerus fractures are best managed with open reduction and internal fixation using medial and lateral plates using an olecranon osteotomy to facilitate articular reconstruction.
- The coronoid, although small, plays an important role in elbow stability. Anteromedial coronoid facet fractures are difficult to diagnose. If treated inappropriately, varus posteromedial instability may result.
- The treatment of Mason III radial head fractures is controversial; however, good outcomes may be achieved with rigid internal fixation with or without bone grafting and/or collateral ligament repair or reconstruction.
- Elbow ulnar collateral ligament and lateral collateral ligament injuries commonly occur in conjunction with elbow fractures. These soft tissue injuries should be managed with surgical repair or reconstruction. Restoration of stability is as important as anatomic fracture repair.

ANATOMY OF THE ELBOW JOINT

The brachial artery and median nerve cross the elbow joint anteriorly, and the radial nerve crosses from the posterior aspect of the humerus through the anterolateral musculature as it passes across the joint. The ulnar nerve curves under the medial epicondyle into the cubital fossa in close proximity to bone and is thus exposed to compromise with elbow fractures and dislocations.

Careful neurovascular examination is mandatory when examining patients with suspected elbow injuries. The posterior interosseus branch of the radial nerve enters the

[a] The Steadman Clinic, Steadman Philippon Research Institute, 181 West Meadow Drive, Suite 400, Vail, CO 81657, USA; [b] Oslo University Hospital, Division of Orthopaedic Surgery, Kirkeveien 166, Oslo 0450, Norway; [c] Norwegian Armed Forces Joint Medical Services, Forsvarsvegen 75, Sessvollmoen 2058, Norway
* Corresponding author.
E-mail address: rv@thesteadmanclinic.com

Clin Sports Med 39 (2020) 623–636
https://doi.org/10.1016/j.csm.2020.03.002   sportsmed.theclinics.com
0278-5919/20/© 2020 Elsevier Inc. All rights reserved.

supinator muscle distal to the annular ligament and is at risk when the radial neck is fractured. The ulnar nerve is easily palpated in the cubital fossa and is vulnerable in distal humerus fractures and proximal ulna fractures, especially in fracture-dislocations. The median nerve has better protection due to surrounding soft tissue but may be injured in distal humerus fractures, specifically supracondylar fractures in children.

The elbow collateral ligaments are pivotal to elbow stability. The anterior band of the medial collateral ligament (ulnar collateral ligament [UCL]) originates from the inferolateral aspect of the medial epicondyle and inserts on the sublime tubercle of the ulna.[1] The UCL is the primary stabilizer against valgus forces. The lateral ligament complex consists of the radial collateral ligament and lateral UCL (LUCL).[2] The ligaments weave into the annular ligament, which encases the radial head. The LUCL and radial collateral ligament originate from the isometric center of the elbow joint on the distal aspect of the lateral epicondyle.[3] The fibers of the LUCL insert distally on the supinator crest of the ulna. The LUCL is the primary varus stabilizer of the elbow joint.[4]

The bony architecture of the elbow joint is complex, which, in the setting of trauma, can create several challenges. The distal humerus consists of medial and lateral columns. The medial column supports the trochlea, which articulates with the ulna. The lateral column supports the spherical capitellum, which articulates with the concave radial head. The lesser sigmoid notch articulates with the radial head and facilitates rotation of the forearm. The significance of the coronoid process as the main anterior buttress cannot be overstated, because it plays a critical role in elbow stability.

The joint capsule also contributes significantly to elbow stability. Anteriorly, the joint capsule is taut in extension and the posterior capsule is taut in flexion. Posttraumatic thickening of the capsule contributes significantly to elbow stiffness. Postoperative rehabilitation protocols should focus on aggressive elbow and forearm range of motion.

DISTAL HUMERUS FRACTURES

Distal humerus fractures are associated with high-energy injuries in young men and lower energy falls in older, osteoporotic women. Distal humerus fractures can be divided into extra-articular, partial intra-articular, and intra-articular (**Fig. 1**). Nonoperative treatment can be attempted in minimally displaced fractures or if the patient is noncompliant or medically unfit for surgery. However, the risk of elbow stiffness increases with prolonged immobilization, and operative treatment with open reduction and plate fixation is usually recommended.

Plate fixation is the most commonly used fixation method for distal humerus fractures, and double plating is preferred because it neutralizes the rotational forces.[5] An extensive posterior approach with or without olecranon osteotomy is the most commonly used approach to treat distal humerus fractures. The ulnar nerve should be identified and protected throughout such procedures. The paratricipital approach is well suited for extra-articular and simple intra-articular fractures.[6–8] In complex intra-articular fractures, an olecranon osteotomy can be performed to visualize the posteroinferior aspects of the joint and allow for unimpeded placement of hardware (**Fig. 2**). Several olecranon-sparing approaches have also been described that preserve the integrity of the olecranon. However, the latter necessitate that the medial and/or lateral ligament is released, and these structures must be restored following fixation.

A subset of distal humerus fractures are the coronal shear fractures (**Fig. 3**). The coronal shear fragment is very difficult to address from the posterior approach and should

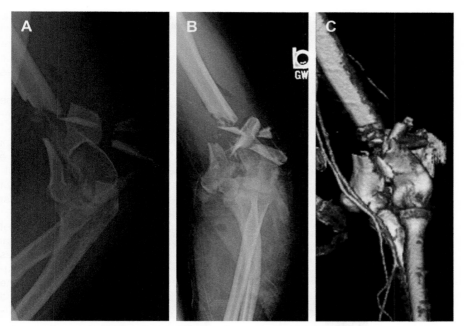

Fig. 1. (*A*) Lateral radiograph, (*B*) oblique radiograph, and (*C*) three-dimensional (3D) reconstruction images of a severely comminuted intra-articular distal humerus fracture.

be addressed from a separate lateral or medial interval for anatomic reduction. The fragment can be fixed through a posterolateral plate or with isolated headless compression or countersunk screws (**Fig. 4**).[9]

The rate of complications and secondary surgery is high following distal humerus fractures.[7,10–14] Ulnar neuritis is a common complication and evaluation of the ulnar nerve following fixation is important. If there is a risk of hardware irritation or instability of the ulnar nerve in its sulcus, the nerve should be transposed anteriorly. The latter should be tested intraoperatively by passively flexing and extending the elbow. However, the ulnar nerve should not be routinely transposed.[15] Furthermore, the risk of heterotopic ossification is high following these injuries, especially following high-energy injuries. Prophylaxis with indomethacin should be considered in severe cases. Patients should be carefully counseled on the risk of elbow stiffness, ulnar neuritis, and hardware-related problems that may require secondary surgery.

FRACTURES OF THE MEDIAL EPICONDYLE

Isolated fractures of the medial epicondyle are uncommon and associated with adolescent boys. The fracture is the result of excess valgus force and is an avulsion fracture of the flexor-pronator mass that inserts on the medial epicondyle. The injury is prevalent among adolescent baseball pitchers and presents as an epiphysiolysis.

Displacements of less than 5 mm are commonly treated nonoperatively. Those fractures with greater than 5 mm of displacement should be treated with open reduction and internal fixation (ORIF). Screw fixation is preferred.

Both the insertion of the UCL and the activities of the patient must be considered when evaluating medial epicondyle fractures. Because the UCL origin detaches with

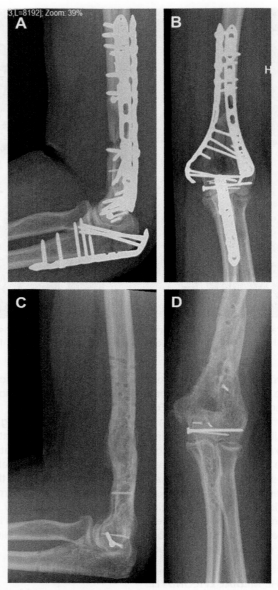

Fig. 2. (*A*) Lateral and (*B*) anteroposterior radiographs of open reduction and internal fixation (ORIF) of the fracture seen in **Fig. 1**. (*C*) Lateral and (*D*) anteroposterior radiographs of the fracture from (*A*, *B*) after healing and plate removal.

the avulsion fragment, injuries with as little as 2 mm may result in elbow instability in throwing athletes. Operative treatment restores native function of the UCL. Fixation with 2 isolated screws often provides adequate stability with high union rates and excellent outcomes. Operative fixation should be considered in throwing athletes with medial epicondyle fractures with as little as 2 mm of displacement.

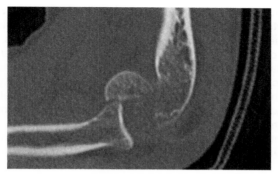

Fig. 3. Sagittal computed tomography (CT) scan showing a capitellum shear fracture.

RADIAL HEAD FRACTURES

Radial head fractures are the most common elbow fracture and constitute one-third of all elbow injuries.[16] The radial head is an important restraint to valgus forces in concert with the UCL. Biomechanical studies have shown that the radius contributes significantly to force transmission in the extended elbow because 40% of total force is transmitted over the radiocapitellar joint, with peak loads shown in supination.[17,18]

Radial head fractures occur as isolated bony injuries or in conjunction with other stabilizing structures that result in fracture-dislocations of the elbow. Radial head fractures are most commonly caused following valgus trauma.[19,20] Therefore, the integrity of the UCL must also be assessed in the setting of a radial head fracture.

The Mason classification is commonly used to classify radial head fractures with types I through IV. Computed tomography (CT) evaluation is recommended, especially to evaluate the articulation of the proximal radioulnar joint. Minimally displaced fractures that do not cause impairment of rotation may be treated nonoperatively and patients can start immediate mobilization.[21] Failure to initiate early active range of motion can cause elbow stiffness.[22] Larger fragments that interfere with rotation

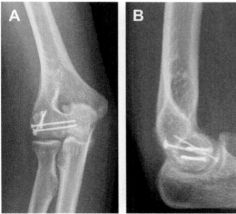
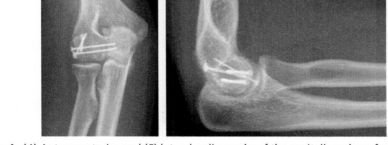

Fig. 4. (A) Anteroposterior and (B) lateral radiographs of the capitellum shear fracture from **Fig. 3** after ORIF.

can be treated with open reduction and isolated screw fixation (**Fig. 5**). Mason 3 fractures can be treated with ORIF or radial head arthroplasty.[23] Resection is not recommended because this may result in shortening of the radius, rapid arthritic development, and chronic wrist pain.[24] Whether Mason 3 fractures should be treated with ORIF or radial head arthroplasty is debated. It is the senior author's opinion that these fractures can be treated with ORIF as long as the integrity of the UCL is restored, either through primary repair or graft reconstruction. Usually, plate fixation is necessary in addition to isolated screws (**Fig. 6**). The patients should be informed that plate removal may be necessary to restore functional rotation. However, ORIF avoids the potential disadvantages associated with radial head arthroplasty, such as overstuffing and osteolysis of the proximal radius, and does not preclude its future use.[25]

Radial head fractures associated with elbow dislocation are classified as Mason 4 fractures.[26] These fractures are treated similarly to Mason 3 fractures with ORIF with concomitant UCL repair or reconstruction. However, the overall bone quality and vascular integrity of the reconstructed radial head must be considered when attempting ORIF, and radial head replacement is a reasonable solution for elderly and/or low-demand patients.

OLECRANON FRACTURES

Fractures of proximal ulna range from simple isolated transverse olecranon process fractures to complex highly comminuted fractures in which the articular surface is nearly unreconstructable. Olecranon fractures typically result from either a fall on an outstretched arm or a direct trauma to the olecranon. Minimally displaced fractures (<2 mm) can be treated nonoperatively; however, this treatment option, which requires prolonged extension immobilization, may lead to elbow stiffness. Olecranon fractures with more than 2 mm of displacement should be treated with ORIF unless the patient is unfit for surgery. Options include either tension band wiring (TBW) or plate fixation.[27] (**Fig. 7**) In the past, TBW has been used to treat simple fracture patterns, whereas plate fixation is the treatment of choice in multifragmented olecranon fractures. Given that plate fixation allows more aggressive postoperative rehabilitation and avoids the frequent hardware complications seen with TBW, plate fixation has become the preferred treatment option. The functional outcomes of the two methods seem to be comparable.[28] However, the true rate of simple fracture patterns is much lower than suspected by just plain radiographs alone.[29] In addition, the rates of complication and hardware removal are significantly higher after TBW, and biomechanical studies

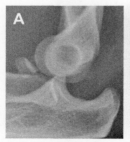
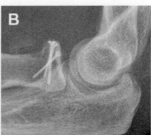
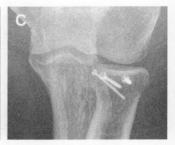

Fig. 5. (*A*) Lateral radiograph showing a Mason II elbow fracture of the radial head with a posterior elbow dislocation. (*B*) Lateral and (*C*) anteroposterior radiographs of (*A*) after ORIF.

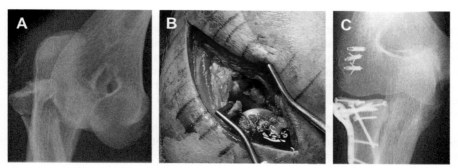

Fig. 6. (*A*) Oblique radiograph showing a Mason III comminuted radial head fracture and elbow dislocation. (*B*) Intraoperative view showing severe comminution and bone loss. (*C*) Anteroposterior radiograph showing (*A*) after ORIF.

have shown better fracture-retaining capabilities when olecranon fractures are treated with plate fixation.

Operative treatment of olecranon fractures is designed to restore the extension mechanism of the elbow and the bony architecture of the olecranon articular surface.

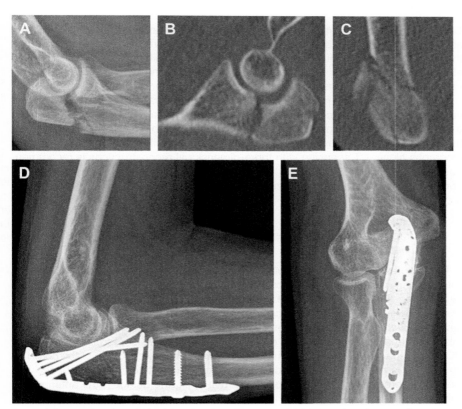

Fig. 7. (*A*) Lateral radiograph, (*B*) sagittal CT image, and (*C*) coronal CT image of a comminuted olecranon fracture. (*D*) Lateral and (*E*) anteroposterior radiographs of the fracture from (*A–C*) after ORIF with an olecranon plate.

The olecranon fossa is challenging to evaluate with fluoroscopy because of the double concavity in the axial plane. Therefore, the authors recommend a medial and/or lateral joint arthrotomy to visualize the articular reduction. The subcutaneous location of these fractures allows the posterior, medial, and lateral aspects of the fracture to be easily evaluated and reduced. However, many olecranon fractures involve marginal impaction of the articular surface, which may be difficult to detect even with CT images. Medial and lateral arthrotomies are necessary to achieve anatomic repair of the olecranon articular surface.

Although operative treatment is recommended for young and active patients, there is some data that low-demand and noncompliant patients with displaced olecranon fractures can be treated nonoperatively.[30] The authors recommend that a splint or cast is applied for 2 to 3 weeks for pain relief. The result of this treatment is usually a pain-free fibrous nonunion, but without the potential wound and hardware complications.

Rehabilitation following operative treatment of displaced olecranon fractures can commence with active range of motion with weights up to 1 kg. The patients are usually permitted mobilization without restrictions after 6 to 8 weeks but should be counseled that hardware removal is required in up to 50%.

CORONOID FRACTURES

Coronoid fractures are less common than other elbow fractures and often dismissed as clinically insignificant because of the small size of the fracture fragment. However, these fractures are frequently associated with concomitant ligament injuries and elbow instability. Failure to recognize these fractures and associated injuries may result in chronic elbow instability, stiffness, pain, and poor function.

The mechanisms that result in coronoid fractures are varus posteromedial forces, valgus posterolateral forces, and/or hyperextension. Regan and Morrey[31] described a classification of coronoid fractures based on the size of the fracture fragment on the lateral radiograph. However, these fractures are difficult to evaluate using plain radiographs alone. CT scanning with three-dimensional reconstructions is recommended for most injuries. O'Driscoll and colleagues[32] published a classification of coronoid fractures based on the size and anatomic location of the fracture, describing 3 categories:

1. Tip fractures
2. Large fractures (basilar fractures)
3. Anteromedial fractures

Tip fractures are observed following valgus posterolateral injury. Coronoid fractures with concomitant radial head fracture and posterior dislocation are known as the terrible triad (**Fig. 8**).[33] The terrible triad has been associated with poor clinical outcomes. However, over the past decade, improved recognition and fixation techniques have improved treatment outcomes by recognizing and treating all 3 components of this triad: repair or reconstruction of the radial head, repair or reconstruction of the UCL, and repair of the coronoid injury. Whether reduction and fixation of the coronoid tip fracture is necessary remains debated. Larger tip fractures can be reduced and fixed with screws (**Fig. 9**). If the tip is too small to fix, the defect in the anterior joint capsule can be repaired through drill holes from the dorsal aspect of the ulna.[34] Traditionally, it has been thought that the injury that causes a terrible triad originates on the lateral side and progresses to the medial side.[32] However, this has been challenged in recent studies showing that UCL injury is more prevalent in valgus posterolateral

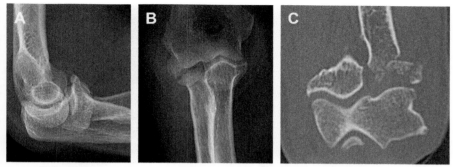

Fig. 8. (*A*) Lateral radiograph, (*B*) anteroposterior radiograph, (*C*) coronal CT image of a terrible triad injury.

injuries.[35] UCL repair or reconstruction is controversial. Some clinicians advocate UCL reconstruction only when instability remains following repair of the coronoid/anterior capsule, LUCL, and radial head.[36] However, the importance of elbow stability in the management of these injuries is increasingly recognized. Medial elbow stabilization should always be considered. In cases where the UCL has been avulsed from the medial epicondyle or sublime tubercle, it may be repaired using anchor techniques. In cases where there is inadequate tissue for ligament repair, UCL reconstruction is necessary.

Large coronoid fractures are associated with varus posteromedial injury and in most cases also involve rupture of the LUCL.[37] Radial head involvement is rarely observed. The coronoid fracture can be simple or multifragmented. Anatomic reduction of large coronoid fractures can be performed through small incisions with a bone hook.[38] Following reduction, fixation can be achieved with screws inserted from the dorsal aspect of the ulna. Multifragmented fractures should be addressed via a medial approach. Restoration of the anterior coronoid buttress is pivotal to restore elbow stability when the coronoid fracture involves more than the tip. Multifragmented fractures can be addressed with small plates that buttress the coronoid process. After reduction and fixation of the coronoid fragment, if clinical examination reveals UCL and/or LUCL instability, repair or reconstruction should be performed.

Fractures of the anteromedial coronoid facet are difficult to diagnose (**Fig. 10**).[39] This fracture pattern is uncommon, but it is important to identify because overlooked facet fractures lead to rapid anteromedial arthritis. As seen following posteromedial

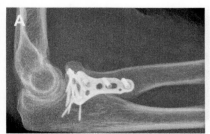
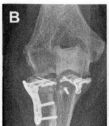
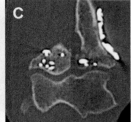

Fig. 9. (*A*) Lateral and (*B*) anteroposterior radiographs, and (*C*) axial CT image of the terrible triad from **Fig. 8** after ORIF of the coronoid and comminuted radial head fractures.

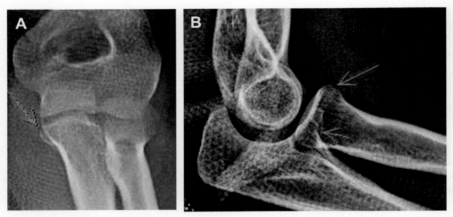

Fig. 10. (*A*) Anteroposterior and (*B*) lateral radiographs showing an anteromedial facet coronoid fracture. The green arrows show the subtleties of the fracture.

rotatory injuries, the LUCL is often injured and the radial head is intact. These fractures may involve the sublime tubercle and cause disruption of the UCL as well (**Fig. 11**).

WHAT TO DO IF RESIDUAL INSTABILITY PERSISTS

Residual instability following repair or reconstruction of elbow fracture-dislocation poses a conundrum to orthopedic surgeons. Following repair and reconstruction of the injured structures, elbow stability has to be tested before the patient leaves the operating room. Testing varus and valgus stability following repair can be hazardous

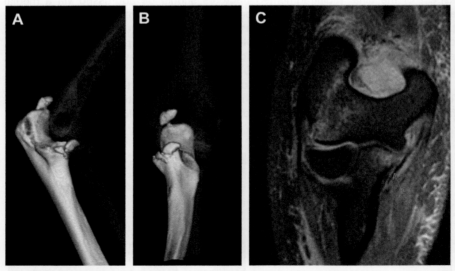

Fig. 11. (*A, B*) 3D reconstruction images of the anteromedial coronoid facet fracture seen in **Fig. 10**. (*C*) Coronal MRI of the fracture seen in (*A, B*) showing an associated UCL tear (*green arrow*).

and is of limited value. Instead, authors recommend that the congruity of the elbow joint is examined with fluoroscopy. A folded towel bump is placed under the humerus and a perfect lateral view of the elbow joint is obtained. The elbow is extended from the fully flexed position and extended. The "drop sign" is considered an increased distance between the olecranon fossa and distal humerus, which may indicate residual instability.[40] The test should be performed while putting the hand in supination and pronation, and the fluoroscopy checked for joint incongruence.

The repair has to be reevaluated if residual instability is suspected. The placement of anchors or burr holes for the repaired or reconstructed ligaments must be carefully evaluated, because misplaced anchors may affect isometry.

The ligaments may also have been attenuated from the initial trauma. It is important that repair is performed as soon as possible because the quality of the ligaments is diminished after 2 to 3 weeks. Attempts to repair the damaged UCL or LUCL prove futile and the authors recommend that the ligaments are reconstructed with autograft or allograft if surgery is performed in the subacute setting.

A hinged external fixator has been proposed as an adjunct when residual instability persists following adequate repair of the elbow stabilizers. However, the application is technically challenging. With anatomic reconstruction of all fractures patterns and appropriate soft tissue repair and/or reconstruction, hinged external fixator use is rarely necessary. It does have a role in high-energy and or open injures where anatomic bone and soft tissues injury is impossible. In this setting, cross-pinning the ulnohumeral joint with 2-mm Kirschner wires drilled from the dorsal cortex of the ulna has been suggested as an acceptable alternative for temporary provisional fixation.[41]

REHABILITATION

The initial rehabilitation focus after elbow fracture fixation is restoration of elbow motion. The elbow is predisposed to both capsular stiffness and heterotopic ossification. In order to prevent these complications, aggressive range-of-motion exercises are initiated immediately postoperatively. Typically, most rehabilitation protocols use static progressive splinting only when there is failure to progress and/or restore motion with manual exercises. With recent improvements in fixation techniques, static progressive splinting may be used immediately postoperatively. When fracture fixation is adequate, gentle strengthening may also be initiated immediately postoperatively. In addition, because many surgical approaches to the elbow require exposure of the radial, median, and/or ulnar nerves, nerve gliding exercises should be used for at least 6 to 8 weeks postoperatively.

RETURN TO SPORTS

Advances in fracture fixation, aggressive range-of-motion rehabilitation, and early strengthening have all improved outcomes of elbow fractures. Functional elbow range of motion and strength may resume after several weeks after elbow fracture fixation. However, return to sports and competition depends on fracture healing and strength. For most elbow fractures, return to competition is allowed when the fracture is clinically and radiographically healed and the strength has returned to 80% to 90% of the normal limb. If fracture healing is difficult to assess, serial CT scans may be necessary. In some cases, prominent hardware may interfere with sports activities. In these cases, the symptomatic hardware is removed at 1 year postoperatively. For some, including competitive athletes, hardware may be removed as early as 6 months or immediately after the competition season ends to allow for full rehab before next season. However, reports of return to play after elbow fracture fixation are limited in the literature. One study detailed 25 baseball players who previously underwent ORIF for olecranon stress fractures and reported that 94% of athletes return to their prior levels of baseball ability at an average of 29 weeks postoperatively.[42]

DISCLOSURE

R.W. Viola: Consulting and royalties from OsteoMed and Conmed/Linvatec. The rest of the authors have nothing to disclose.

REFERENCES

1. Frangiamore SJ, Moatshe G, Kruckeberg BM, et al. Qualitative and quantitative analyses of the dynamic and static stabilizers of the medial elbow: an anatomic study. Am J Sports Med 2018;46:687–94.
2. Capo JT, Collins C, Beutel BG, et al. Three-dimensional analysis of elbow soft tissue footprints and anatomy. J Shoulder Elbow Surg 2014;23:1618–23.
3. Barnes JW, Chouhan VL, Egekeze NC, et al. The annular ligament—revisited. J Shoulder Elbow Surg 2018;27:e16–9.
4. Morrey BF, An KN. Functional anatomy of the ligaments of the elbow. Clin Orthop Relat Res 1985;201:84–90.
5. Galano G, Ahmad CS, Levine WN. Current treatment strategies for bicolumnar distal humerus fractures. J Am Acad Orthop Surg 2010;18:20–30.
6. Chen G, Liao Q, Luo W, et al. Triceps-sparing versus olecranon osteotomy for ORIF: Analysis of 67 cases of intercondylar fractures of the distal humerus. Injury 2011;42:366–70.
7. Iwamoto T, Suzuki T, Matsumura N, et al. Lateral Para-Olecranon Approach for the Treatment of Distal Humeral Fracture. J Hand Surg Am 2017;42:344–50.
8. Schildhauer TA, Nork SE, Mills WJ, et al. Extensor mechanism-sparing paratricipital posterior approach to the distal humerus. J Orthop Trauma 2003;17:374–8.
9. Dubberley JH, Faber KJ, Macdermid JC, et al. Outcome after open reduction capitellar and trochlear fractures. J Bone Joint Surg Am 2006;88A:46–54.
10. Wang C, Meng JH, Zhang YW, et al. Suture button versus hook plate for acute unstable acromioclavicular joint dislocation: a meta-analysis. Am J Sports Med 2019;1–8. https://doi.org/10.1177/0363546519858745.
11. Tunalı O, Erşen A, Pehlivanoğlu T, et al. Evaluation of risk factors for stiffness after distal humerus plating. Int Orthop 2018;42:921–6.
12. Varecka TF, Myeroff C. Distal humerus fractures in the elderly population. J Am Acad Orthop Surg 2017;25:673–83.
13. Neuman P, Dahlberg LE, Englund M, et al. Concentrations of synovial fluid biomarkers and the prediction of knee osteoarthritis 16 years after anterior cruciate ligament injury. Osteoarthr Cartil 2017;25:492–8.
14. Lawrence TM, Ahmadi S, Morrey BF, et al. Wound complications after distal humerus fracture fixation: Incidence, risk factors, and outcome. J Shoulder Elbow Surg 2014;23:258–64.
15. Ruan HJ, Liu JJ, Fan CY, et al. Incidence, management, and prognosis of early ulnar nerve dysfunction in type C fractures of distal humerus. J Trauma 2009; 67:1397–401.
16. Kaas L, van Riet RP, Vroemen JPAM, et al. The epidemiology of radial head fractures. J Shoulder Elbow Surg 2010;19:520–3.
17. Morrey BF, An KN, Stormont TJ. Force transmission through the radial head. J Bone Joint Surg Am 1988;70:250–6.

18. Hwang JT, Kim Y, Bachman DR, et al. Axial load transmission through the elbow during forearm rotation. J Shoulder Elbow Surg 2018;27:530–7.

19. Duckworth AD, Clement ND, Jenkins PJ, et al. The epidemiology of radial head and neck fractures. J Hand Surg Am 2012;37:112–9.

20. Mason ML. Some observations on fractures of the head of the radius with a review of one hundred cases. Br J Surg 1954;42:123–32.

21. Egol KA, Haglin JM, Lott A, et al. Minimally displaced, isolated radial head and neck fractures do not require formal physical therapy: Results of a prospective randomized trial. J Bone Joint Surg Am 2018;100:648–55.

22. Pettersen PM, Eriksson J, Bratberg H, et al. Increased ROM and high patient satisfaction after open arthrolysis: A follow-up-study of 43 patients with posttraumatic stiff elbows. BMC Musculoskelet Disord 2016;17:1–6.

23. Vannabouathong C, Akhter S, Athwal GS, et al. Interventions for displaced radial head fractures: network meta-analysis of randomized trials. J Shoulder Elbow Surg 2019;28:578–86.

24. Nestorson J, Josefsson PO, Adolfsson L. A radial head prosthesis appears to be unnecessary in Mason-IV fracture dislocation. Acta Orthop 2017;88:315–9.

25. Jung M, Groetzner-Schmidt C, Porschke F, et al. Low return-to-sports rate after elbow injury and treatment with radial head arthroplasty. J Shoulder Elbow Surg 2019;28:1441–8.

26. Johnston GW. A follow-up of one hundred cases of fracture of the head of the radius with a review of the literature. Ulster Med J 1962;31:51–6.

27. He M, Aa A, Buckley S, et al. Surgical interventions for treating fractures of the olecranon in adults (Review) SUMMARY OF FINDINGS FOR THE MAIN COMPARISON. Cochrane Database Syst Rev Surg 2014. https://doi.org/10.1002/14651858.CD010144.pub2.www.cochranelibrary.com.

28. Duckworth AD, Clement ND, White TO, et al. Plate Versus tension-band wire fixation for olecranon fractures. J Bone Joint Surg Am 2017;99:1261–73.

29. Wellman DS, Lazaro LE, Cymerman RM, et al. Treatment of olecranon fractures with 2.4-and 2.7-mm plating techniques. J Orthop Trauma 2015;29:36–43.

30. Duckworth AD, Bugler KE, Clement ND, et al. Nonoperative management of displaced olecranon fractures in low-demand elderly patients. J Bone Joint Surg Am 2014;96:67–72.

31. Regan W, Morrey BF. Fractures of the coronoid process of the ulna. J Bone Joint Surg Am 1989;71:1348–54.

32. O'Driscoll S, Jupiter J, Cohen M, et al. Difficult elbow fractures: pearls and pitfalls. Instr Course Lect 2003;52:113–34.

33. Pugh DMW, McKee MD. Terrible triad fracture-dislocations of the elbow. Oper Tech Orthop 2013;23:198–204.

34. Reichel LM, Milam GS, Reitman CA. Anterior approach for operative fixation of coronoid fractures in complex elbow instability. Tech Hand Up Extrem Surg 2012;16:98–104.

35. Schreiber JJ, Warren RF, Hotchkiss RN, et al. An online video investigation into the mechanism of elbow dislocation. J Hand Surg Am 2013;38:488–94.

36. McKee MD, Pugh DMW, Wild LM, et al. Standard surgical protocol to treat elbow dislocations with radial head and coronoid fractures. J Bone Joint Surg Am 2005;87:22–32.

37. Rhyou IH, Kim YS. New mechanism of the posterior elbow dislocation. Knee Surg Sports Traumatol Arthrosc 2012;20:2535–41.

38. Ring D, Jupiter JB, Sanders R, et al. Transolecranon fracture-dislocation of the elbow. J Orthop Trauma 1997;11:545–50.

39. Rhyou IH, Lee JH, Kim KC, et al. What injury mechanism and patterns of ligament status are associated with isolated coronoid, isolated radial head, and combined fractures? Clin Orthop Relat Res 2017;475:2308–15.

40. Rhyou IH, Lim KS, Kim KC, et al. Drop sign of the elbow joint after surgical stabilization of an unstable simple posterolateral dislocation: Natural course and contributing factors. J Shoulder Elbow Surg 2015;24:1081–9.

41. Ring D, Bruinsma WE, Jupiter JB. Complications of hinged external fixation compared with cross-pinning of the elbow for acute and subacute instability. Clin Orthop Relat Res 2014;472:2044–8.

42. Paci JM, Dugas JR, Guy JA, et al. Cannulated screw fixation of refractory olecranon stress fractures with and without associated injuries allows a return to baseball. Am J Sports Med 2013;41(2):306–12.

Elbow Dislocation

Nima Rezaie, MD*, Sunny Gupta, MD, Benjamin C. Service, MD,
Daryl C. Osbahr, MD

KEYWORDS

- Simple elbow dislocation • Complex elbow dislocation • Posterolateral instability
- Posteromedial instability • Chronic dislocation

KEY POINTS

- Acute simple elbow dislocations largely are treated conservatively. If surgical intervention is required, then early motion rehabilitation is advocated.
- Some elbow dislocations with ligament-only injuries may be considered complex dislocations due to the extent of the soft tissue trauma.
- Complex elbow fracture-dislocations are treated first with management of bony injuries, followed by assessment of ligamentous stability if instability persists.
- Starting an appropriate early range of motion rehabilitation helps achieve optimal outcomes with both surgical and nonsurgical treatments of elbow dislocations.

INTRODUCTION

The elbow is the second most commonly dislocated joint[1,2] representing 11% to 28% of elbow injuries,[3,4] with an annual incidence of 5.21 per 100,000.[5] Historically, acute dislocations without accompanying bony pathology were considered "simple" and ones with bony involvement referred to as "complex" dislocations. Simple elbow dislocations, the most common, represent approximately 74% of all elbow dislocations.[6] Complex dislocations should be subdivided into ligamentous dislocations and fracture-dislocations, with recognition that certain ligamentous injury patterns can also represent complex injuries.

Elbow stability is sustained by bony, capsuloligamentous, and musculotendinous components. The primary stabilizers of the elbow are the ulnohumeral articulation, the anterior band of the medial collateral ligament (aMCL), and the lateral ulnar collateral ligament (LUCL) complex.[7,8] They have fixed positions relative to one another through the elbow's arc of motion and function as static stabilizers. The congruent anatomy of the distal humerus and proximal ulna provide inherent stability to the joint. The radial head and the medial collateral ligament (MCL) complex contribute to the valgus stability of the elbow. The muscles across the elbow produce joint compressive

Orlando Health, 1222 South Orange Street, Orlando, FL 32806, USA
* Corresponding author.
E-mail address: Nima8806@gmail.com

Clin Sports Med 39 (2020) 637–655
https://doi.org/10.1016/j.csm.2020.02.009
0278-5919/20/© 2020 Elsevier Inc. All rights reserved.

forces and function as dynamic stabilizers. Most elbow dislocations are simple dislocations and occur in the posterior or posterolateral direction. Anterior dislocations are less common, and divergent dislocations are rare.[9]

SIMPLE ELBOW DISLOCATIONS

Simple elbow dislocations traditionally were thought to be caused by falling onto an outstretched hand, resulting in an externally rotated, valgus, and axially directed load to the elbow.[9–11] Multiple theories have tried to explain the sequence of soft tissue injury. Historically, O'Driscoll and colleagues[12] described that the typical injury pattern involves a sequential disruption of anatomic structures from lateral to medial, termed the *Horii circle*. First, the lateral collateral ligament (LCL) complex usually avulses off its origin on the lateral epicondyle of the humerus, leading to posterolateral instability of the elbow. It is followed by disruption of anterior and posterior capsule with the coronoid perched under the trochlea. The aMCL is the next to be injured followed by the entire MCL complex and possibly the common flexor origin. In some injury patterns, the MCL complex can remain intact, acting as a pivot for a posterolateral dislocation of the elbow.[7]

Newer studies evaluating magnetic resonance imaging (MRI) scans after reduction of a simple elbow dislocation show a higher rate of injury to the anterior bundle of the MCL when compared with the lateral side.[13,14] Schreiber and colleagues,[15] in a video review study from YouTube videos of elbow dislocations, found that the most common mechanism involves hyperextension, valgus force and an axial load; the extremity usually was positioned in forearm pronation, shoulder abduction, and forward flexion. According to their article, the injury first starts medially with the MCL, then proceeds with anterior capsular tearing, and then progresses laterally. Further cadaveric studies simulating posterior elbow dislocations showed similarities to these findings, with a higher incidence of damage to medial-sided ligaments compared with the lateral ligaments.[16] Additionally, common to all of these newer studies is a spectrum of soft tissue injury starting from the medial side up the injury ladder to the lateral side with avulsion of the common extensor tendon.[17] Realistically, the pattern of soft tissue injury largely depends on the position of the limb at the time of impact, direction of the force, and the variations in soft tissue laxity of the patient.[18]

Evaluation

A patient usually presents complaining of severe elbow pain after a trauma, such as a fall onto an outstretched hand. Patients often present with persistent deformity, but there may be situations where the elbow has reduced prior to orthopedic evaluation. After obtaining a thorough history, a comprehensive orthopedic examination is vital when evaluating patients with a possible elbow dislocation, including the contralateral upper extremity. Assessment of neurovascular status, bone and joint deformity, and limitations of elbow motion is necessary for a complete work-up. The most cost-effective initial imaging should start with plain anteroposterior and lateral radiographs of the elbow.[9] Oblique views can help detect intra-articular fractures[19] (**Fig. 1**). Computed tomography (CT) is helpful to detect occult fractures that may be missed on plain radiographs and to identify intra-articular fracture fragments causing mechanical symptoms after reduction[20] (**Fig. 2**). MRI is more useful in chronic elbow instability to evaluate the integrity of the ligaments.[21] MRI can be helpful in the evaluation of acute dislocations when the postreduction imaging demonstrates nonconcentric reduction but no fractures. MRI helps determine the extent of injury to the ligaments as well as show interposed cartilage and soft tissue, such as the annular ligament,

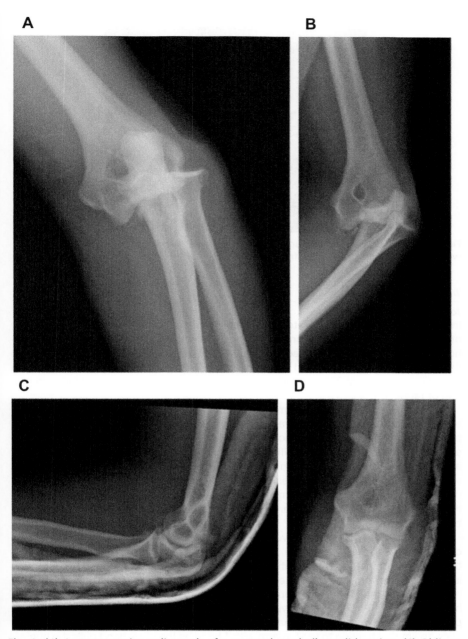

Fig. 1. (*A*) Anteroposterior radiograph of a posterolateral elbow dislocation. (*B*) Oblique radiograph of a posterolateral elbow dislocation. (*C*) Post reduction lateral radiograph with posterior splint. (*D*) Post reduction anteroposterior radiograph with posterior splint.

which can contribute to persistent instability.[22] Diagnostic elbow arthroscopy can provide useful information to detect radial head subluxation, articular damage, ligamentous disruption, or loose bodies.[23,24]

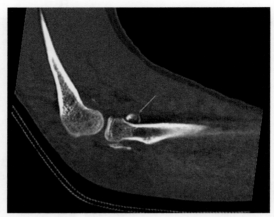

Fig. 2. Sagittal CT scan after reduction of an elbow dislocation with an arrow pointing toward a concomitant radial head fracture.

Treatment Algorithm

Joint reduction

In the setting of an injured athlete on the sideline, clinical evaluation is paramount. The athlete should be taken to a controlled environment away from the sideline. A reduction attempt should be performed using any one of the several techniques described in this section, using traction and countertraction. The elbow should be placed into a posterior slab splint at 90°, and radiographic imaging should be obtained for confirmation of reduction.

A patient in the emergency room must have emergent injuries ruled out. Once evaluated from a clinical and radiographic perspective, reduction of the joint should be performed next. Muscle relaxation usually is required during an elbow reduction attempt. If the reduction is too difficult or cannot be achieved in a safe manner with analgesics or conscious sedation, then it can be performed in the operating room with general or regional anesthesia.[9] An intra-articular lidocaine injection may be used to assist in reduction and may reduce the need for sedation or general anesthesia.[24] Fluoroscopic imaging can be used to guide the reduction and to assess stability after the reduction.[9]

Three different techniques have been described for reducing a posterior elbow dislocation. In the first technique, the patient lies supine with the elbow flexed and the forearm supinated. Traction then is applied to the forearm while countertraction is applied to the arm. Then, the medial or lateral displacement of the olecranon is corrected. Finally, the olecranon is pushed distally to engage the olecranon fossa of the humerus[7,9,12,25] **(Fig. 3)**. The Parvin method can be performed with the patient lying prone with the arm and forearm hanging over the side of the table. The physician applies downward traction to the forearm with 1 hand as the other hand pulls the humerus upward and laterally. The thumb of the hand pulling on the humerus is used to push the olecranon distally into the olecranon fossa[26] **(Fig. 4)**. A third technique places the patient supine with the arm across the chest, the elbow flexed to 90°, and the forearm fully supinated. The physician applies traction to the forearm with 1 hand, while the other pulls the arm in the opposite direction. The elbow is gently flexed and the thumb pushes the olecranon into the olecranon fossa.[27] Forearm supination during reduction is important to clear the coronoid under the trochlea in order to minimize additional

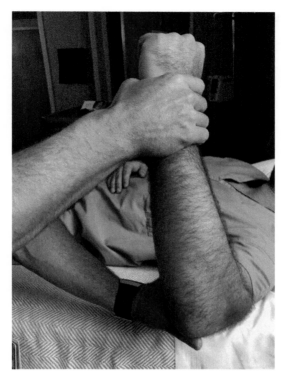

Fig. 3. Supine elbow reduction maneuver.

trauma to the intact medial structures.[12] A modified version of the cross-arm technique can be used if there is an assistant available to help get better control of the olecranon as it is pushed over into the olecranon fossa (**Fig. 5**).

Assessment of joint stability
Next, the elbow is flexed and extended through a full range of motion in neutral rotation to assess for stability. Historically, a posterior splint was applied for comfort until the patient returned to clinic 1 week later, with follow-up visits every 5 days to 7 days for a total of 3 weeks after injury.[7] If the joint is stable throughout the range of motion, without any subluxation or crepitus, an argument can be made for early active range of motion with a sling for comfort. Iordens and colleagues[28] compared early mobilization to plaster immobilization in a multicenter randomized clinical trial, showing that patients recover faster and return to work earlier without increasing complications. Another retrospective study showed that the return to work between the 2 groups can be cut in half,[17] with return to work in the early mobilization group at 3.2 weeks compared with the plaster immobilization group returning to work at 6.6 weeks.[29] Any immobilization longer than 1 week consistently has shown poor patient outcomes with specific regard to elbow stiffness.[28–30] Advances in rehabilitation have allowed for the great patient outcomes that avoid complications. An overhead motion protocol, described by Schreiber and colleagues,[31] can be implemented within 1 week of injury converting gravity from a distracting force to a stabilizing force (**Fig. 6**).

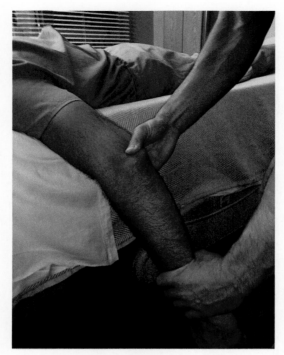

Fig. 4. Parvin prone elbow dislocation reduction maneuver.

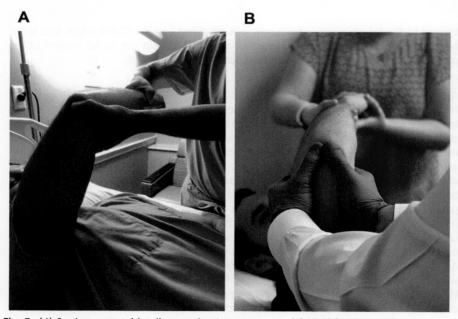

Fig. 5. (*A*) Supine cross-table elbow reduction maneuver. (*B*) Modification with assistant.

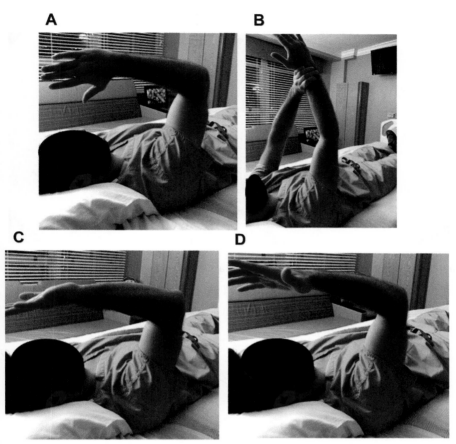

Fig. 6. Overhead motion protocol for early rehabilitation. (*A*) Patient supine with shoulder adducted and flexed to 90° with forearm in neutral rotation. (*B*) Active assistance to achieve elbow extension. (*C*) Patient supine with shoulder adducted and flexed to 90° with forearm in full pronation. (*D*) Patient supine with shoulder adducted and flexed to 90° with forearm in full supination.

If there is elbow subluxation or dislocation in extension, Watts[32] argues for the use of MRI to determine the extent of soft tissue injury. Although the authors of this article do not advocate for routine use of MRI for acute simple dislocation, they acknowledge that it can be helpful, especially in elbow dislocations that do not involve fracture but that have questionable joint congruency. Those with grade 3 or grade 4 injuries, elbows with recurrent dislocation in extension, and subluxation on postreduction imaging can be managed with examination under anesthesia using fluoroscopic imaging[32]:

1. Patient supine with forearm in pronation at full extension and 30° of flexion
2. Varus stress applied → if >10° of joint widening seen → lateral ligament complex repair (**Fig. 7**)
3. Forearm supinated with elbow in full extension and 30° of flexion
4. Valgus stress applied → if >10° of joint widening seen → medial ligament complex repair. Please see **Fig. 8** for a simplified algorithm.

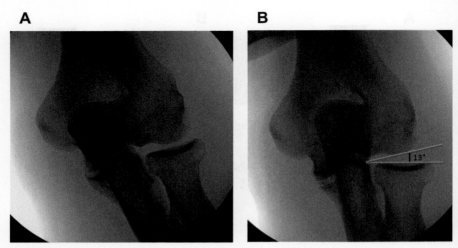

Fig. 7. (*A*) Anteroposterior fluoroscopic image of a concentric elbow joint. (*B*) Varus stress applied with the elbow in extension showing a 13° widening of the radiocapitellar joint.

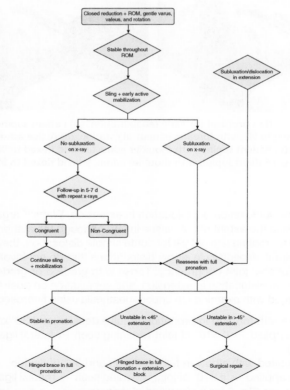

Fig. 8. Simple elbow dislocation algorithm. ROM, range of motion.

Surgical Intervention

Indications for surgical treatment of simple dislocations include residual instability in more than 45° of flexion, joint incongruence on postreduction radiographs, or an open dislocation.[24] The LCL is addressed first before considering repair of the MUCL. The MCL should be repaired only if there is gross instability after LCL repair.[3,24,33]

If a previous repair has failed or if the tissue integrity and quality are poor, then a ligamentous reconstruction should be considered. The use of an external fixator in cases of persistent elbow instability for cases without fracture is rare; furthermore, recently developed internal joint fixation systems are able to stabilize the elbow without transcutaneous pins, which further decreases the need for external fixation.[34] Regardless of the ligament treatment, attention also should be directed toward potential missed cartilaginous or osseous injuries in cases where combined MCL and LCL repairs are insufficient in restoring stability.

Postoperative Rehabilitation

Early understanding of postoperative rehabilitation after a reduction and collateral ligament repair/reconstruction was to immobilize the elbow in a posterior splint for 1 week before beginning active range of motion.[24,35] With the progression of nonsurgical management for early active range of motion, postoperative rehabilitation also has shown positive outcomes with earlier mobilization. Based on the ligaments that are repaired, the elbow can be placed in a hinged braced within 1 week to allow for active assisted range of motion as tolerated. At 6 weeks, the brace is used intermittently to begin daily activities.[36] The brace can be discontinued at 3 months to begin strengthening exercises. The patient may begin to participate in sporting activities while in the brace; the brace is recommended to be used for sports activities for a total of 3 months to 6 months postoperatively.[3,24]

Progressive static splinting is started 4 weeks to 8 weeks after injury if contracture develops and the range of active motion is less than 30° to 130°.[37] If ongoing elbow stiffness is present, then a turnbuckle orthosis can be used.[38,39] Contracture release surgery should be considered if no remarkable improvement occurs despite using a turnbuckle orthosis for 3 months.

COMPLEX ELBOW DISLOCATIONS

This section overviews the topic of complex elbow dislocations with a discussion covering coronoid fractures, terrible triad injuries, and posterior Monteggia fracture dislocations (**Fig. 9**). Each topic is introduced briefly, followed by an overall treatment algorithm. The overall theme in the management of these injuries is to obtain bony healing and stability first and then to address and treat the ligamentous injury present. Treatment protocols and postoperative rehabilitation on how to achieve best patient outcomes are discussed.

Coronoid Fractures

Coronoid fractures can be small but can contribute significantly to elbow instability[40] (**Fig. 10**). The anteromedial facet of the coronoid, 50% of which is unsupported by ulnar metaphysis, is prone to fractures secondary to varus/posteromedial injuries of the elbow with axial loading. Coronoid fractures almost always present with an associated injury to the LCL. Additionally, the posterior band of the MCL typically is ruptured while the anterior band is intact and attached to the anteromedial coronoid facet. The lateral

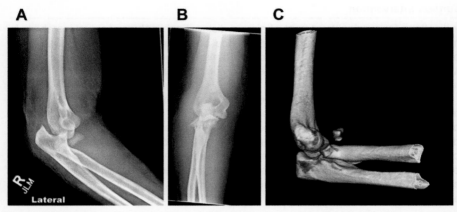

Fig. 9. (*A*) Lateral radiograph of a terrible triad elbow dislocation. (*B*) Anteroposterior radiograph of a terrible triad elbow dislocation. (*C*) A 3-dimensional CT reconstruction post-reduction image showing the extent of radial head fracture and displacement.

joint space usually is widened. Together with the radial head, coronoid also provides posterolateral rotatory stability.[41]

There is a lack of a universally accepted physical examination maneuver to detect posteromedial rotatory injury. The most useful test is the gravity varus stress test. The patient is asked to place the shoulder in 90° abduction with the forearm in neutral rotation. The test is considered positive if the patient experiences instability or crepitation, while the elbow is actively moved from flexion to extension (**Fig. 11**).

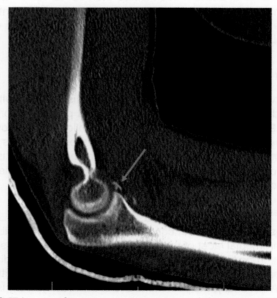

Fig. 10. A sagittal CT image of an arrow pointing toward the coronoid tip fracture.

A   **B**

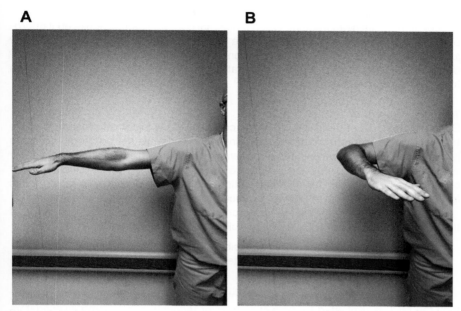

Fig. 11. (*A*) Gravity varus stress test to assess for posteromedial varus rotatory instability with the patient's shoulder at 90° and forearm in neutral rotation and elbow extended. (*B*) Patient maintains neutral forearm rotation and flexes elbow.

Additionally, the hyperpronation test can be used to assess for ulnohumeral subluxation with hyperpronation of the forearm.[42]

Monteggia Fracture-Dislocation

The Monteggia fracture is a fracture of proximal third of ulna with dislocation of radial head. Mechanism of injury can be a fall on an outstretched hand with forearm in excessive pronation or direct blow on the back of the upper forearm. Bado[43] described a 4-category classification of Monteggia fractures based on the direction of radial head displacement and whether or not an associated fracture of the radial diaphysis was present. Monteggia fracture types IIB and IID commonly are associated with coronoid fractures and ligamentous injury with posterior dislocation of radial head. Type I Monteggia usually can be managed with restoring the ulnar length without any complex reconstruction.

Terrible Triads

The term, *terrible triad of the elbow,* was used by Hotchkiss to describe the constellation of a traumatic elbow dislocation, radial head fracture, and associated coronoid fracture.[44] This dislocation pattern along with its associated bony fractures historically has poor outcomes, with a tendency for early recurrent instability, chronic instability, and posttraumatic arthritis.[45–48] Without an algorithmic approach, the historical treatment of patients with elbow dislocations associated with radial head and coronoid fractures resulted in poor outcomes in 64% of patients.[49,50]

These injuries may occur due to high-energy trauma and thus a thorough work-up to rule out concomitant musculoskeletal and visceral injuries must be performed. The distal radioulnar joint and forearm should be specifically evaluated for tenderness or instability as a longitudinal injury of the forearm needs to be ruled out if there is a concomitant radial head fracture. Good functional outcome can be achieved if appropriate repairs are performed that result in a stable, concentric reduction of the elbow joint. This usually is accomplished via open reduction and internal fixation or arthroplasty of all injured osseous structures that contribute to elbow stability, in addition to necessary ligamentous repairs.[45,47,49,51]

Treatment algorithm

Generally, the goal of treating a traumatic complex elbow injury is to restore a stable trochlear notch and to maintain proper joint alignment while the collateral ligaments heal.[40] The exact indications for nonoperative treatment remain controversial for each of these injury patterns and must be reserved for the appropriate patient. Patient compliance is pertinent during rehabilitation. Both serial clinical and radiographic follow-ups are necessary to monitor for recurrent joint incongruence and instability.

The type of surgical procedures for coronoid fractures depends on the subtype of the fracture according to O'Driscoll and colleagues' classification.[52]

- Subtype 1: nonoperative versus possible repair of LCL
- Subtypes 2 and 3: open reduction internal fixation (ORIF) using a buttress plate and/or LCL repair

If residual elbow valgus instability is identified after coronoid ORIF and LCL repair, then the MCL is evaluated for possible repair or reconstruction. Some investigators advocate suture fixation through capsular attachments if the fracture is too small for plate and screw fixation because it adds to anterior capsular stability.[40,53] Alternatively, in cases of a larger anteromedial facet fracture without comminution where solid bony stability can be obtained with ORIF, repair of the LCL is not absolutely necessary.

Treatment of Monteggia injuries is directed at restoration of ulnar length and alignment to indirectly achieve radial head reduction. It rarely is necessary that the proximal radiocapitellar joint be opened to achieve radial head reduction but may be necessary in some cases as a result of annular ligament interposition.[53,54] The posterior Monteggia injury has been shown to have more concomitant injuries involving either the radial head, coronoid process, or LUCL complex, with resultant ulnohumeral instability.[55-57]

Advances in contemporary techniques have improved surgical outcomes using internal fixation.[58] When dealing with the multitude of injuries in a posterior Monteggia fracture dislocation or a terrible triad, a stepwise surgical approach aids in addressing all the critical components of this injury. This includes

1. Anatomic fixation of proximal ulna fracture, fixation or replacement of the radial head fracture[58-63] (Fig. 12)
2. Fixation of the coronoid fragment[40,64,65]
3. Repair of the LCL at the center of the arc of the capitellum[66] (Fig. 13)
4. Assessment of stability to determine the need for adjunctive treatment such repair of the MCL[67]
5. Finally, if necessary, placement of an external fixator or internal joint stabilization implant

In most terrible triad injuries, the lateral ligament complex (LUCL and radial collateral ligament) and common extensor origin are avulsed from the lateral epicondyle. Multiple successful repair techniques, including suture repair using transosseous tunnels and suture anchors, have been described.[68] Fig. 14 shows a detailed algorithm to manage complex elbow dislocations.

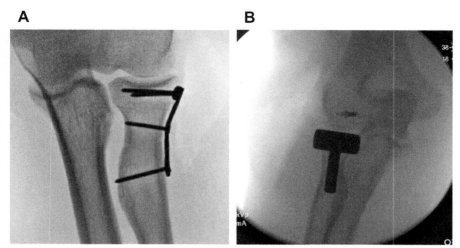

Fig. 12. (*A*) Radial head fracture status post-ORIF. (*B*) Comminuted radial head fracture with LUCL injury status post–radial head replacement and LUCL repair.

Postoperative protocol

Postoperatively, patients may be immobilized between 2 days and 3 weeks, depending on the severity of the injury and the mode of surgical intervention used.[69] Radiographs are taken throughout the postoperative care to verify fracture healing. Elbow range of motion is initiated as early as possible in a hinged brace. Shoulder abduction is avoided to minimize varus stress on the elbow. Unlimited flexion of the elbow is allowed immediately. Some protocols limit extension of

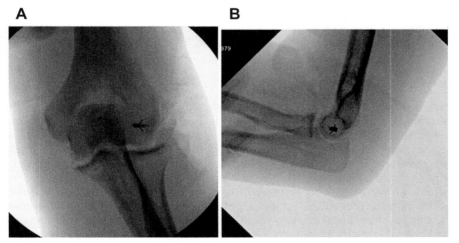

Fig. 13. (*A*) An anteroposterior fluoroscopic image after LUCL repair. (*B*) A lateral fluoroscopic image after an LUCL repair.

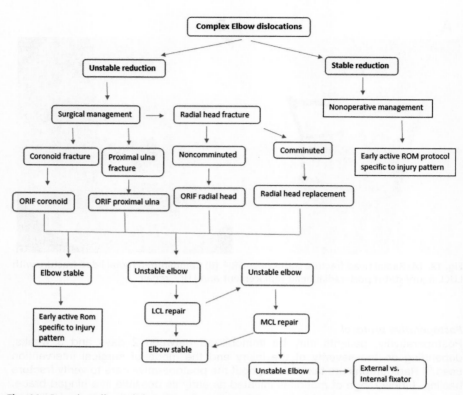

Fig. 14. Complex elbow dislocation algorithm. ROM, range of motion.

the elbow to 30° until approximately 5 weeks; however, due to concerns for loss of extension, some surgeons will progress extension quicker. Forearm position is determined by whether or not a repair was performed on the LCL or MCL.[70] Strengthening exercises may be started once satisfactory healing has occurred, typically at approximately 12 weeks.

CHRONIC ELBOW INSTABILITY

There is no established classification for chronic instability, but this entity can be classified according to the pattern of injury as posterolateral rotatory, varus, posteromedial varus, valgus, anterior, or global instability with injury of both collateral ligament complexes and circumferential capsular stripping of the elbow. The treatment of chronic elbow dislocation is a challenging problem. Postoperative complications, including stiffness, recurrent instability, and/or dysfunction related to violation of the extensor mechanism, have led some surgeons to recommend against surgical procedures for older patients and patients who are more than 3 months out from initial injury.[71] For the elderly, low-demand patients or patients with severe posttraumatic arthritis, elbow arthroplasty can be considered in appropriately selected situations.[72] **Fig. 15** illustrates the authors' recommended treatment algorithm.

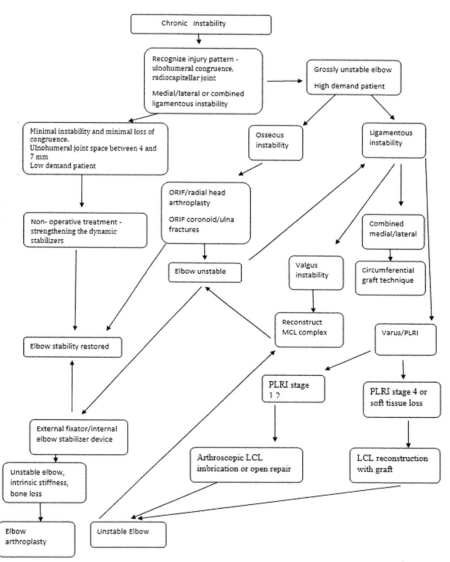

Fig. 15. Chronic elbow dislocation algorithm.[76] PLRI, posterolateral rotatory instability. (*From* Hackl M, Müller LP, Wegmann K. The Circumferential Graft Technique for Treatment of Chronic Multidirectional Ligamentous Elbow Instability. JBJS Essent Surg Tech. 2017;7(1); with permission.)

SUMMARY

Elbow dislocations are the second most commonly dislocated joint, with a majority receiving nonoperative management. The most common athletes who sustain this injury are those in contact and tumbling sports. In a study observing National Collegiate Athletic Association athletes, men's wrestling had the highest incidence of elbow dislocation, followed by women's gymnastics and men's football.[73] The most common complication with nonoperative management has been elbow stiffness. With new advances with early motion rehabilitation protocols, such as early overhead motion protocols, patients have seen a significant improvement in their outcomes. Simple elbow dislocations in an athlete should be treated with return to play on a case-by-case basis. The athlete should demonstrate full painless range of motion with strength equal to contralateral extremity. Return to play can be considered in as early as 2 weeks to 4 weeks in a hinged elbow brace with a contact athlete.[74] Even in elite-level athletes, a study observing National Football League players treated nonoperatively showed a mean return to play in 25 days.[75] Although complex injuries previously were described as elbow dislocations with an associated fracture, the authors believe that complex elbow dislocations should include elbow dislocations that involve serious ligamentous injury that require surgical intervention for stabilization. Advanced imaging and improved understanding of the mechanism of injury have helped address concomitant injuries that can lead to continued instability if missed on initial examination. An advance toward early motion for complex injuries also has been made specific to each injury pattern and mode of operative fixation. As fixation techniques continue to develop and advance, alongside the vast improvement in rehabilitation protocols, patient outcomes will continue to improve.

REFERENCES

1. De Haan J, Schep NWL, Tuinebreijer WE, et al. Simple elbow dislocations: a systematic review of the literature. Arch Orthop Trauma Surg 2010;130(2):241–9.
2. Coonrad RW, Roush TF, Major NM, et al. The drop sign, a radiographic warning sign of elbow instability. J Shoulder Elbow Surg 2005;14(3):312–7.
3. Heo YM, Yi JW, Lee JB, et al. Unstable simple elbow dislocation treated with the repair of lateral collateral ligament complex. Clin Orthop Surg 2015;7(2):241–7.
4. Sheps DM, Hildebrand KA, Boorman RS. Simple dislocations of the elbow: evaluation and treatment. Hand Clin 2004;20(4):389–404.
5. Stoneback JW, Owens BD, Sykes J, et al. Incidence of elbow dislocations in the United States population. J Bone Joint Surg Am 2012;94(3):240–5.
6. Josefsson PO, Nilsson BE. Incidence of elbow dislocation. Acta Orthop Scand 1986;57(6):537–8.
7. O'Driscoll SW, Jupiter JB, King GJW, et al. The unstable elbow. Instr Course Lect 2001;50:89–102.
8. O'Driscoll SW, Bell DF, Morrey BF. Posterolateral rotatory instability of the elbow. J Bone Joint Surg Am 1991;73(3):440–6.
9. Hildebrand KA, Patterson SD, King GJW. Acute elbow dislocations: simple and complex. Orthop Clin North Am 1999;30(1):63–79.
10. Murthi AM, Keener JD, Armstrong AD, et al. The recurrent unstable elbow: diagnosis and treatment. Instr Course Lect 2011;60:215–26.
11. Mehlhoff TL, Noble PC, Bennett JB, et al. Simple dislocation of the elbow in the adult. Results after closed treatment. J Bone Joint Surg Am 1988;70(2):244–9.
12. O'Driscoll SW, Morrey BF, Korinek S, et al. Elbow subluxation and dislocation. A spectrum of instability. Clin Orthop Relat Res 1992;(280):186–97.
13. Schreiber JJ, Potter HG, Warren RF, et al. Magnetic resonance imaging findings in acute elbow dislocation: insight into mechanism. J Hand Surg Am 2014;39:199–205.
14. Rhyou IH, Kim YS. New mechanism of the posterior elbow dislocation. Knee Surg Sports Traumatol Arthrosc 2012;20:2535–41.

15. Schreiber JJ, Warren RF, Hotchkiss RN, et al. An online video investigation into the mechanism of elbow dislocation. J Hand Surg Am 2013;38(3):488–94.
16. Søjbjerg JO, Helmig P, Kjaersgaard-Andersen P. Dislocation of the elbow: an experimental study of the ligamentous injuries. Orthopedics 1989;12:461–3.
17. Robinson PM, Griffiths E, Watts AC. Simple elbow dislocation. Shoulder Elbow 2017;9(3):195–204.
18. Luokkala T, Temperley D, Basu S, et al. Analysis of magnetic resonance imaging-confirmed soft tissue injury pattern in simple elbow dislocations. J Shoulder Elbow Surg 2019;28(2):341–8.
19. Cohen MS, Hastings H. Acute elbow dislocation: evaluation and management. J Am Acad Orthop Surg 1998;6(1):15–23.
20. Sanchez-Sotelo J, O'Driscoll SW, Morrey BF. Medial oblique compression fracture of the coronoid process of the ulna. J Shoulder Elbow Surg 2005;14(1):60–4.
21. Potter HG, Weiland AJ, Schatz JA, et al. Posterolateral rotatory instability of the elbow: usefulness of MR imaging in diagnosis. Radiology 1997;204(1):185–9.
22. Hotchkiss R. Displaced fractures of the radial head: internal fixation or excision? J Am Acad Orthop Surg 1997;5(1):1–10.
23. Modi CS, Lawrence E, Lawrence TM. Elbow instability. J Orthop Trauma 2012; 26(5):316–27.
24. McCabe M, Savoie F. Simple elbow dislocations: evaluation, management, and outcomes. Phys Sportsmed 2012;40(1):62–71.
25. Kuhn MA, Ross G. Acute elbow dislocations. Orthop Clin North Am 2008;39(2): 155–61.
26. Parvin RW. Closed reduction of common shoulder and elbow dislocations without anesthesia. AMA Arch Surg 1957;75(6):972–5.
27. Kumar A, Ahmed M. Closed reduction of posterior dislocation of the elbow: a simple technique. J Orthop Trauma 1999;13(1):58–9.
28. Iordens GIT, Van Lieshout EMM, Schep NWL, et al, on behalf of FuncSiE Trial Investigators. Early mobilisation versus plaster immobilisation of simple elbow dislocations: results of the FuncSiE multicentre randomised clinical trial. Br J Sports Med 2017;51:531–8.
29. Maripuri SN, Debnath UK, Rao P, et al. Simple elbow dislocation among adults: a comparative study of two different methods of treatment. Injury 2007;38(11): 1254–8.
30. Panteli M, Pountos I, Kanakaris NK, et al. Cost analysis and outcomes of simple elbow dislocations. World J Orthop 2015;6(7):513–20.
31. Schreiber JJ, Paul S, Hotchkiss RN, et al. Conservative management of elbow dislocations with an overhead motion protocol. J Hand Surg Am 2015;40(3): 515–9.
32. Watts AC. Primary ligament repair for acute elbow dislocation. JBJS Essent Surg Tech 2019;9(1):e8.
33. Hobgood ER, Khan SO, Field LD. Acute dislocations of the adult elbow. Hand Clin 2008;24(1):1–7.
34. Sochol KM, Andelman SM, Koehler SM, et al. Treatment of traumatic elbow instability with an internal joint stabilizer. J Hand Surg Am 2019;44(2):161.e1–7.
35. Jeon IH, Kim SY, Kim PT. Primary ligament repair for elbow dislocation. Keio J Med 2008;57(2):99–104.
36. Lee JH, Lee JH, Kim KC, et al. Treatment of posteromedial and posterolateral dislocation of the acute unstable elbow joint: a strategic approach. J Shoulder Elbow Surg 2019;28(10):2007–16.
37. Linscheid RL, Wheeler DK. Elbow dislocations. JAMA 1965;194(11):1171–6.

38. Royle SG. Posterior dislocation of the elbow. Clin Orthop Relat Res 1991;269: 201–4.
39. Green DP, McCoy H. Turnbuckle orthotic correction of elbow-flexion contractures after acute injuries. J Bone Joint Surg Am 1979;61(7):1092–5.
40. Ring D, Horst TA. Coronoid fractures. J Orthop Trauma 2015;29(10):437–40.
41. Schneeberger AG, Sadowski MM, Jacob HA. Coronoid process and radial head as posterolateral rotatory stabilizers of the elbow. J Bone Joint Surg Am 2004; 86A(5):975–82.
42. Ramirez MA, Stein JA, Murthi AM. Varus posteromedial instability. Hand Clin 2015;31(4):557–63.
43. Bado JL. The monteggia lesion. Clin Orthop Relat Res 1967;50:71–86.
44. Hotchkiss RN. Fractures and dislocations of the elbow. In: Rockwood CA, Green DP, Bucholz RW, et al, editors. Rockwood and Green's fractures in adults. 4th edition. Philadelphia: Lippincott-Raven; 1996. p. 929–1024.
45. Tashjian RZ, Katarincic JA. Complex elbow instability. J Am Acad Orthop Surg 2006;14(5):278–86.
46. Giannicola G, Sacchetti FM, Greco A, et al. Management of complex elbow instability. Musculoskelet Surg 2010;94(Suppl 1):S25–36.
47. Bohn K, Ipaktchi K, Livermore M, et al. Current treatment concepts for "terrible triad" injuries of the elbow. Orthopedics 2014;37(12):831–7. Johnson DL, editor, SLACK Incorporated.
48. Xiao K, Zhang J, Li T, et al. Anatomy, definition, and treatment of the "terrible triad of the elbow" and contemplation of the rationality of this designation. Orthop Surg 2015;7(1):13–8.
49. Ring D, Jupiter JB, Zilberfarb J. Posterior dislocation of the elbow with fractures of the radial head and coronoid. J Bone Joint Surg Am 2002;84-A(4):547–51.
50. Fitzgibbons PG, Louie D, Dyer GSM, et al. Functional outcomes after fixation of "terrible triad" elbow fracture dislocations. Orthopedics 2014;37(4):e373–6.
51. Pierrart J, Bégué T, Mansat P, GEEC. Terrible triad of the elbow: treatment protocol and outcome in a series of eighteen cases. Injury 2015;46(Suppl 1):S8–12.
52. O'Driscoll SW, Jupiter JB, Cohen MS, et al. Difficult elbow fractures: pearls and pitfalls. Instr Course Lect 2003;52:113–34.
53. Ring D, Jupiter JB, Simpson NS. Monteggia fractures in adults. J Bone Joint Surg Am 1998;80(12):1733–44.
54. Ring D. Monteggia fractures. Orthop Clin North Am 2013;44(1):59–66.
55. Jupiter JB, Leibovic SJ, Ribbans W, et al. The posterior Monteggia lesion. J Orthop Trauma 1991;5(4):395–402.
56. Konrad GG, Kundel K, Kreuz PC, et al. Monteggia fractures in adults: long term results and prognostic factors. J Bone Joint Surg Br 2007;89(3):354–60.
57. Ring D, Jupiter JB. Fracture-dislocation of the elbow. J Bone Joint Surg Am 1998; 80(4):566–80.
58. Ring D. Open reduction and internal fixation of fractures of the radial head. Hand Clin 2004;20(4):415–27, vi.
59. Watters TS, Garrigues GE, Ring D, et al. Fixation versus replacement of radial head in terrible triad: is there a difference in elbow stability and prognosis? Clin Orthop Relat Res 2014;472(7):2128–35.
60. Witt J. Toward safe exposure of the proximal part of the radius: landmarks and measurements. J Bone Joint Surg Am 2001;83-A(10):1589–90.
61. Diliberti T, Botte MJ, Abrams RA. Anatomical considerations regarding the posterior interosseous nerve during posterolateral approaches to the proximal part of the radius. J Bone Joint Surg Am 2000;82(6):809–13.

62. Caputo AE, Mazzocca AD, Santoro VM. The non-articulating portion of the radial head: anatomic and clinical correlations for internal fixation. J Hand Surg Am 1998;23(6):1082–90.
63. Ikeda M, Sugiyama K, Kang C, et al. Comminuted fractures of the radial head. Comparison of resection and internal fixation. J Bone Joint Surg Am 2005; 87(1):76–84.
64. Doornberg JN, Ring D. Coronoid fracture patterns. J Hand Surg Am 2006;31(1): 45–52.
65. Ring D. Fractures of the coronoid process of the ulna. J Hand Surg Am 2006; 31(10):1679–89.
66. Cohen MS, Bruno RJ. The collateral ligaments of the elbow: anatomy and clinical correlation. Clin Orthop Relat Res 2001;383:123–30.
67. Beingessner DM, Stacpoole RA, Dunning CE, et al. The effect of suture fixation of type I coronoid fractures on the kinematics and stability of the elbow with and without medial collateral ligament repair. J Shoulder Elbow Surg 2007;16(2): 213–7.
68. Cohen MS. Lateral collateral ligament instability of the elbow. Hand Clin 2008; 24(1):69–77.
69. Galbiatti JA, Cardoso FL, Ferro JAS, et al. Terrible triad of the elbow: evaluation of surgical treatment. Rev Bras Ortop 2018;53(4):460–6.
70. Liu G, Ma W, Li M, et al. Operative treatment of terrible triad of the elbow with a modified Pugh standard protocol: Retrospective analysis of a prospective cohort. Medicine (Baltimore) 2018;97(16):e0523.
71. Fowles JV, Kassab MT, Douik M. Untreated posterior dislocation of the elbow in children. J Bone Joint Surg Am 1984;66:921–6.
72. Ramesh M, Foead AI, Ali AB, et al. Salvage of elbow function in chronic complex elbow fracture dislocation with total elbow arthroplasty: a case report. Med J Malaysia 2013;68(4):353–5.
73. Goodman AD, Lemme N, DeFroda SF, et al. Elbow dislocation and subluxation injuries in the National Collegiate Athletic Association, 2009-2010 Through 2013-2014. Orthop J Sports Med 2018;6(1). 2325967117750105.
74. Morris MS, Ozer K. Elbow dislocations in contact sports. Hand Clin 2017;33(1): 63–72.
75. Chang ES, Bishop ME, Dodson CC, et al. Management of elbow dislocations in the National Football League. Orthop J Sports Med 2018;6(2). 2325967118755451.
76. Hackl M, Müller LP, Wegmann K. The circumferential graft technique for treatment of chronic multidirectional ligamentous elbow instability. JBJS Essent Surg Tech 2017;7(1):e6.

Lateral Epicondylitis/ Extensor Tendon Injury

Matthew Meunier, MD

KEYWORDS

- Tennis elbow • Lateral epicondylitis • Extensor carpi radialis brevis
- Extensor digitorum communis

KEY POINTS

- Lateral epicondylitis is a common complaint in patients between 40 years and 60 years of age.
- It is frustrating and may have a prolonged course. Multiple treatment options have been proposed.
- Many can be effective in the short term, but none has demonstrated a clear long-term benefit over simple activity modification and forearm rehabilitation or even simple observation.
- Irrespective of intervention, nearly all report durable relief at approximately 12 months. Surgical treatment has been proposed, but, again, scant evidence exists for any superiority in outcome.
- The most effective aspect of surgical intervention may be a period of enforced immobility and rehabilitation after the chosen treatment.

Pain over the lateral aspect of the elbow, without nerve injury or elbow instability, often is diagnosed as lateral epicondylitis or, colloquially, tennis elbow. It is a common complaint, seen most frequently in women between ages 40 years and 60 years, although it is common in men too. Typical presenting symptoms include pain with prolonged wrist extension activities, pain with resisted wrist or elbow extension, and pain at rest radiating from the elbow along the dorsum of the forearm.

The proposed etiology of lateral epicondylitis is repetitive microtrauma to the origin of the long wrist extensors, in particular, the extensor carpi radialis brevis (ECRB) and the extensor digitorum communis (EDC). Nirschl[1] proposed histologic findings of angiofibroblastic tendinosis. There may be an early inflammatory stage; however, after the presentation of symptoms, there is degeneration and ultimately fibrosis.

DIAGNOSIS

The typical patient presents with a complaint of pain over the lateral aspect of the elbow, particularly with resisted wrist extension activities or activities with the forearm

Orthopedic Surgery, UC San Diego Health System, 350 West Dickinson Avenue, Suite 121, San Diego, CA 92103, USA
E-mail address: mmeunier@ucsd.edu

Clin Sports Med 39 (2020) 657–660
https://doi.org/10.1016/j.csm.2020.03.001
0278-5919/20/© 2020 Elsevier Inc. All rights reserved.

sportsmed.theclinics.com

in pronation. Symptoms may present acutely or may have a lingering progression. Using a keyboard, gardening, sports activities, and writing often are presenting complaints. Exacerbating factors should be discussed, along with sports and recreational activities. Care should be taken to determine whether there is a history of elbow injury or instability.

PHYSICAL EXAMINATION

Physical examination findings are related to determining the area of discomfort and eliminating confounding findings. Palpation over the lateral condylar ridge, just proximal to the lateral epicondyle, often elicits pain, particularly when combined with resisted wrist extension. Active range of motion often is limited by pain, but passive motion usually is normal. The path of the radial nerve should be palpated, particularly along the span of the supinator muscle to differentiate from radial tunnel syndrome or a palsy of the posterior interosseous nerve. Nerve symptoms, in particular, loss of active digital or thumb extension, are not part of the diagnosis of lateral epicondylitis.

IMAGING

Radiographs do not prove lateral epicondylitis; however, they may help determine or eliminate other causes of lateral elbow pain.

Magnetic resonance imaging often is ordered by referring primary care physicians. Frequently there are findings of signal change over the lateral elbow; however, the true importance of this is not known. Cadaver studies have shown degenerative changes with age. Recent ultrasound studies also have shown an incidence of damage to the extensor origin in 21% of scanned patients.[2,3]

TREATMENT

Treatment of lateral epicondylitis has been controversial for a long time. As far back as 1936, Cyriax[4] proposed simply avoiding provocative movements and that it could take as long as 12 months to resolve. Nirschl[1] on the other hand proposed excision of the degenerative portion and repair of the extensor origin.

In the author's practice, patients with signs consistent with lateral epicondylitis are treated with forearm stretches and eccentric ECRB strengthening. The author has found this to be a physical therapy modality that has been effective as part of a treatment program when occupational therapy is required.[5] Counterforce bracing can be helpful[6] but the author typically uses wrist extension splinting to offload the extensors. Patients are counseled that symptoms may be present for approximately 9 months to 12 months. Proximal strengthening and core activation also can help decrease symptoms.

Injections and other interventions also are controversial. Steroid injections can provide early improvement in symptoms, although they may not prove more durable than any other treatment.[7] Injection at the site of pain (epicondyle) or within muscle both have appeared effective. Normal saline injections have an approximately 30% efficacy by themselves, which implies there are multiple confounding factors associated with symptoms. Prolotherapy and platelet-rich plasma have had some anecdotal success, but there is no large-scale benefit to either modality and the expense makes their value dubious. A comparison of corticosteroid, autologous blood, and normal saline showed no difference in outcome between any of the modalities at 2 months and at 6 months.[8] There are multiple studies in the literature regarding multiple treatment interventions. The overwhelming majority do not have a comparison to physical therapy, which makes assessment of true efficacy difficult.[9] A meta-analysis of the literature found 22 studies comparing nonsurgical intervention with either a nonintervention or observation arm and found no discernible difference in outcome between any of the treatment modalities.[10]

SURGERY

Surgical treatment has been proposed as a successful treatment of lateral epicondylitis. The reported outcomes are in line with nonsurgical interventions as well as with nontreatment. As described by Nirschl,[1] the incision is made laterally directly over the common extensor origin. The ECRB and EDC are effectively confluent at the origin from the lateral column, and a longitudinal incision is made in the extensor tendon. The muscle is split rather than being elevated from the lateral column and the degenerative tissue, if identified, is excised. The lateral epicondyle then is débrided of fibrinous tissue and the extensor tendon then is repaired. Arthroscopic débridement is reported as a possible treatment, with débridement of the capsule and undersurface of the ECRB.[11] Buchbinder and colleagues[12] in a Cochran review determined that there is insufficient evidence that any specific surgical intervention, or even surgery in general, is supported compared with any other treatment or even with simple observation.

If surgery is pursued, the operative surgeon should be careful with release and cognizant of the location of the lateral collateral complex of the elbow. There are reports of exuberant débridement resulting in disruption of the lateral collateral complex and creating an iatrogenic posterolateral rotatory instability of the elbow. Multiple corticosteroid injections can lead to thinning or depigmenting of the skin as well as to failure of the lateral collateral complex and posterolateral rotatory instability.[11]

RETURN TO ACTIVITY

As Drake and Ring[13,14] have discussed, the most important factor in treating lateral epicondylitis is communicating that this is a self-limited process. Once the acute pain has been stabilized, either with counterforce bracing or wrist extension splinting, patients may be counseled to return to activities as symptoms allow. Patients should be counseled that pain is likely to be present, particularly after a period activity, but, provided it is within acceptable limits and there are no symptoms of instability, they may return to sports activities.

SUMMARY

Lateral epicondylitis is a common complaint in patients between 40 years and 60 years of age. It is frustrating and may have a prolonged course. Multiple treatment options have been proposed. Many can be effective in the short term but none has demonstrated a clear long-term benefit over simple activity modification and forearm rehabilitation or even simple observation. Irrespective of intervention, nearly all report durable relief at approximately 12 months. Surgical treatment has been proposed, but, again, scant evidence exists for any superiority in outcome. The most effective aspect of surgical intervention may be a period of enforced immobility and rehabilitation after the chosen treatment.

REFERENCES

1. Nirschl RP. The etiology and treatment of tennis elbow. J Sports Med 1974;2(6): 308–23.

2. Kajita Y, Iwahori Y, Harada Y, et al. Ultrasonographic analysis of the extensor carpi radialis brevis in asymptomatic individuals. J Orthop Sci 2020 [pii:S0949-2658(19)30352-5].

3. Lindenhovius A, Henket M, Gilligan BP, et al. Injection of dexamethasone versus placebo for lateral elbow pain: a prospective, double-blind, randomized clinical trial. J Hand Surg Am 2008;33(6):909–19.

4. Cyriax JH. The pathology and treatment of tennis elbow. J Bone Joint Surg 1936; 18(4):921–40.

5. Cullinane FL, Bocock MG, Trevelyan FC. Is eccentric exercise an effective treatment for lateral epicondylitis? A systematic review. Clin Rehabil 2014;28(1):3–19.

6. Garg R, Adamson GJ, Dawson PA, et al. A prospective randomized study comparing a forearm strap brace versus a wrist splint for the treatment of lateral epicondylitis. J Shoulder Elbow Surg 2010;19(4):508–12.

7. Claessen FMAP, Heesters BA, Chan JJ, et al. A meta-analysis of the effect of corticosteroid injection for enthesopathy of the extensor carpi radialis brevis origin. J Hand Surg Am 2016;41(10):988–98.

8. Wolf JM, Ozer K, Scott F, et al. Comparison of autologous blood, corticosteroid, and saline injection in the treatment of lateral epicondylitis: a prospective, randomized, controlled multicenter study. J Hand Surg Am 2011;36(8):1269–72.

9. Cowan J, Lozano-Calderone S, Ring D. Quality of prospective controlled randomized trials. Analysis of trials of treatment for lateral epicondylitis as an example. J Bone Joint Surg Am 2007;89(8):1693–9.

10. Sayegh E. Does nonsurgical treatment improve longitudinal outcomes of lateral epicondylitis over no treatment? A meta-analysis. Clin Orthop Relat Res 2015; 473(3):1093–107.

11. Cohen MS, Romeo AA, Hennigan SP, et al. Lateral Epicondylitis: anatomic relationships of the extensor tendon origins and implications for arthroscopic treatment. J Shoulder Elbow Surg 2008;17(6):954–60.

12. Buchbinder R, Johnston RV, Barnsley L, et al. Surgery for lateral elbow pain. Cochrane Database Syst Rev 2011;(3):CD003525.

13. Drake ML, Ring DC. Enthesopathy of the Extensor Carpi Radialis Brevis Origin: Effective Communication Strategies. J Am Acad Orthop Surg 2016;24(6):365–9.

14. Dunn JH, Kim JJ, Davis L, et al. Ten to 14-year follow-up of the Nirschl technique for lateral epicondylitis. Am J Sports Med 2008;36(2):261–6.

Distal Biceps Injuries

Fotios Paul Tjoumakaris, MD[a], James P. Bradley, MD[b],*

KEYWORDS

- Biceps • Distal • Rupture • Repair • Reconstruction

KEY POINTS

- Injury to the distal biceps typically occurs in middle aged, higher demand patients who often require surgical reconstruction to optimize outcome and performance.
- Although MRI is not required to make the diagnosis, it is often performed to confirm a complete rupture and plan surgical management.
- There exists significant controversy regarding the best method of treatment of distal biceps injuries, namely, single-incision versus two-incision surgical techniques.
- Most studies demonstrate good clinical outcomes, regardless of surgical technique chosen.

INTRODUCTION

The treatment of distal biceps tendon injuries has evolved considerably over the past several decades. Initially, early reports advocated tenodesis of the biceps to the brachialis because of the high risk of neurovascular injury. With a greater appreciation and understanding of the regional anatomy of the elbow, there has been increased attention on anatomic repair of the biceps tendon. Most orthopedic surgeons advocate for early repair of the distal biceps tendon in young, active patients. There are several studies detailing different methods of fixation, approaches to the radial tuberosity, and patient selection criteria. The following article details the epidemiology, pathoanatomy and biomechanics, and clinical presentation and treatment of distal biceps injuries.

EPIDEMIOLOGY

Distal biceps tendon ruptures account for approximately 3% of biceps brachii injuries. The incidence of these injuries has slowly risen and is estimated at 2.55 per 100,000 population per year.[1] The average age of patients with distal biceps tears is 50 years (range, 18–72; most commonly between ages 40 and 60), and most patients who

[a] Orthopaedic Surgery, Sidney Kimmel College of Medicine, Thomas Jefferson University, Rothman Institute Orthopaedics, 2500 English Creek Avenue, Building 1300, Egg Harbor Township, NJ 08234, USA; [b] University of Pittsburgh Medical Center, Pittsburgh Steelers, Burke and Bradley Orthopaedics, 200 Delafield Road, Suite 4010, Pittsburgh, PA 15215, USA
* Corresponding author.
E-mail address: bradleyjp@upmc.edu

Clin Sports Med 39 (2020) 661–672
https://doi.org/10.1016/j.csm.2020.02.004
0278-5919/20/© 2020 Elsevier Inc. All rights reserved.

sportsmed.theclinics.com

present with this injury are male. Although the injury can occur in either extremity, it is far more common in the dominant arm and these injuries typically occur in active people. Tobacco use, anabolic steroid use, and elevated body mass index have been associated with an increased risk of distal biceps tendon injuries to variable degrees.[2]

ANATOMY AND BIOMECHANICS

The biceps brachii muscle originates proximally in the upper arm at the level of the deltoid tuberosity. The muscle is contained in the anterior compartment of the arm and is comprised of two heads, the long head and the short head. The long head of the biceps has its' proximal attachment at the shoulder where it attaches to the superior glenoid tubercle. The short head attaches proximally more medially at the coracoid process of the scapula. After converging in the upper arm, the distal tendon gives rise to the bicipital aponeurosis (lacertus fibrosus), which spreads out in an ulnar direction and blends with the forearm fascia.[3,4] With rupture of the distal biceps tendon, is not uncommon for the lacertus fibrosus to remain intact, tethering the biceps tendon in the antecubital fossa and preventing superior migration. Distal to the lacertus fibrosus, the distal biceps tendon then travels deep into the antecubital fossa before attaching to the bicipital (radial) tuberosity of the radius. The distal tendon has been found to have two distinct attachment sites. The tendon of the short head attaches more distal on the tuberosity and is thought to be primarily a flexor of the elbow. The tendon of the long head inserts farther from the axis of rotation of the forearm and acts primarily as a supinator of the elbow. The biceps muscle is innervated by the musculocutaneous nerve, which travels down the arm between the biceps and the brachialis. The most distal continuation of the musculocutaneous nerve is the lateral antebrachial cutaneous nerve, which supplies sensation to the volar and lateral aspect of the forearm.[5] This nerve traverses the antecubital fossa and is easily injured during surgical dissection or retraction at the time of surgery. Vital neurovascular structures (median nerve, radial and ulnar arteries, radial recurrent artery, radial nerve) are in close proximity to the antecubital fossa during surgical approaches to the tendon.

Because of the dual insertion of the distal biceps tendon, the biceps provides power to the elbow in flexion and supination. The biceps contributes more to flexion power as the elbow is supinated. In addition, the biceps contributes maximum supination strength with the elbow at or greater than 90° of flexion. In a prior study by Morrey and colleagues,[6] it was shown that patients who received conservative treatment of distal biceps tendon ruptures demonstrated a 40% loss of supination strength and a 30% loss of flexion strength. Other studies have demonstrated similar findings, with one study demonstrating an 86% decrease in supination endurance in patients treated nonoperatively.[7] Anatomic restoration of the insertion site during repair of the distal biceps tendon is likely critical to achieve optimum power after surgery. In a cadaveric study evaluating one-incision and two-incision techniques, the authors found that the two-incision approach was able to restore the anatomy closer to the native state.[8] This resulted in a 15% increase in supination torque at neutral rotation and 40% more supination power at 45° supination than the nonanatomic, one-incision approach. The optimal method of biceps tendon fixation continues to be hotly debated.

CLINICAL PRESENTATION
History

Most patients who present with distal biceps tendon ruptures will not have had prior pain around the elbow. Often times, the history is one of a forceful, eccentric contraction of the elbow. Patients report their arm being driven or forced into extension while they forcefully contract their elbow to prevent dropping something (ie, carrying a heavy piece of furniture and it is heavier than anticipated). Distal biceps ruptures can occur in competitive weight-lifters during eccentric biceps contractile exercises in addition to football players attempting to make a tackle with one arm as another player is running away, causing an eccentric pattern of contraction to the muscle. Patients often describe a pop or tearing sensation in their arm or forearm. There is often localized swelling around the elbow and antecubital fossa. Days after the injury, patients may notice bruising in the fossa or around the forearm. Once swelling subsides, typically there is a cosmetic deformity of the biceps as it retracts proximally in the upper arm. Patients may report weakness or pain with attempted flexion or supination of the elbow and/or forearm. Once the acute inflammation and swelling subsides, the pain is minimal in some cases, causing a minority of patients to forego prompt medical treatment. Patients who sustain a partial tear to the tendon may report more vague symptoms, such as soreness after activities or pain in the forearm that is poorly localized and deep.

Physical Examination

Patients with distal biceps tendon ruptures may have obvious bruising or swelling around the forearm. There may be an abnormal flexion crease proximal to the elbow where the biceps has retracted. There may also be an obvious cosmetic deformity (commonly referred to as a "Popeye" deformity) (**Fig. 1**). Palpation of the bicep elicits tenderness at the distal portion of the muscle and the tendon can often be palpated in the forearm or upper arm. If the lacertus fibrosus is intact, the tendon can sometimes be palpated deep to the lacertus, but there may be less of a deformity in these cases. Weakness and pain can often be elicited with resisted forearm flexion and supination. Full range of motion of the elbow is typically the norm for most patients. Patients who present with chronic ruptures (>4 weeks) may no longer have tenderness or overt signs of rupture but likely demonstrate atrophy of the biceps muscle and diminished strength. In cases of complete rupture such tests as the biceps squeeze test or the hook test can further help to make the diagnosis. In the squeeze test, with the forearm

A   **B**

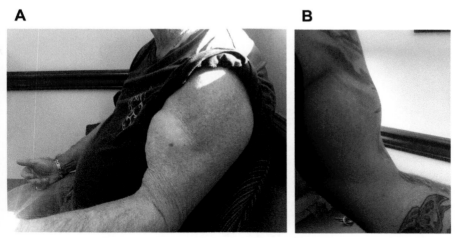

Fig. 1. (*A, B*) Clinical photographs of the classic "Popeye" deformity from a distal biceps tendon rupture. The biceps muscle retracts proximally into the upper arm resulting in this classic appearance.

in neutral rotation, the examiner squeezes the biceps brachii muscle.[9] If the biceps is intact, the forearm supinates (similar to the Thompson test for Achilles rupture). The hook test is performed by placing the arm at 90° of flexion and the examiner attempts to hook the lateral edge of the biceps tendon with the index finger (pulling from a lateral to a medial direction) (**Fig. 2**).[10] A positive test elicits a cordlike, intact tendon. An abnormal test (positive rupture) does not elicit a palpable tendon in the antecubital fossa. Comparing the injured extremity with the opposite extremity is helpful in less obvious cases. In patients with a partial tear, direct compression of the radial tuberosity during pronation and supination may elicit tenderness and could help to raise suspicion of a partial tear in patients with an otherwise normal clinical examination.[11]

IMAGING

Imaging typically starts with a routine radiographic elbow series (anteroposterior, lateral, oblique views). Most patients have no evidence of fracture or other osseous injury. There may be soft tissue swelling in the antecubital fossa on radiographs and, in rare cases, a bony avulsion off the radial tuberosity. MRI is a useful adjunct to confirm the diagnosis but is not often necessary when the clinical picture is as described previously for acute ruptures (**Figs. 3** and **4**). Specialized imaging protocols, such as the elbow flexed, shoulder abducted, and forearm supinated view (FABS view), allow for complete imaging of the distal biceps on MRI.[12] MRI is especially helpful in cases of partial tendon injury and in patients who have a body habitus that precludes an accurate clinical assessment. Although ultrasound is not routinely used for diagnosis of distal biceps tendon injuries, it is a useful tool in the hands of experienced ultrasonographers.

TREATMENT
Conservative Treatment

Conservative, or nonoperative treatment, is typically reserved for low demand and elderly patients who are not good candidates for surgery. This may also be a

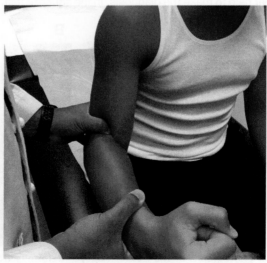

Fig. 2. Clinical demonstration of the hook test. With the patient actively supinating, the examiner can hook their finger under the biceps tendon from the lateral side.

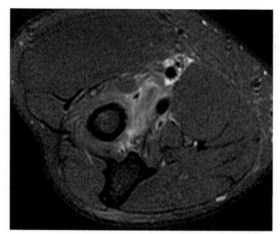

Fig. 3. Axial T2 MRI sequence of a patient with a distal biceps tendon rupture. This image is at the level of the radial tuberosity where the tendon is seen separated from the radial tuberosity with a hematoma at the site of tendon injury.

reasonable treatment option for patients with low-grade (<50%) partial tears of the distal biceps. A brief period of immobilization with a splint, followed by gentle range of motion and progression to strengthening with physical therapy can result in a significant improvement in clinical symptoms. It is critical that patients who elect nonsurgical treatment of complete ruptures understand the likelihood of supination and flexion strength loss in addition to fatigue-related pain when activating the biceps. Supination strength loss has been shown in some studies to be 40% to 60% relative to the uninjured arm, whereas flexion strength loss can be 30%.[13,14] Patients who decide on late repair (>4 weeks) after failing nonoperative management should be made aware of the inferior results of delayed treatment or the need for alternative surgical techniques (tendon grafting or biceps to brachialis tenodesis).

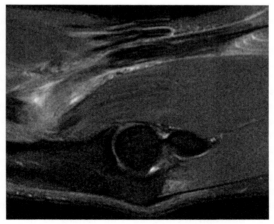

Fig. 4. Sagittal T2 MRI sequence of a patient with a distal biceps tendon rupture. The tendon is seen proximally migrated away from the radial tuberosity.

Operative Treatment

Most patients who sustain a rupture of the distal biceps tendon require operative fixation to restore strength to the biceps and elbow. Perhaps the most important factor when determining surgical treatment is timing. Patients who rupture their distal biceps tendon have more successful outcomes if they are attended to within 4 weeks of their injury. Delay beyond this time frame can result in the tendon migrating proximally in the arm and scarring to the adjacent brachialis muscle. More extensive surgical dissection might then be required and reapproximation of the tendon stump to bone is difficult or impossible in some instances, necessitating autograft or allograft reconstruction. In cases where the lacertus is intact, the biceps tendon stump may not migrate as proximally and late repair is more easily achievable; however, the reliability of an intact lacertus fibrosus after biceps rupture is variable. Patients who present for delayed treatment or who decide to have surgery after failing a protracted course of nonoperative management may be candidates for either allograft (Achilles, semitendinosus most common) or autograft (fascia lata, semitendinosus) reconstruction. Although there are reports of successful outcomes after late reconstruction, these results are less reliable than early primary repair and so are reserved for patients with significant disability. Nonanatomic repair (biceps to brachialis tenodesis) is performed in chronic injuries with activity-related pain and cramping. Patients may report improvement in flexion strength after this technique; however, no improvement is achieved in supination or with respect to loss of endurance.

Although patient selection (younger, active, and high-demand individuals) and acute treatment of ruptures (<4 weeks) are established principles of surgical treatment, perhaps the most controversial aspect of distal biceps treatment is the operative technique. There is significant debate as to the best method of treatment of distal biceps tendon ruptures, namely between single-incision and two-incision techniques. Both techniques offer strong fixation of the ruptured tendon stump to the radial tuberosity with transosseous tunnels (two-incision), suture anchors (either technique), interference screws (single-incision), or cortical fixation buttons/suspension devices (single-incision). Boyd and Anderson[15] popularized the two-incision technique to decrease the risk of iatrogenic nerve injury. The main advantage of this technique was that it achieved more anatomic restoration of the native footprint of the distal biceps tendon. Hasan and coworkers[16] demonstrated that with a single-incision technique, only 9.7% of the repair site was within the original bicipital footprint, whereas the two-incision technique demonstrated 73.4% of the repair site to be within the original footprint. With a single incision technique, the forearm is maximally supinated during the exposure and the tendon attachment is at the far ulnar aspect of the tuberosity. The technique requires fixation within a cortical tunnel and creating the tunnel too close to the edge could cause cortical blowout or "falling-off" the edge of the tuberosity. For this reason, a less anatomic insertion is favored to accommodate the technique. Critics of the two-incision technique popularized by Boyd and Anderson[15] point to the increased risk of radioulnar synostosis because of exposure along the posterolateral border of the ulna. This risk is likely increased because of exposure of the ulna periosteum.[17] This risk has been minimized, however, with the evolution of the technique. Currently, most surgeons using the two-incision technique favor the posterolateral incision over the common extensor muscle with dissection carried out between the common extensor and the supinator.[18] Proponents of each technique have demonstrated their respective merits and multiple studies have demonstrated near equivalent outcomes between techniques with regard to strength and patient-reported outcome measures.

COMPLICATIONS

Distal biceps repair has a low complication rate and a high success rate. Most complications are nerve related (lateral antebrachial cutaneous nerve, posterior interosseous nerve) or related to loss of rotation and strength.[19] Heterotopic ossification is more commonly seen with the two-incision technique but is much less frequent in the muscle splitting approach. Heterotopic ossification, when present, is rarely clinically meaningful and is rarely the cause of rotation or strength loss. Nerve injuries may be more common with the single-incision approach because distal retraction is required to visualize the radial tuberosity and may put the neurovascular structures at risk of stretch. Most nerve injuries resolve spontaneously with supportive treatment alone. When present beyond 3 months, an electromyography/nerve conduction study is helpful to evaluate the extent of nerve injury and provide some guidance regarding prognosis. Managing complications appropriately with routine follow-up, modification of the rehabilitation program when necessary, and clear communication can help to minimize patient apprehension and dissatisfaction. Effective patient communication and managing expectations is as important to the success of surgery as the operative plan chosen.

POSTOPERATIVE REHABILITATION

Patients who undergo distal biceps tendon repair are often splinted or immobilized for a short period of time after surgery. Gentle, passive range of motion is then permitted fairly early in the postoperative period to decrease the risk of scar tissue and

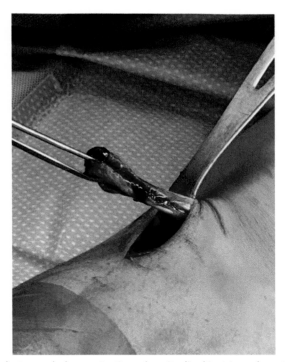

Fig. 5. A clinical photograph demonstrating a longitudinal incision where the biceps tendon stump is retrieved and clamped for whipstitch placement.

arthrofibrosis of the elbow joint. Once the splint is removed (usually Week 2), a hinged elbow brace is applied, which can be set to block terminal extension of the elbow beyond 30°, putting less stress on the repair. Weekly, the brace is allowed more terminal extension and active assisted range of motion exercises are initiated by 3 to 4 weeks postsurgery. By 6 weeks, patients should have nearly normal passive range of motion and approaching normal active assisted range of motion. Full active range of motion is typically achieved by 8 weeks postsurgery in flexion/extension and pronation/supination. Resistive exercises are typically initiated at 8 weeks and graduated slowly to minimize stress on the repair. Strengthening of the biceps is continued well into 3 to 4 months postsurgery and most patients are graduated to full activity by 6 months after surgery. Return to sports and strenuous use of the elbow during forceful flexion and extension activities is typically acceptable between 5 and 6 months after surgical repair. Patients undergoing allograft reconstruction of the distal biceps tendon may require a more protracted phase of protection and may take an additional 3 months to achieve similar gains relative to acute repair patients.

OUTCOMES/RESULTS

Regardless of technique chosen, distal biceps repair has shown excellent results with regard to function (flexion/supination) and overall patient outcome scores (disabilities of the arm shoulder and hand [DASH]). McKee and coworkers[20] compared one-incision technique patients with those undergoing a two-incision repair and found no difference in DASH scores, with flexion and supination strength almost equal to the uninjured limb at final follow-up. Additionally, Grewal and coworkers[21] performed

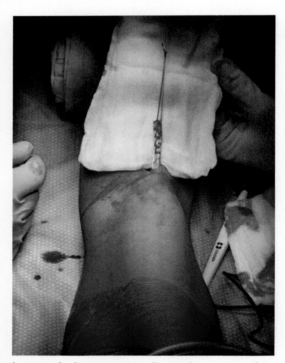

Fig. 6. A clinical photograph demonstrating the tendon stump adequately stitched and secured to a clinical button for later deployment.

a direct comparison between one-incision (suture anchors) and two-incision (bone tunnels) techniques and found no differences in reported outcomes at 2 years. The one-incision cohort had slightly better flexion but an overall higher complication rate (mostly lateral antebrachial cutaneous nerve palsies). In a similar study by Shields and coworkers,[22] similar functional scores were found between groups; however, Schmidt and coworkers[23] demonstrated superior strength restoration after a two-incision repair for the distal biceps. In a systematic review evaluating 22 studies, Watson and colleagues[24] found that single- and two-incision techniques had excellent outcomes; however, the authors found more nerve injuries in the single-incision patients and lower complication rates in patients who were fixed with bone tunnels and cortical buttons (relative to suture anchors and intraosseous screws).

For chronic ruptures requiring autograft reconstruction, Frank and colleagues[25] compared 19 patients undergoing reconstruction with 16 patients receiving a primary repair. DASH and SANE scores demonstrated no difference between groups with equal complication rates between both cohorts. Although the authors concluded that direct repair is preferable for most patients, near equal results were achieved in this select group of patients when undergoing autograft reconstruction. Darlis and Sotereanos[26] evaluated seven patients after allograft reconstruction (Achilles tendon repaired with suture anchors) and found an 87% return of supination strength when compared with the contralateral arm. Although acute repair is still preferable to optimize outcome and minimize complications, these results suggest that patients can still be treated successfully when undergoing a delayed reconstruction procedure.

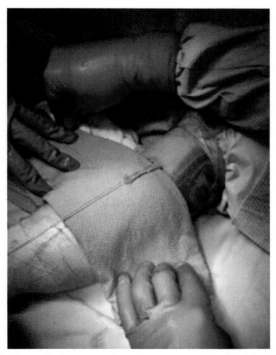

Fig. 7. A clinical photograph demonstrating a transverse antecubital incision demonstrating the whipstitch technique in the distal biceps tendon stump.

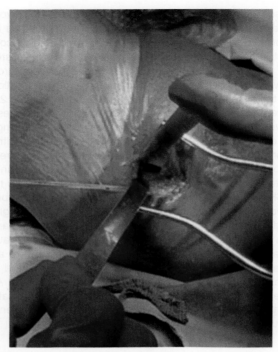

Fig. 8. A clinical photograph of the posterolateral incision with retractors placed around the radial tuberosity. Deep within the wound the trough for the biceps tendon is visualized, which was created with a small round burr.

AUTHOR'S PREFERRED TECHNIQUE

Our preferred technique for distal biceps repair is a single-incision technique using a fixation button and interference screw for tuberosity fixation of the tendon. Typically a transverse (or alternatively, a longitudinal incision can be used) incision is created just distal to the biceps crease. The lateral antebrachial cutaneous nerve is identified in the surgical field and gently retracted lateral to the biceps tendon, which is typically migrated proximally in the upper arm. If the lacertus fibrosus is intact, the tendon will not retract as proximally and may lie fairly close to the surgical field. The tendon is delivered into the wound, mobilized fully ("water skiing technique"), and whipstitched with a No. 2 nonabsorbable suture (**Fig. 5**). The radial tuberosity is then exposed with the elbow in full extension and maximum supination to minimize risk to the posterior interosseous nerve. Deep retractors are placed medially and laterally around the tuberosity. Care must be taken when retracting laterally to minimize stretch injury to the nerve. A 3.2-mm guide pin is then drilled bicortically through the tuberosity and a reamer is placed over the guide pin to create an unicortical tunnel for the tendon. The suture limbs are then passed through a cortical button and the button is passed through the tuberosity and flipped on the far cortex (**Fig. 6**). The tendon is advanced into the tunnel and the suture is tied securing the tendon to the radial tuberosity. If necessary, additional fixation with a small interference screw can then be used to "push" the tendon more distal and ulnar in the tunnel (creating a more anatomic placement). The wounds are then closed in layers and a posterior splint is applied.

For the two-incision technique, a transverse incision is used to retrieve the tendon in the antecubital fossa and a whipstitch is placed in the tendon (**Fig. 7**). A posterolateral incision is then created at the level of the radial tuberosity and a curved clamp is used to pass the sutures through the antecubital incision and laterally around the radius with the forearm pronated to minimize the risk of nerve injury. A trough is created in the tuberosity and the tendon is delivered into the trough with the assistance of drill holes (**Fig. 8**). The sutures are then tied down over a bone tunnel finalizing the repair.

DISCLOSURE

The authors report nothing to disclose.

REFERENCES

1. Kelly MP, Perkinson SG, Ablove RH, et al. Distal biceps tendon ruptures: an epidemiological analysis using a large population database. Am J Sports Med 2015;43(8):2012–7.
2. Miyamoto RG, Elser F, Millett PJ. Distal biceps tendon injuries. J Bone Joint Surg Am 2010;92(11):2128–38.
3. Bhatia DN, Kandhari V, DasGupta B. Cadaveric study of insertional anatomy of the distal biceps tendon and its' relationship to the dynamic proximal radioulnar space. J Hand Surg Am 2017;42(1):e15–23.
4. Kulshreshtha R, Singh R, Sinha J, et al. Anatomy of the distal biceps brachii tendon and its' clinical relevance. Clin Orthop Relat Res 2007;456:117–20.
5. Pacha Vicente D, Forcada Calvet P, Carrera Burgaya A, et al. Innervation of the biceps brachii and brachialis: anatomical and surgical approach. Clin Anat 2005;18:186–94.
6. Morrey BF, Askew LJ, An KN, et al. Rupture of the distal biceps tendon of the biceps brachii. A biomechanical study. J Bone Joint Surg Am 1985;67:418–21.
7. Baker BE, Bierwagen D. Rupture of the distal tendon of the biceps brachii. Operative versus non-operative treatment. J Bone Joint Surg Am 1985;67:414–7.
8. Prud'homme-Foster M, Louati H, Pollock JW, et al. Proper placement of the distal biceps tendon during repair improves supination strength: a biomechanical analysis. J Shoulder Elbow Surg 2015;24(4):527–32.
9. Ruland RT, Dunbar RP, Bown JD. The biceps squeeze test for diagnosis of distal biceps tendon ruptures. Clin Orthop Relat Res 2005;437:128–31.
10. O'Driscoll SW, Goncalves LB, Dietz P. The hook test for distal biceps tendon avulsion. Am J Sports Med 2007;35:1865–9.
11. Abboud JA, Ricchetti E, Tjoumakaris FP, et al. The direct radial tuberosity compression test: a sensitive method for diagnosing partial distal biceps tendon ruptures. Curr Orthop Pract 2011;22(1):76–80.
12. Giuffre BM, Moss MJ. Optimal positioning for MRI of the distal biceps brachii tendon: flexed abducted supinated view. AJR Am J Roentgenol 2004;182(4):944–6.
13. Chillemi C, Marinelli M, De Cupis V. Rupture of the distal biceps brachii tendon: conservative treatment versus anatomic reinsertion-clinical and radiological evaluation after 2 years. Arch Orthop Trauma Surg 2007;127:705–8.
14. Hetsroni I, Pilz-Burstein R, Nyska M, et al. Avulsion of the distal biceps brachii tendon in middle-aged population: is surgical repair advisable? A comparative study of 22 patients treated with either non-operative management or early anatomical repair. Injury 2008;39:753–60.

15. Boyd HB, Anderson HL. A method for reinsertion of the distal biceps brachii tendon. J Bone Joint Surg Am 1961;43:1041–3.
16. Hasan SA, Cordell CL, Rauls RB, et al. Two-incision versus one-incision repair for distal biceps rupture: a cadaveric study. J Shoulder Elbow Surg 2012;21(7): 935–41.
17. Failla JM, Amadio PC, Morrey BF, et al. Proximal radioulnar synostosis after repair of distal biceps brachii rupture by the two-incision technique. Report of four cases. Clin Orthop Relat Res 1990;253:133–6.
18. Austin L, Mathur M, Simpson E, et al. Variables influencing successful two-incision distal biceps repair. Orthopedics 2009;32:88.
19. Amin NH, Volpi A, Lynch TS, et al. Complications of distal biceps tendon repair: a meta-analysis of single-incision versus double incision surgical technique. Orthop J Sports Med 2016;4(10). 2325967116668137.
20. McKee MD, Hirji R, Schemitsch EH, et al. Patient-oriented functional outcome after repair of distal biceps tendon ruptures using a single-incision technique. J Shoulder Elbow Surg 2005;14:302–6.
21. Grewal R, Athwal GS, MacDermid JC, et al. Single versus double-incision technique for the repair of acute distal biceps tendon ruptures: a randomized clinical trial. J Bone Joint Surg 2012;94:1166–74.
22. Shields E, Olsen JR, Williams RB, et al. Distal biceps brachii tendon repairs: a single-incision technique using a cortical button with interference screw versus a double-incision technique using suture fixation through bone tunnels. Am J Sports Med 2015;43(5):1072–6.
23. Schmidt CC, Brown BT, Qvick LM, et al. Factors that determine supination strength following distal biceps repair. J Bone Joint Surg Am 2016;98(14): 1153–60.
24. Watson JN, Moretti VM, Schwindel L, et al. Repair techniques for acute distal biceps tendon ruptures: a systematic review. J Bone Joint Surg Am 2014;96(24): 2086–90.
25. Frank T, Seltser A, Grewal R, et al. Management of chronic distal biceps tendon ruptures: primary repair vs. semitendinosus autograft reconstruction. J Shoulder Elbow Surg 2019;28(6):1104–10.
26. Darlis NA, Sotereanos DG. Distal biceps tendon reconstruction in chronic ruptures. J Shoulder Elbow Surg 2006;15(4):440–4.

Distal Triceps Tendon Injuries

Clark Monroe Walker, MD[a], Thomas John Noonan, MD[b,c],*

KEYWORDS

- Triceps rupture • Distal triceps • Triceps tendon injury • Treatment • Elbow

KEY POINTS

- Distal triceps ruptures are uncommon injuries, usually caused by a fall on an outstretched hand or a direct blow.
- Eccentric loading of a contracting triceps has been associated with injury as well, particularly in professional athletes.
- Other common factors linked to injury are anabolic steroid use, weightlifting, and traumatic laceration.
- Some local and systemic risk factors include local steroid injection, hyperparathyroidism, and olecranon bursitis.
- The initial diagnosis can be complicated by pain and swelling, and a palpable defect is not always present.

INTRODUCTION

In contrast with distal biceps tendon injuries, distal triceps tendon injuries are relatively rare. Anzel and colleagues[1] reviewed more than 1000 cases of tendon injuries and found triceps tendon injuries to be the least common, accounting for less than 1% of the cases. The triceps muscle is the primary and most important elbow extensor and is critical for normal upper extremity function.

Triceps tendon injuries are most commonly the result of a discrete injury and typically appreciated by the patient. There are several known risk factors for this injury. The tendon tear can be partial or complete. Complete tears are optimally treated with surgical repair, with the best results obtained with acute repair. Significant injuries may present with relative preservation of strength, sometimes resulting in a delay in diagnosis.

[a] UCHealth Steadman Hawkins Clinic – Denver, 175 Inverness Drive West Suite 200, Englewood, CO 80112, USA; [b] UCHealth Steadman Hawkins Clinic – Denver, 175 Inverness Drive West Suite 200, Englewood, CO 80112, USA; [c] Department of Orthopedic Surgery, University of Colorado, Aurora, CO, USA
* Corresponding author. UCHealth Steadman Hawkins Clinic – Denver, 175 Inverness Drive West Suite 200, Englewood, CO 80112.
E-mail address: thomas.noonan@cuanschutz.edu

Clin Sports Med 39 (2020) 673–685
https://doi.org/10.1016/j.csm.2020.03.003
0278-5919/20/© 2020 Elsevier Inc. All rights reserved.

sportsmed.theclinics.com

ANATOMY

The triceps muscle is a pennate muscle with 3 heads: long, lateral, and medial. It is the only muscle located in the posterior compartment of the arm and is innervated by the radial nerve. The long head takes origin from the infraglenoid tubercle of the scapula as well as the inferior glenohumeral joint capsule.[2] The lateral head originates from the posterior humerus lateral to the teres minor insertion, extending distally from the superior aspect of the spiral groove and the lateral intermuscular septum. The medial head originates from the posterior humerus distal to the spiral groove and medial intermuscular septum.

The insertion of the triceps tendon consists of a central tendon insertion onto the olecranon process as well as a lateral triceps extension (**Fig. 1**).[3] The lateral tendon expansion is continuous with the anconeus fascia and has a mean width of 16.8 mm. The total width of the triceps tendon is approximately 4 cm. The mean thickness of the central tendon insertion is 6.8 mm. The medial triceps tendon has a distinct, rolled medial edge and an insertion consistently confluent with the central tendon. The mean insertional width and length of the tendon proper are 20.9 mm and 13.4 mm, respectively. The mean distance from the olecranon tip to the tendon is 14.8 mm. The tendon width, thickness, and insertional dimensions correlate with the olecranon width. One study demonstrated a mean area of the footprint insertion of 466 mm^2, whereas a second study used a 3-dimensional modeling process to calculate the insertion area as 646 mm^2.[4,5] A more recent study from Barco and colleagues[6] found 3 distinct insertional areas of the triceps tendon on the olecranon. These were the posterior capsular insertion, the deep muscular portion, and the superficial tendinous portion of the triceps with areas of 1.5, 1.2, and 2.8 cm,^{2} respectively (**Fig. 2**). The deep muscular head corresponded to the medial head of the triceps and the tendinous portion corresponded to the long and lateral heads and correlated with the height of the specimen. The triceps inserted at a mean of 1.1 cm from the tip of the olecranon.

RISKS FACTORS

Triceps tendon injuries are most common in athletes. They have been found to be especially common in football players.[7] They are most common in men[8] and have

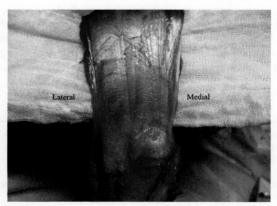

Fig. 1. Posterior view of a left elbow showing typical appearance of expansive lateral triceps in continuity with anconeus fascia. (*From* Keener JD, Chafik D, Kim HM, et al. Insertional anatomy of the triceps brachii tendon. J Shld Elbow Surg 2010;19(3):399–405; with permission.)

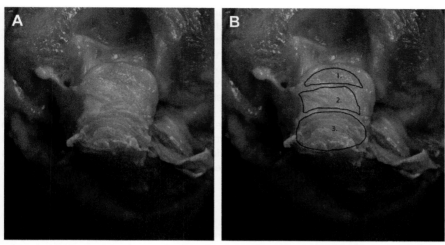

Fig. 2. After resection of the complete triceps insertion and posterior capsule, the bare olecranon shows 3 insertional areas corresponding to the posterior capsular insertion (1), the deep muscular head of the triceps (2), and the superficial tendinous head of the triceps (3). (*From* Barco R, Sánchez P, Morrey ME, Morrey BF, Sánchez-Sotelo J. The distal triceps tendon insertional anatomy-implications for surgery. JSES Open Access. 2017 Jul 25;1(2):98-103; with permission.)

found to be associated with anabolic steroid use.[9] Local corticosteroid injection has also been linked an increased risk of triceps tendon rupture.[9,10] Other factors that may play a role in triceps tendon injury include hyperparathyroidism, renal osteodystrophy, hypocalcemic tetany, Marfan syndrome, osteogenesis imperfecta, rheumatoid arthritis, type 1 diabetes mellitus, and olecranon bursitis.[11,12] In a systematic review of 262 patients, the most common medical comorbidity was renal disease, being present in 10% of the patients with triceps tendon ruptures.[13] Other common comorbidities included anabolic steroid use (7%) and local steroid injection (5%).

MECHANISM OF INJURY

Triceps tendon injuries usually occur as the result of a forceful eccentric contraction. Examples include weightlifting as well as the use of the arms by football lineman to push opponents. Direct blunt trauma to the posterior aspect of the arm is a less common mechanism. Rarely, a laceration to the posterior arm can cause a rupture of the tendon. A recent study[14] showed triceps tendon tears occurring with the following frequency owing to different mechanisms: direct elbow trauma (44.9%), extension/lifting exercises (20.3%), overuse (17.4%), and hyperflexion or hyperextension (17.4%). An additional study[15] showed similar results with the most common mechanisms of injury being fall (56.5%) and weightlifting (19%). The injury usually involves avulsion of the tendon from the bone but can occur at the muscle tendon junction.

CLINICAL EVALUATION

An accurate history is critical in diagnosing a triceps tendon rupture. The patient most commonly reports a discrete injury to the elbow, oftentimes with an associated sensation of tearing or a pop. They often complain of a loss of elbow extension strength. On physical examination, ecchymosis and swelling are often present over the posterior aspect of the arm in the case of an acute injury. A palpable divot may be present adjacent to the olecranon in the case of a retracted tear. Range of motion is typically full, although potentially limited by pain. Strength testing typically yields some degree of weakness with resisted elbow extension. In the case of a complete central tendon rupture with a preserved lateral triceps expansion, strength may be deceptively good. As a result, an accurate diagnosis by clinical examination only may be challenging. In fact, van Riet and colleagues,[16] showed that approximately 50% of acute triceps tendon ruptures were missed on the initial examination. Viegas[17] described a test similar to the Thompson test used for the diagnosis of Achilles tendon ruptures. In this variation, the patient is placed prone with the affected arm hanging over the edge of the examination table. The triceps muscle belly is squeezed and if the tendon is intact, the elbow should extend slightly. If the elbow fails to extend, the test is positive for a triceps tendon rupture.

DIAGNOSTIC IMAGING

In the case of a suspected triceps tendon rupture, plain radiographs should be obtained. In many patients, these images are normal. In the setting of preexisting tendinopathy, there are often enthesophytes present at the tip of the olecranon. These structures can fracture with a triceps tendon rupture. The flake sign is the presence of an avulsion fracture from the olecranon process and is felt to be pathognomonic of a triceps rupture (**Fig. 3**). A recent systematic review showed presence of bony avulsion in 61% of patients with triceps tendon rupture.[13]

Advanced imaging is usually obtained to confirm the presence of a triceps tendon rupture. For most practitioners, MRI is the modality of choice. Ultrasound examination can also be used to evaluate the integrity of the tendon. Both MRI and ultrasound examination are capable of distinguishing between partial and complete tendon injuries.[7,11,18–21] A triceps tendon rupture is best visualized on sagittal images (**Fig. 4**). A complete tear will be evident on T2-weighted images with high signal seen between the tendon and the olecranon. Chronic partial tears show an area of increased signal on T1-weighted or proton density images. Acute partial tears also show increased

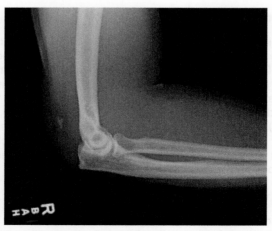

Fig. 3. A lateral radiograph showing the flake sign, representing a displaced traction spur from the olecranon in the setting of a full-thickness triceps tendon tear. (*From* Keener JD, Sethi P. Distal triceps tendon injuries. Hand Clinics 2015;31(4):641-50; with permission.)

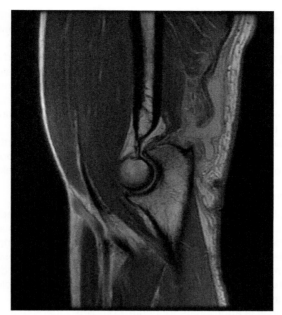

Fig. 4. Sagittal MRI clearly showing a complete rupture of the central triceps tendon.

signal on T2-weighted images.[19] Partial tears can involve the deep or superficial layers and are more common at the medial aspect of the tendon.[7,22] A recent study did find that MRI may overestimate the presence of full-thickness tears.[23] Of the 3 surgically confirmed complete tears, MRI correctly reported a complete tear in all patients. Of the 6 partial tears confirmed at surgery, MRI correctly identified 4 tears. In 2 cases, MRI described a complete tear, but only a partial tear was noted at surgery.

Nonsurgical Treatment

The management of distal triceps tears is generally guided by tear location and functional extension strength of the extremity. Assessment of functional extension strength is important because complete anatomic ruptures do not necessarily cause full loss of function.[24] If intact, the lateral triceps expansion or anconeus may compensate adequately for the loss of triceps function. The patient with complete anatomic rupture but with some function remaining should be identified and treated according to goals set specifically for that patient.[11] Treatment decisions should be based on the patient's medical and functional status on an individualized level. In general, any tear of less than 50% can be treated nonsurgically with satisfactory results.[24] Tears of greater than 50% are treated nonsurgically in the sedentary person; however, in the active person, surgical intervention may be appropriate.[7,25] Complete tears are generally managed surgically.[16,26,27]

Partial tears at the muscle belly, musculotendinous junction, and tendon insertion with insignificant loss of extension strength can be managed nonsurgically.[28] Tears of the triceps occurring within the muscle or musculotendinous junction are thought to have good healing potential and are generally treated conservatively. Muscle belly tears tend to heal with scar tissue rather than with newly regenerated muscle.

Outcomes are relatively similar with these tears regardless of treatment. Thus, even complete tears within the muscle belly can typically be managed nonsurgically.

Good results have been reported with nonsurgical management, with published studies indicating a return to preinjury level of function.[7,29,30] Mair and colleagues[7] reported that of 10 professional football players with partial tears, 6 healed with nonsurgical treatment and experienced no residual pain or weakness. Three players were treated with bracing for the remainder of the season, after which they received surgical treatment to correct residual pain and weakness. One player sustained a complete rupture on return to play despite bracing.

Nonsurgical management routinely includes a brief period of splint immobilization (3–4 weeks) at 30° of flexion. This period is followed by progressive elbow flexion mobilization. Progression of elbow motion is allowed as tolerated after 4 weeks.[11,24,26,28,29,31]

Surgical Treatment

Almost all complete triceps tendon injuries should be managed with surgical repair.[11,32] The exceptions include very low demand patients or those not medically fit for surgery. Partial tendon injuries that are high grade (involving >50% of the tendon), associated with tendon retraction and extension weakness, or that have failed conservative treatment also benefit from surgical repair by decreasing pain and improving strength.[22] These indications are particularly applicable in active individuals and athletes.

Early primary repair is appropriate for acute, complete triceps tear at the tendinous insertion with significant loss of triceps strength.[25] Ideally, repair should be performed within 2 to 3 weeks, although primary repair has been described as late as 8 months after injury.[33] A 2003 study showed that repair is most successful when performed in the first 3 weeks, with all patients regaining four-fifths manual strength, but a mean of 10° of terminal extension was lost.[16]

A variety of surgical techniques have been described for triceps tendon repair. There is no clear superior technique in terms of clinical outcomes, but each has theoretic advantages. All techniques focus on reattachment of the torn central tendon to the olecranon. In addition, any disruption of the lateral triceps expansion should be addressed because this strategy helps to augment the primary repair.

One of the historically popular repair techniques involves the use of the Bunnell or Krackow whipstitch technique, which includes placement of nonabsorbable sutures through the tendon. The sutures are then passed through transosseous drill holes in the olecranon and are tied over a bone bridge (**Figs. 5** and **6**).[16,34–36] The transosseous drill hole technique can also be used in skeletally immature patients.[37] Alternatively, the triceps may be reattached with the use of suture anchors placed within the olecranon in a single or double row configuration.[27,31,38,39] With both of these techniques, side-to-side sutures are recommended to reinforce the edges of the repair. Other repair techniques found in the literature include direct tendon repair to a periosteal flap raised from the olecranon.[27,39]

An alternative technique involves the creation of 3 parallel drill holes in the olecranon. The drill holes are angled in an oblique and dorsal fashion from proximal to distal through the olecranon, avoiding the joint surface. Using nonabsorbable sutures, 2 parallel Krackow-type stitches are placed through the detached tendon, leaving 4 tails. The 2 middle tails are passed through the central hole, and the medial and lateral tails are passed through the medial and lateral holes, respectively. The arm is held in approximately 35° to 40° of flexion for tensioning, and the sutures are tied.[40]

Modified repair techniques have recently become more popular in attempts to restore a larger, native anatomic footprint and improve the mechanical strength of

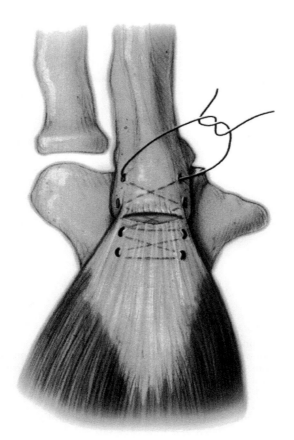

Fig. 5. Traditional bone tunnel repair of the triceps tendon. Bunnell-type suture configuration securing the central triceps tendon through crossing tunnels in the olecranon. (*Used with* permission of Mayo Foundation for Medical Education and Research. All rights reserved.)

the repair. The strength of the native triceps tendon has been shown to be roughly 1700 N in cadavers.[41,42] Yeh and colleagues[4] showed significantly greater repair strength, under cyclical loading, with a transosseous-equivalent repair compared with both traditional bone tunnel and suture anchor repairs. In addition, the transosseous-equivalent repair gave a better recreation of the native triceps footprint qualitatively compared with the other techniques, although this finding was not quantified. With the transosseous equivalent repair, 2 anchors are positioned in the proximal olecranon approximately 12 mm from the olecranon tip. Sutures from these anchors are then passed through the tendon creating horizontal mattress stitches. These sutures, along with the tails of a Krackow-type suture weaved through the triceps tendon, are then secured to 2 anchors placed more distally on the dorsal aspect of the ulna. This arrangement effectively compresses the distal tendon footprint against the bone, creating a larger area of boney apposition and better recreating the large area of the native triceps footprint. Alternatively, medial mattress stitches from anchors can be combined with a central tendon Bunnell-type suture secured through crossing bone tunnels.[43]

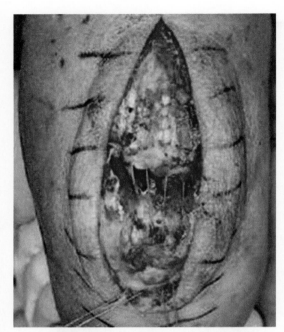

Fig. 6. Modified bone tunnel repair of the triceps tendon. Krackow-type suture configuration in the triceps tendon. The tendon is secured through 3 parallel tunnels passed through the olecranon tip. (*From* Sierra RJ, Weiss NG, Shrader MW, et al. Acute triceps ruptures: case report and retrospective chart review. J Shld Elbow Surg 2006;15(1):131; with permission.)

Knotless repair constructs have recently been studied and show favorable biomechanical strength.[44,45] In addition, this type of repair can be performed with 1 anchor and is less expensive than transosseous repair techniques. Clark and colleagues[45] studied an anatomic knotless repair compared with a traditional cruciate bone tunnel repair in cadaveric elbows. The knotless repair showed significantly less displacement under cyclic loading and better peak load to failure and yield strength than the traditional repair. With the anatomic knotless repair, 2 core high-tensile, braided sutures are woven through the central triceps tendon, creating 4 repair strands (2 medial and lateral suture ends). A shuttle suture is passed through the distal tendon on both the medial and lateral aspects of the tendon as well. Two parallel bone tunnels are created at the medial and lateral aspects of the olecranon, exiting the dorsal aspect of the ulna. The 3 strands of suture are passed through the olecranon bone tunnel on both the medial and lateral sides. Next, each shuttle suture is used to repass the free ends of the Krackow suture back through each of the bone tunnels, creating a cruciate repair (1 limb from the medial and lateral sides are crossed into the opposite tunnel). All slack is taken out of the 4 Krackow strands and the elbow is extended. All 4 strands are then secured to an interference fit-type anchor placed after predrilling into the dorsal apex of the olecranon, angled away from the articular surface.

A subset of patients will present with a torn triceps in which a portion of the olecranon has avulsed with the attached tendon on a bony fragment. This type of injury is more commonly seen in skeletally immature patients whose ossification center of the olecranon has yet to fuse. In these cases, the olecranon fracture can be reduced and fixed either with a screw and washer or with stainless steel wires via a tension band construct.[17] Smaller fragments can be reduced and fixed with suture fixation or can be excised with primary reattachment of the tendon to the olecranon.[31]

Triceps rupture at the myotendinous junction can be challenging to manage because of the poor quality of tissue available for primary repair. Wagner and Cooney[46] described the use of a V-Y triceps tendon advancement technique in which strength was augmented by interweaving an autologous plantaris tendon with the remaining proximal and distal triceps tissue.

In the setting of chronic, revision, or difficult acute tears, multiple procedures have been described to address deficient tissue, poor tissue quality, and a fixed retracted tendon. Reported reconstruction techniques include the use of Achilles tendon allograft (with or without a bone block), semitendinosus allograft or autograft, and anconeus rotation flap. With these techniques, the remaining triceps tendon and muscle are mobilized, and the allograft is secured distally at the olecranon. In the setting of bone deficiency, an Achilles allograft with attached calcaneal bone is affixed to the olecranon with a screw. In the setting of adequate bone stock, the allograft is secured to the triceps tendon using bone tunnel repair, anchor repair, or hybrid repair technique. With the allograft expansion proximally, the tendon is wrapped around the musculotendinous junction of the triceps tendon and sutured in place with the elbow in 40° to 60° of flexion.[47] Using the anconeus rotation flap reconstruction technique, the Kocher interval between the extensor carpi ulnaris muscle and the anconeus is used. The anconeus is mobilized from the ulnar and humeral attachments and is rotated over the proximal olecranon and then is repaired with drill holes and/or suture anchors. In scenarios with deficient or poor quality tissue, hamstring augmentation can be used to reinforce the repair or gain tendon length. The tendon is woven in a Bunnell fashion through the residual tendon. A transverse bicortical tunnel is drilled 1 cm from the olecranon tip. The free ends of the graft are passed through the tunnel from opposite directions (**Fig. 7**). An interference screw is placed, securing the graft within the tunnel with the elbow in extension.[48] The use of an interference screw, rather

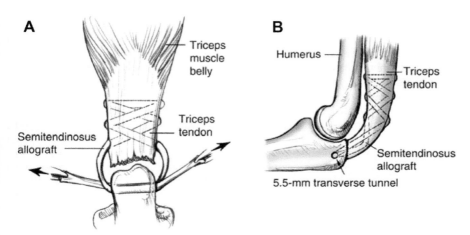

Fig. 7. Anteroposterior (*A*) and lateral (*B*) views of the hamstring allograft technique used to augment distal triceps repair. The allograft semitendinosus tendon is woven through the remaining proximal triceps tendon edge. The transverse tunnel is drilled through the olecranon 1 cm from the tip. The tunnel is centered between the articular surface and the posterior cortex. (*From* Yeh PC, Dodds SD, Smart LR, et al. Distal triceps rupture. J Am Acad Orthop Surg 2010;18(1):31–40; with permission.)

than suturing the tendon to itself, improves the fixation strength and resistance to displacement. Improved fixation strength at the repair site may allow for earlier initiation of active motion and may decrease potential elbow stiffness or joint contracture.[11]

Postoperative Care

Most postoperative protocols recommend immobilization of the elbow in 30° to 45° of flexion for 2 weeks to allow for wound healing and to protect the repair. The initial splint can then be replaced with a static thermoplastic splint in 30° to 60° of flexion or a hinged elbow brace if so desired. Therapy, consisting of passive or gravity-assisted extension and guided active flexion, is initiated at 2 weeks after immobilization. At 4 weeks postoperatively, active range of motion is initiated, and efforts are centered on regaining full elbow motion by 6 to 8 weeks postoperatively. Light strengthening begins at 6 weeks with slow progression until 3 months. Heavy lifting and weight training should be delayed until 4 to 6 months after surgery.[16]

Results and Complications

The clinical results of acute distal triceps tendon repairs are generally very good. Successful repair has been found to be more predictable when performed within 2 to 3 weeks of injury. Most studies reporting the outcomes of triceps tendon repair are retrospective and consist of small case series without control groups or direct comparisons of various repair constructs. In addition, outcomes are not reported in a consistent fashion and often lack validated scales of upper extremity function.[48] Van Riet and colleagues[16] showed peak strength of 92% (range, 75%–106%) and loss of extension of 8° compared with the uninjured side at 1 year postoperatively in 14 acute tears (average of 63 days before surgery) that were primarily repaired using the transosseous cruciate technique. Bava and colleagues[38] noted good results in 5 acute tears repaired with suture anchors at a mean of 32 months after surgery. Function was nearly normal in these patients with a mean Disabilities of the Arm, Shoulder, and Hand score of 1.4, and American Shoulder and Elbow Surgeons elbow score of 99.2, and a mean Mayo Elbow Performance Index of 95.8. The results of more anatomic repair constructs are largely unknown. Kokkalis and colleagues[43] reported the results of 11 acute triceps tendon tears repaired with a double row technique at a mean of 21 months after surgery. All repairs were performed within 3 weeks of injury. The mean visual analog scale pain score decreased from 8.5 preoperatively to 2.4 at follow-up. The mean loss of elbow extension was 7° and the mean arc of elbow motion was 136°. Elbow extension strength was significantly improved but not quantified. Nine of the 11 patients were completely satisfied with the surgery and had returned to full activity.

Reports of chronic or difficult rupture repairs are often lacking quantitative data and subjective outcome measures. However, Van Riet and colleagues[16] measured the outcomes of 9 chronic ruptures, an average of 163 days before surgery, that underwent reconstructions. These patients showed, on average, 66% peak elbow extension strength (range, 35%–100%) and loss of elbow extension of 13°. Despite the wide range of peak strength, this report shows that reconstructions of chronic tears are inferior to primary repairs of acute tears. The results of repairs and reconstructions from 3 recurrent rupture cases were functionally equivalent to results of first-time primary repairs. Other studies have shown that augmentation of primary repairs with hamstring autograft results in good outcomes. Case reports indicate that patients have returned to manual labor as well as competitive weightlifting with 5 of 5 manual strength testing in the clinic.[47,49]

Potential postoperative complications include olecranon bursitis secondary to wire suturing, flexion contractures ranging from 5° to 20°, irritation from underlying internal fixation, and rerupture.[36] Rerupture is rare and usually results from a traumatic fall after complete recovery from the first rupture.[16] However, rerupture is a concern, especially with poor quality tissue or delayed repairs performed under tension.

REFERENCES

1. Anzel SH, Covey KW, Weiner AD, et al. Disruption of muscles and tendons; an analysis of 1,014 cases. Surgery 1959;45(3):406–14.
2. Handling MA, Curtis AS, Miller SL. The origin of the long head of the triceps: a cadaveric study. J Shoulder Elbow Surg 2010;19(1):69–72.
3. Keener JD, Chafik D, Kim HM, et al. Insertional anatomy of the triceps brachii tendon. J Shoulder Elbow Surg 2010;19(3):399–405.
4. Yeh PC, Stephens KT, Solovyova O, et al. The distal triceps tendon footprint and a biomechanical analysis of 3 repair techniques. Am J Sports Med 2010;38(5):1025–33.
5. Capo JT, Collins C, Beutel BG, et al. Three-dimensional analysis of elbow soft tissue footprints and anatomy. J Shoulder Elbow Surg 2014;23(11):1618–23.
6. Barco R, Sánchez P, Morrey ME, et al. The distal triceps tendon insertional anatomy-implications for surgery. JSES Open Access 2017;1(2):98–103.
7. Mair SD, Isbell WM, Gill TJ, et al. Triceps tendon ruptures in professional football players. Am J Sports Med 2004;32(2):431–4.
8. Stucken C, Ciccotti MG. Distal biceps and triceps injuries in athletes. Sports Med Arthrosc 2014;22(3):153–63.
9. Sollender JL, Rayan GM, Barden GA. Triceps tendon rupture in weight lifters. J Shoulder Elbow Surg 1998;7(2):151–3.
10. Stannard JP, Bucknell AL. Rupture of the triceps tendon associated with steroid injections. Am J Sports Med 1993;21(3):482–5.
11. Yeh PC, Dodds SD, Smart LR, et al. Distal triceps rupture. J Am Acad Orthop Surg 2010;18(1):31–40.
12. Clayton ML, Thirupathi RG. Rupture of the triceps tendon with olecranon bursitis: a case report with a new method of repair. Clin Orthop Relat Res 1984;184:183–5.
13. Dunn JC, Kusnezov N, Fares A, et al. Triceps tendon ruptures: a systematic review. Hand (N Y) 2017;12(5):431–8.
14. Waterman BR, Dean RS, Veera S, et al. Surgical repair of distal triceps tendon injuries: short-term to midterm clinical outcomes and risk factors for perioperative complications. Orthop J Sports Med 2019;7(4). 2325967119839998.
15. Mirzayan R, Acevedo DC, Sodl JF, et al. Operative management of acute triceps tendon ruptures: review of 184 cases. Am J Sports Med 2018;46(6):1451–8.
16. van Riet RP, Morrey BF, Ho E, et al. Surgical treatment of distal triceps ruptures. J Bone Joint Surg Am 2003;85-A(10):1961–7.
17. Viegas SF. Avulsion of the triceps tendon. Orthop Rev 1990;19(6):533–6.
18. Downey R, Jacobson JA, Fessell DP, et al. Sonography of partial-thickness tears of the distal triceps brachii tendon. J Ultrasound Med 2011;30(10):1351–6.
19. Wenzke DR. MR imaging of the elbow in the injured athlete. Radiol Clin North Am 2013;51(2):195–213.
20. Thornton R, Riley GM, Steinbach LS. Magnetic resonance imaging of sports injuries of the elbow. Top Magn Reson Imaging 2003;14(1):69–86.
21. Kaempffe FA, Lerner RM. Ultrasound diagnosis of triceps tendon rupture. A report of 2 cases. Clin Orthop Relat Res 1996;(332):138–42.

22. Athwal GS, McGill RJ, Rispoli DM. Isolated avulsion of the medial head of the triceps tendon: an anatomic study and arthroscopic repair in 2 cases. Arthroscopy 2009;25(9):983–8.

23. Kholinne E, Al-Ramadhan H, Bahkley AM, et al. MRI overestimates the full-thickness tear of distal triceps tendon rupture. J Orthop Surg (Hong Kong) 2018;26(2). 2309499018778364.

24. Vidal AF, Drakos MC, Allen AA. Biceps tendon and triceps tendon injuries. Clin Sports Med 2004;23:707–22.

25. Strauch RJ. Biceps and triceps injuries of the elbow. Orthop Clin North Am 1999; 30:95–107.

26. Sharma SC, Singh R, Goel T, et al. Missed diagnosis of triceps tendon rupture: a case report and review of literature. J Orthop Surg (Hong Kong) 2005;13:307–9.

27. Pina A, Garcia I, Sabater M. Traumatic avulsion of the triceps brachii. J Orthop Trauma 2002;16:273–6.

28. Harris PC, Atkinson D, Moorehead JD. Bilateral partial rupture of triceps tendon: case report and quantitative assessment of recovery. Am J Sports Med 2004;32: 787–92.

29. Bos CF, Nelissen RG, Bloem JL. Incomplete rupture of the tendon of triceps brachii: a case report. Int Orthop 1994;18:273–5.

30. Aso K, Torisu T. Muscle belly tear of the triceps. Am J Sports Med 1984;12:485–7.

31. Farrar EL 3rd, Lippert FG 3rd. Avulsion of the triceps tendon. Clin Orthop Relat Res 1981;161:242–6.

32. Tom JA, Kumar NS, Cerynik DL, et al. Diagnosis and treatment of triceps tendon injuries: a review of the literature. Clin J Sport Med 2014;24(3):197–204.

33. Inhofe PD, Moneim MS. Late presentation of triceps rupture: a case report and review of the literature. Am J Orthop 1996;25:790–2.

34. Tsourvakas S, Gouvalas K, Gimtsas C, et al. Bilateral and simultaneous rupture of the triceps tendons in chronic renal failure and secondary hyperparathyroidism. Arch Orthop Trauma Surg 2004;124:278–80.

35. Langenhan R, Weihe R, Kohler G. Traumatic rupture of the triceps brachii tendon and ipsilateral Achilles tendon [German]. Unfallchirurg 2007;110:977–80.

36. Esenyel CZ, Oztürk K, Ortak O, et al. Rupture of the triceps brachii tendon: a case report [Turkish]. Acta Orthop Traumatol Turc 2003;37:178–81.

37. Kibuule LK, Fehringer EV. Distal triceps tendon rupture and repair in an otherwise healthy pediatric patient: a case report and review of the literature. J Shoulder Elbow Surg 2007;16:e1–3.

38. Bava ED, Barber FA, Lund ER. Clinical outcome after suture anchor repair for complete traumatic rupture of the distal triceps tendon. Arthroscopy 2012; 28(8):1058–63.

39. Bach BR Jr, Warren RF, Wickiewicz TL. Triceps rupture. A case report and literature review. Am J Sports Med 1987;15(3):285–9.

40. Sierra RJ, Weiss NG, Shrader MW, et al. Acute triceps ruptures: case report and retrospective chart review. J Shoulder Elbow Surg 2006;15:130–4.

41. Petre BM, Grutter PW, Rose DM, et al. Triceps tendons: a biomechanical comparison of intact and repaired strength. J Shoulder Elbow Surg 2011;20(2):213–8.

42. Adams DJ, Mazzocca AD, Fulkerson JP. Residual strength of the quadriceps versus patellar tendon after harvesting a central free tendon graft. Arthroscopy 2006;22(1):76–9.

43. Kokkalis ZT, Mavrogenis AF, Spyridonos S, et al. Triceps brachii distal tendon reattachment with a double-row technique. Orthopedics 2013;36(2):110–6.

44. Paci JM, Clark J, Rizzi A. Distal triceps knotless anatomic footprint repair: a new technique. Arthrosc Tech 2014;3(5):e621–6.

45. Clark J, Obopilwe E, Rizzi A, et al. Distal triceps knotless anatomic footprint repair is superior to transosseous cruciate repair: a biomechanical comparison. Arthroscopy 2014;30(10):1254–60.

46. Wagner JR, Cooney WP. Rupture of the triceps muscle at the musculotendinous junction: a case report. J Hand Surg Am 1997;22:341–3.

47. Sanchez-Sotelo J, Morrey BF. Surgical techniques for reconstruction of chronic insufficiency of the triceps: rotation flap using anconeus and tendo achillis allograft. J Bone Joint Surg Br 2002;84(8):1116–20.

48. Keener JD, Sethi P. Distal triceps tendon injuries. Hand Clin 2015;31(4):641–50.

49. Weistroffer JK, Mills WJ, Shin AY. Recurrent rupture of the triceps tendon repaired with hamstring tendon autograft augmentation: a case report and repair technique. J Shoulder Elbow Surg 2003;12:193–6.

Rehabilitation of Elbow Injuries
Nonoperative and Operative

Check for updates

Kevin E. Wilk, PT, DPT[a,b,*], Christopher A. Arrigo, MS, PT, ATC[c,d]

KEYWORDS

- Overhead athlete • Ulnar collateral ligament • Elbow • Rehabilitation

KEY POINTS

- Multiphased rehabilitation programs allow individualized progression of the athlete as determined by successful completion of each phase.
- A complete and thorough evaluation allows the rehabilitation specialist to properly design an effective treatment program for each athlete.
- The rehabilitation programs are designed to gradually introduce forces and stresses through functional and sport-specific drills to prepare the athlete to a return to their prior level of function.
  - Youth baseball players injure their elbows because of improper throwing mechanics, throwing when fatigued, and not enough rest between games, and the end of the season.
  - Elite baseball players injure their elbow because of high-velocity throwing and effort.
  - Correcting throwing mechanics is critical to the successful treatment of the overhead throwing athlete.

Athletic elbow injuries occur in virtually every sport affecting all ages and activity levels. They can be caused by a wide range of circumstances from acute trauma to chronic overuse and range in severity from catastrophic to minor. The frequency of repetitive stress injuries in the overhead athlete, particularly baseball pitchers, continues to increase.[1–4] In Major League Baseball, pitchers are the most injured players, and although shoulder injuries have decreased in the past 5 years, elbow injuries have increased, accounting for 22% to 26% of all pitching injuries.[5–7] Unlike injuries produced by traumatic forces, the high injury rate seen in pitchers is the result of the

[a] Champion Sports Medicine-Physiotherapy Associates, Birmingham, AL, USA; [b] American Sports Medicine Institute, 805 St. Vincent's Drive, Suite G100, Birmingham, AL, USA; [c] Advanced Rehabilitation, 4539 South Dale Mabry, Suite 100, Tampa, FL 33611, USA; [d] MedStar Sports Medicine, Washington, DC, USA
* Corresponding author. 805 St. Vincent's Drive, Suite G100, Birmingham, AL.
E-mail address: kwilkpt@hotmail.com

Clin Sports Med 39 (2020) 687–715
https://doi.org/10.1016/j.csm.2020.02.010
0278-5919/20/© 2020 Elsevier Inc. All rights reserved.

sportsmed.theclinics.com

biomechanics of overhead throwing whereby elbow extension occurs at more than 2300°/s, producing a medial sheer force of 300 N and a compressive force of 900 N, creating a valgus elbow stress 64 N m^2 during the acceleration phase of throwing, which exceeds the ultimate tensile strength of the ulnar collateral ligament (UCL), causing osteophytes posteriorly, olecranon stress fractures, and physeal injuries.[2,8,9]

An effective elbow rehabilitation program must identify the causative factors of the condition, be designed to specifically address these factors, and appropriately advance the program controlling all elements involved in a positive fashion to systematically return the athlete to their prior level of function as quickly and safely as possible. A team approach to treatment and rehabilitation is a critical element with the physician, physical therapist, athletic trainer, and strength and conditioning specialist all being included in treatment planning. Communication among each of the team members is vital and invaluable to ensure everyone remains on the same page throughout the process. A systematic, multiphased approach presented here is designed to follow a gradual progression of exercises and stresses applied sequentially to restore joint mobility, motion, motor control, strength, dynamic stability, and neuromuscular control not only to the elbow but also to the entire kinetic chain. Guidelines for this rehabilitation approach following elbow injury (**Box 1**) are outlined in detail, and the postoperative rehabilitation programs for specific pathologic conditions and for surgical interventions are also presented.

NONSURGICAL REHABILITATION
Phase I: Acute Phase

This first phase is designed to reduce pain and inflammation, normalize range of motion (ROM) and muscle balance, correct postural adaptations, and reestablish baseline dynamic joint stability. The athlete may be prescribed nonsteroidal anti-inflammatory drugs (NSAIDs) and/or local injections and local therapeutic modalities, such as ice, laser, iontophoresis, and electrical stimulation, to reduce pain and inflammation. The athlete is also educated about activity avoidance and modification during exercise and strenuous activities.

ROM activities are initiated to normalize elbow motion. It is common for athletes to exhibit a loss of elbow extension after injury or surgery, particularly throwers.[10,11] The elbow is predisposed to flexion contractures because of the intimate congruency of the joint articulations, the tightness of the joint capsule, and the tendency of the anterior capsule and brachialis to develop adhesions and scar following injury.[10] ROM activities should be performed for all planes of elbow and wrist motions to prevent the formation of scar tissue and adhesions by providing nourishment to the articular cartilage and assisting in the synthesis, alignment, and organization of collagen tissue.[10,12,13] Restoring full elbow extension is the primary goal of early ROM activities.[14]

Joint mobilizations are performed to minimize the occurrence of joint contractures and improve joint mobility. Grade I and II mobilization techniques are used to neuromodulate pain by stimulating type I and type II articular receptors. Posterior glides of the humeroulnar joint are performed at end range of available joint mobility to assist in regaining full elbow extension (**Fig. 1**), along with mobilizations of the radiocapitellar and radioulnar joints.

The aggressiveness of the stretching and mobilization techniques is determined by the healing constraints of the involved tissues, the specific pathologic condition or surgery, and the amount of available motion and end feel. If the athlete presents with a reduction in motion and a hard end feel without pain, aggressive stretching and

---

Box 1
Nonsurgical rehabilitation program for elbow injuries

I. Acute phase (week 1)
 Goals: To improve motion, diminish pain and inflammation, retard muscle atrophy
 Exercises
 1. Stretches for wrist, elbow, and shoulder joint
 2. Strengthening exercises; isometrics for wrist, elbow, and shoulder musculature
 3. Pain and inflammation control: cryotherapy, HVGS, ultrasound, and whirlpool

II. Intermediate phase (weeks 2–4)
 Goals: To normalize motion; improve muscular strength, power, and endurance
 Week 2
 1. Initiate isotonic strengthening for wrist and elbow muscles
 2. Initiate exercise tubing exercises for shoulder
 3. Continue using cryotherapy and other pain-control modalities
 Week 3
 1. Initiate rhythmic stabilization drills for elbow and shoulder joint
 2. Progress isotonic strengthening for entire upper extremity
 3. Initiate isokinetic strengthening exercises for elbow flexion/extension
 Week 4
 1. Initiate Thrower's Ten Program
 2. Emphasize work on eccentric biceps, concentric triceps, and wrist flexor
 3. Progress endurance training
 4. Initiate light plyometric drills
 5. Initiate swinging drills

III. Advanced strengthening phase (weeks 4–8)
 Goals: To prepare athlete for return to functional activities
 Criteria: To progress to advanced phase
 1. Full nonpainful ROM
 2. No pain or tenderness
 3. Satisfactory isokinetic test
 4. Satisfactory clinical examination
 Weeks 4 to 5
 1. Continue daily strengthening exercises, endurance drills, and flexibility exercises
 2. Continue Thrower's Ten Program
 3. Progress plyometric drills
 4. Emphasize maintenance program based on pathologic condition
 5. Progress swinging drills (such as hitting)
 Weeks 6 to 8
 1. Initiate interval sport program as determined by physician
 2. Begin phase I program

IV. Return-to-activity phase (weeks 6–9)
 Return to play depends on the athlete's condition and progress; physician determines when it is safe
 1. Continue strengthening program and Thrower's Ten Program
 2. Continue flexibility program
 3. Progress functional drills to unrestricted play

Abbreviation: HVGS, high-voltage galvanic stimulation.
 Data from Wilk KE, Reinhold MM, Andrews JR: Rehabilitation of the thrower's elbow. *Tech Hand Up Extrem Surg* 2003;7(4):197-216.

---

mobilization techniques may be used. Conversely, an athlete who exhibits pain before resistance or an empty end feel should be progressed slowly with gentle stretching.

At times it can be difficult to regain full elbow extension, and low-load, long duration (LLLD) stretch is needed to produce deformation or creep of the collagen tissue. This

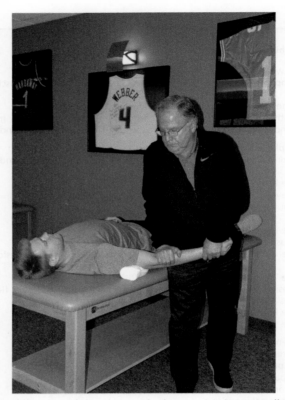

Fig. 1. Posterior mobilization of the ulna on the humerus to improve elbow extension.

stretch can be performed by having the athlete lie supine with a towel roll placed under the distal humerus to act as a cushion and fulcrum. Light resistance exercise tubing is applied to the athlete's wrist and secured to the table or to a dumbbell on the ground (**Fig. 2**) as the athlete is instructed to relax for the duration of 10 to 15 minutes of LLLD treatment. The amount of resistance applied should be of low magnitude to enable the athlete to perform the stretch for the entire duration of the treatment without pain or muscle spasm. Athletes are instructed to perform the LLLD stretches several times per day, equaling at least 60 minutes of total end range time to improve extension and reduce joint stiffness.[15]

During this phase, the voluntary activation of muscle and the retardation of muscular atrophy are also addressed via pain-free submaximal isometrics for the elbow flexors and extensors, wrist flexors and extensors, as well as the forearm pronators and supinators. Shoulder isometrics also may be performed during this phase, with caution against internal rotation and external rotation exercises if they are painful. Rhythmic stabilization drills are also incorporated for the elbow and shoulder to begin reestablishing proprioception and neuromuscular control of the upper extremity.

Phase II: Intermediate Phase

This phase is initiated when the athlete has achieved full ROM, experiences minimal pain and tenderness, and has a good (4/5) manual muscle strength of the elbow flexor and extensor musculature. The goals of this phase are to progress the strengthening

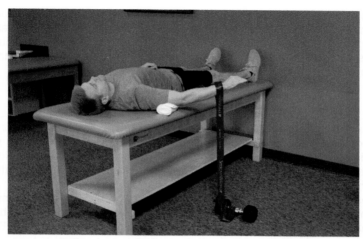

Fig. 2. LLLD stretch to increase elbow extension. The stretch is performed using light resistance while the shoulder is placed in internal rotation, with the forearm pronated to minimize compensation and best isolate the stretch on the elbow joint.

program, maintain normal physiologic flexibility, mobility, and ROM of the elbow, and enhance neuromuscular control of the upper quarter.

A combination of stretching and ROM exercises as well as grade III/IV joint mobilizations of the elbow, shoulder, and trunk is incorporated throughout this phase of rehabilitation to stretch the joint capsule and improve mobility. Flexibility exercises are continued for the wrist flexors, extensors, pronators, and supinators, with increased emphasis on improving elbow extension and forearm pronation flexibility.

It is common for the overhead athlete to lose internal rotation, horizontal adduction, and at times external rotation. The loss of internal rotation is commonly described as a glenohumeral internal rotation deficit. An 18° loss of internal rotation in the throwing shoulder has been implicated in elbow injuries and shoulder pathologic conditions.[16–18] External rotation should be assessed, because a loss of motion here can result in increased strain on the medial aspect of the elbow during the throwing motion. Because of these potential issues, shoulder flexibility exercises in all planes of movement should be performed in this phase.

Isotonic strengthening exercises begin concentrically and then are advanced to eccentric movements. Emphasis is placed on the elbow and forearm musculature, but exercises for the glenohumeral and scapulothoracic musculature must also be incorporated. The Thrower's Ten Program,[19] which is based on electromyographic (EMG) data to ensure the restoration of muscle balance in the treatment process, can be used as a base comprehensive program for every athlete.[20,21] Also, because the external rotators are commonly weak, particular focus should be placed on this muscle group via the inclusion of side-lying shoulder external rotation and prone rowing into shoulder external rotation exercises, because these movements have been shown to have high EMG activity of the posterior rotator cuff.[22]

The proximal stability needed for effective distal arm mobility is provided via the scapulothoracic musculature.[23,24] Specific exercises for these muscles have been developed to enhance proprioceptive and kinesthetic awareness facilitating improved neuromuscular control of the scapulothoracic joint.[25] Closed kinetic chain exercises, such as table pushups on a tilt board or ball, are incorporated to strengthen the upper and middle trapezius and serratus anterior (**Fig. 3**).[26] Rhythmic stabilization drills can be performed by having the athlete place a hand on a small ball against a wall as the clinician performs perturbation drills to the athlete's arm (**Fig. 4**) in combination with neuromuscular control exercises, including proprioceptive neuromuscular facilitation exercises with rhythmic stabilizations and manual resistance drills (**Fig. 5**).

Phase III: Advanced Strengthening Phase

This phase initiates aggressive strengthening exercises, progressing functional drills to enhance power and endurance, and improve neuromuscular control to prepare for a gradual return to sport. Before advancing to this phase, the athlete should exhibit full nonpainful ROM, have no pain or tenderness, and demonstrate strength that is 70% of the contralateral side.

Athletes are progressed to the Advanced Thrower's Ten Exercise Program, which incorporates high-level endurance and alternating movement patterns to further challenge neuromuscular control and restore muscle balance and symmetry.[27] Because muscle fatigue has been shown to decrease neuromuscular control and diminish proprioceptive sense, the program uses sustained holds and challenges the athlete to maintain a set position while the opposite extremity performs superimposed isotonic exercises.[28] Manual resistance drills can be added to increase muscle excitation and

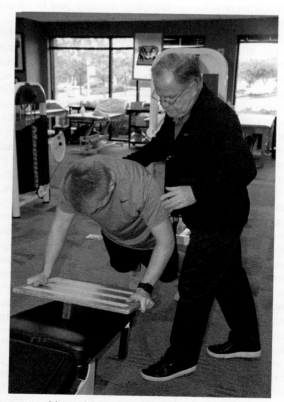

Fig. 3. Pushup on an unstable surface with manual rhythmic stabilizations to facilitate dynamic stability for the shoulder and core musculature.

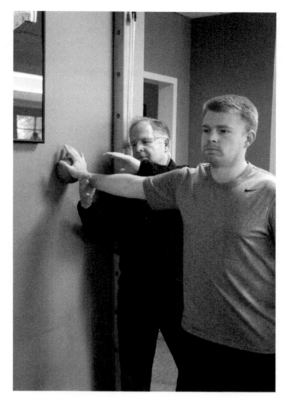

Fig. 4. Dynamic stability training with the patient's hand placed onto a ball against a wall. The arm is in the scapular plane to provide compressive forces into the glenohumeral joint as the clinician provides rhythmic stabilizations.

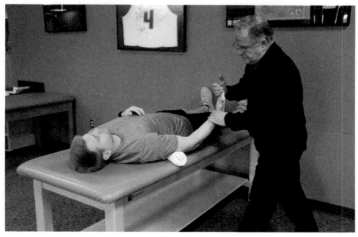

Fig. 5. Manual proprioceptive neuromuscular facilitation using concentric and eccentric resistance with rhythmic stabilizations.

promote endurance, including manual resistance, while seated on a stability ball to augment muscle excitation and improve upper quarter core endurance (**Fig. 6**).

Elbow flexion and extension exercises are progressed to emphasize eccentric control because the biceps is a critical stabilizer in many overhead activities controlling the deceleration of the elbow and preventing pathologic abutment of the olecranon within the fossa.[29] Elbow flexion can be performed manually or with elastic tubing to emphasize slow- and fast-speed concentric and eccentric contractions. Manual external rotation exercises with rhythmic stabilization for enhanced neuromuscular control are incorporated, including side-lying external rotation and standing external rotation with exercise tubing at 0° and finally at 90° (**Fig. 7**).

Resistance exercises with weight machines are incorporated at this time, including bench press, seated rowing, and front latissimus dorsi pull-downs, along with plyometric exercises to further enhance dynamic stability and proprioception, gradually increasing functional stresses on the upper quarter. Enhanced joint position sense, kinesthesia, and power have been demonstrated following 6 to 8 weeks of plyometrics.[30,31] A plyometric program has been described that systematically introduces stresses on the healing tissues, beginning with 2-hand drills, such as the chest pass, side-to-side throws, side throws, and overhead soccer throws, progressing to 1-hand drills, including standing 1-hand throws, wall dribbles, and plyometric step-and-throw exercises (**Figs.8–10**).[32] Specific plyometric drills for the forearm

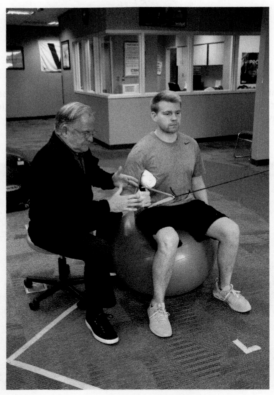

Fig. 6. Manual resistance external rotation using tubing performed on a stability ball to incorporate proximal and core stabilization.

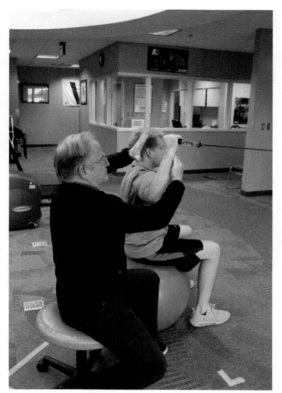

Fig. 7. External rotation at 90° of abduction using exercise tubing. The clinician provides manual resistance and rhythmic stabilizations.

musculature include wrist flexion (**Fig. 11**) and extension flips, which specifically emphasize the forearm and hand musculature.

Endurance training, such as wall dribbles with a medicine ball, prone ball drops (**Fig. 12**), wall arm circles, the upper-body cycle, and the Advanced Thrower's Ten Program, is critical because studies have shown that muscle fatigue decreases proprioception, alters biomechanics, decreases performance, and can contribute to elbow injuries.[33,34]

Phase IV: Return-to-Activity Phase

The last phase of the rehabilitation process focuses on a return to unrestricted full competition and includes implementation of sport-specific interval program. The criteria to enter this phase include full ROM, the absence of pain or tenderness, a satisfactory isokinetic test result, and a satisfactory clinical examination. Isokinetic testing goals for bilateral comparison at 180°/s for elbow flexion of the involved arm are 10% to 20% stronger and the involved extensors typically 5% to 15% stronger than the uninvolved arm.[10]

Interval programs have been developed for a wide variety of sports and activities to gradually introduce the quantity, distance, intensity, and types of activities needed to facilitate the restoration of normal function. The most commonly used upper-extremity interval program is for throwing. An interval throwing program (ITP) is divided into 2

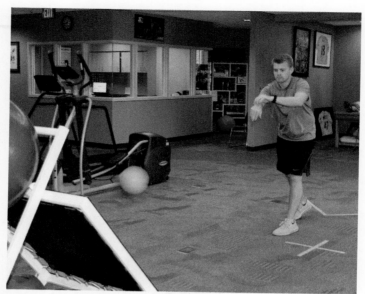

Fig. 8. Plyometric 2-handed chest pass.

phases: phase I is a long-toss program that is initiated at 45 feet (15 m) and is progressed by increasing distance and volume of throws until phase II, throwing from the mound for pitchers is appropriate. During the long-toss program, as intensity and distance increase, the stresses also increase on the athlete's medial elbow and anterior shoulder.[35] The long-toss program is designed to gradually introduce loads and strains and should be completed successfully before throwing from the mound is allowed.

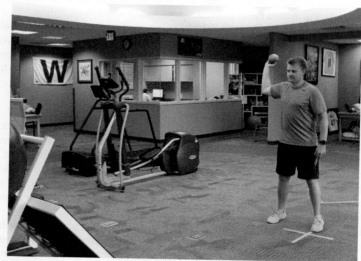

Fig. 9. Plyometric 1-handed Baseball throw.

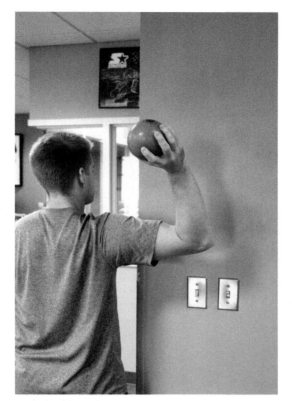

Fig. 10. Endurance wall dribble with medicine ball.

The athlete is instructed to continue with all previously described exercises and drills to maintain and improve upper-extremity, core, and lower-extremity strength, power, and endurance during this phase of rehabilitation. It is also important to teach the athlete a year-round conditioning program, including sport-specific periodization strength-training activities, to help prevent overtraining. Investigators have shown that the incorporation of a dynamic variable resistance exercise program can significantly improve athletic performance, particularly in throwing athletes.[36,37]

REHABILITATION GUIDELINES FOR SPECIFIC CONDITIONS
Ulnar Collateral Ligament Injury

Nonsurgical treatment is generally attempted for partial UCL tears. A brace can be used to restrict motion and minimize valgus stress in a nonpainful arc of motion generally from 10° to 100°, progressing gradually by 5° to 10° per week expecting full ROM in 3 to 4 weeks. Because the flexor carpi ulnaris and flexor digitorum superficialis overlay the UCL, strengthening exercises for these muscles can assist the UCL in resisting valgus stresses at the elbow.[38] In addition, posterior rotator cuff and scapular strengthening exercises are performed to restore proximal stabilization. The advanced strengthening phase usually is initiated at 6 to 7 weeks after injury, with valgus loading monitored throughout the rehabilitation program. An interval return-to-throwing program is initiated after the athlete regains full motion, adequate strength, and dynamic

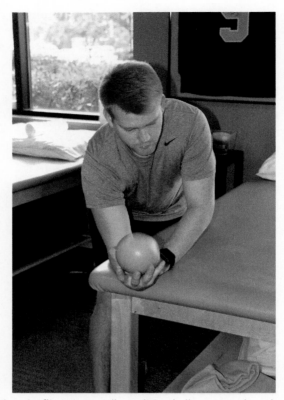

Fig. 11. Plyometric wrist flip using a 2-lb medicine ball to strengthen the wrist flexors.

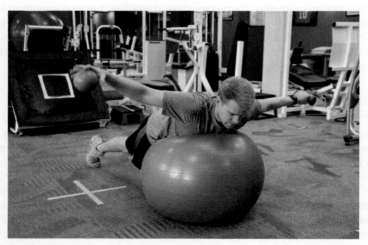

Fig. 12. Athlete performing a prone ball drop and catch, with the shoulder in horizontal abduction for local muscular endurance.

stability of the elbow. The athlete can return to competition following the asymptomatic completion of the interval sport program. If symptoms recur during the ITP, they typically present when throwing at longer distances, with greater intensity, or during throwing from the mound. If symptoms persist, the athlete is reassessed, and surgical intervention is considered.

Ulnar Collateral Ligament Reconstruction Surgery

Surgical reconstruction of the UCL attempts to restore the stabilizing functions of the anterior bundle of the UCL using one of several procedures.[16,39–41] The modified Jobe procedure can be used with either a palmaris longus or gracilis graft passed in a figure-of-8 pattern through drill holes in the sublime tubercle of the ulna and the medial epicondyle.[39] A subcutaneous ulnar nerve transposition is also frequently performed at the time of a UCL reconstruction. The rehabilitation program in current use following UCL reconstruction is outlined in **Box 2**. The athlete's arm is placed in a posterior splint with the elbow immobilized at 90° of flexion for the first 7 days postoperatively to allow early healing of the UCL graft and fascial slings involved in the nerve transposition progressing to a hinged elbow ROM brace to protect the healing tissues from valgus stresses until the beginning of week 5.

Passive ROM activities are initiated immediately to reduce pain and slowly stress the healing tissues. Initially, the focus of the rehabilitation is on obtaining full elbow extension while gradually increasing flexion. Elbow extension is encouraged early, to at least 15°, but full extension is allowed if the patient can comfortably achieve it if no discomfort is present. A recent study demonstrated that passive ROM of the elbow produced 3% or less strain in both bands of the reconstructed ligament and approximately 1% strain for the anterior band of the UCL.[42,43] Therefore, it has been determined that in the immediate postoperative period, full elbow extension is safe and does not place excessive stress on the healing graft. Conversely, elbow flexion to 100° is allowed and should be progressed at about 10° per week until full ROM is achieved by 4 to 6 weeks postoperatively.

Isometric exercises are progressed to include light resistance isotonic exercises at week 4 and the full Thrower's Ten Program by week 6. Progressive resistance exercises are incorporated at week 8 to 9. Again, focus is placed on developing dynamic stabilization of the medial elbow. Because of the anatomic orientation of the flexor carpi ulnaris and the flexor digitorum superficialis overlying the UCL, isotonic and stabilization activities for these muscles can assist the UCL in stabilizing valgus stress at the medial elbow.[38] Thus, concentric and eccentric strengthening of these muscles is routinely performed.

Aggressive exercises involving eccentric and plyometric contractions are included in the advanced phase, usually weeks 12 through 16. The Advanced Thrower's Ten Exercise Program is initiated at week 12 after surgery. Two-hand plyometric drills are performed at week 12, and 1-hand drills are executed at week 14. An ITP is allowed at postoperative week 16. Progression to throwing from a mound may occur within 4 to 6 weeks following the initiation of an ITP, and a return to competitive throwing may commence at approximately 9 months following surgery.

Ulnar Collateral Ligament Internal Brace Repair Surgery

Recent technological advances have sparked renewed interest in repair of the UCL augmented by an internal brace (Internal Brace; Arthrex Inc, Naples, FL, USA) because of the potential for a faster recovery in select instances. Repair of the UCL with Internal Brace is a direct repair of the native ligament with a spanning tape dipped in collagen (Internal Brace) anchored on each end of the UCL.[44] Two 3.5-mm SwiveLocks

Box 2
Postoperative rehabilitation protocol following ulnar collateral ligament reconstruction using autogenous palmaris longus graft (accelerated range of motion)

Immediate postoperative phase (0–3 weeks)
  Goals: To protect healing tissue, reduce pain and inflammation, retard muscular atrophy, protect graft site to allow healing
    Week 1
      Brace: Posterior splint at 90° elbow flexion
      ROM: Wrist AROM extension/flexion immediately after surgery
      Elbow: Postoperative compression dressing 5 to 7 days
      Wrist (graft site) compression dressing 7 to 10 days as needed
      Exercises: Gripping exercises, wrist ROM, shoulder isometrics (no shoulder ER), biceps isometrics
      Cryotherapy to elbow joint and to graft site at wrist
    Week 2
      Brace: Elbow ROM 15°–105° or as tolerated
      Motion to tolerance
      Exercises: Continue all exercises listed above
      Elbow ROM in brace 30°–105°
      Initiate elbow extension isometrics
      Continue wrist ROM exercises
      Initiate light scar mobilization over distal incision (graft)
      Cryotherapy: Continue ice to elbow and graft site
    Week 3
      Brace: Elbow ROM 5°/10°, 115°/120°, motion to tolerance
      Exercises: Continue all exercises listed above
      Elbow ROM in brace
      Initiate AROM wrist and elbow (no resistance)
      Initiate light wrist flexion stretching
      Initiate AROM shoulder
      Full can
      Lateral raises
      ER/IR tubing
      Elbow flexion/extension
      Initiate light scapular strengthening exercises
      May incorporate bicycle for lower-extremity strength, endurance

Intermediate phase (weeks 4–7)
  Goals: Gradual increase to full ROM, promote healing of repaired tissue, regain and improve muscular strength, restore full function of graft site
    Week 4
      Brace: Elbow ROM 0°–135°, motion to tolerance
      Exercises: Begin light resistance exercises for arm (1 lb); wrist curls, extension, pronation, supination; elbow extension/flexion
      Progress shoulder program emphasizing rotator cuff and scapular strengthening
      Initiate shoulder strengthening with light dumbbells
    Week 5
      ROM: Elbow ROM 0°–135°
      Discontinue brace
      Maintain full ROM
      Continue all exercises; progress all shoulder and upper-extremity exercises (progress weight 1 lb)
    Week 6
      AROM: 0°–145° without brace or full ROM
      Exercises: Initiate Thrower's Ten Program, progress elbow strengthening exercises, initiate shoulder ER strengthening, progress shoulder program
    Week 7
      Progress Thrower's Ten Program (progress weights)

Initiate PNF diagonal patterns (light)

Advanced strengthening phase (weeks 8–14)
  Goals: To increase strength, power, endurance; maintain full elbow ROM; gradually initiate sporting activities
    Week 8
      Exercises: Initiate eccentric elbow flexion/extension, continue isotonic program: forearm and wrist, continue shoulder program (Thrower's Ten Program), manual resistance diagonal patterns, initiate plyometric exercise program (2-hand plyometrics close to body only), chest pass, side throw close to body, continue stretching calf and hamstrings
    Week 10
      Exercises: Continue all exercises listed above; program plyometrics to 2-hand drills away from body: side-to-side throws, soccer throws, side throws
    Weeks 12 to 14
      Continue all exercises; initiate isotonic machines strengthening exercises (if desired): bench press (seated), lateral pull down; initiate golf, swimming; initiate interval hitting program

Return-to-activity phase (weeks 14–32)
  Goals: Continue to increase strength, power, endurance of upper-extremity musculature; gradually return to sport activities
    Week 14
      Exercises: Continue strengthening program; emphasize elbow and wrist strengthening and flexibility exercises; maintain full elbow ROM; initiate 1-hand plyometric throwing (stationary throws); initiate 1-hand wall dribble; initiate 1-hand baseball throws into wall
    Week 16
      Exercises: Initiate ITP (phase I, long-toss program); continue Thrower's Ten Program and plyometrics; continue stretching before and after throwing
    Weeks 22 to 24
      Exercises: Progress to phase II throwing (after phase I successfully completed)
    Weeks 30 to 32
      Exercises: Gradually progress to competitive throwing/sports

Abbreviations: AROM, active range of motion; ER, external rotation; IR, internal rotation; PNF, proprioceptive neuromuscular facilitation.
Data from Wilk KE, Arrigo CA, Andrews JR, Azar FM: Rehabilitation following elbow surgery in the throwing athlete. *Oper Tech Sports Med* 1996;4(2):114-132.

spanned with a 2-mm piece of FiberTape (Arthrex, Inc) and size 0 nonabsorbable sutures are used to repair the native ligament back to its anatomic origin, and insertion ensuring that tension of the FiberTape matches that of the native UCL during ROM.

A UCL repair with Internal Brace is reserved for use in cases of partial or complete tears at the origin or insertion of the UCL with good ligament tissue and low-grade midsubstance partial UCL tears.[44] In patients with chronic, attritional damage to the UCL and associated loss of elbow joint stability, reconstruction remains the most appropriate surgical intervention. The decision to perform a surgical repair of the UCL, rather than a reconstruction, can only be made intraoperatively from direct visual assessment of the UCL.

Rehabilitation after UCL repair with Internal Brace surgery is accomplished via a sequential and progressive 5-phased approach, designed to return the athlete to their previous level or higher as quickly and safely as possible[45] (**Box 3**). Initially, rehabilitation interventions are designed to minimize the effects of immobilization, facilitate early healing of the UCL repair, reestablish pain-free ROM, reduce pain and inflammation, and retard muscular atrophy. Early limited passive elbow/forearm ROM exercises and grade I/II joint mobilizations are incorporated in conjunction to neuromodulate pain, promote articular cartilage nutrition, and aid in the synthesis, alignment, and

Box 3
Postoperative rehabilitation after ulnar collateral ligament repair with internal brace

Phase I: Immediate postoperative phase (week 1)
    Goals: Protect healing tissue; reduce pain and inflammation; retard muscle atrophy; full wrist ROM
    Day of surgery
        Elbow ROM brace locked at 90° for 7 days
        Passive ROM (PROM) wrist and hand
    Postoperative day 1 and 2: Add (all performed in locked elbow brace)
        Shoulder PROM: flexion, ER, and IR to tolerance
        Pendulum exercises
        Wrist flexor/extensor stretching
        Putty/gripping exercises
    Postoperative day 3 through 7 (all exercises performed in locked elbow brace)
    1. Continue previous exercises, advancing PROM as tolerated
    2. Add the following exercises:
        a. Shoulder isometrics: ER, IR, abduction, flexion, and extension
        b. Scapular strengthening (seated neuromuscular control drills with manual resistance)

II. Controlled mobility (weeks 2–5)
    Goals: Gradually restore elbow joint ROM; improve muscular strength and endurance; normalize joint arthrokinematics
    Beginning week 2 (day 8)
        Progress elbow ROM brace to 30° to 110°
        Begin elbow PROM and AAROM 30° to 110°
        Initiate AAROM elbow
        Initiate AAROM shoulder joint
        Scapular strengthening exercises
        Progress to light isotonic strengthening at day 10
    Beginning week 3:
        Progress elbow ROM to 10° to 125°
        Initiate Thrower's Ten Exercise Program

III. Intermediate phase (weeks 6–8)
    Goals: Restore full elbow ROM; progress upper-extremity strength, continue with functional progression
    Beginning week 4:
        Progress elbow ROM to 0° to 145°
        Progress to Advanced Thrower's Ten Program
        Progress elbow and wrist strengthening exercises
        Wrist flexion and elbow flexion movements against manual resistance
    Beginning week 6:
        Initiate 2 hand plyometrics
        Discontinue brace at week 6
        Prone planks
    Beginning week 8:
        Progress to 1 hand plyometrics
        Continue with Advanced Thrower's Ten program
        Side planks with ER strengthening

IV. Advanced phase (weeks 9–14)
    Criteria to progress to advanced phase:
    1. Full nonpainful ROM
    2. No pain or tenderness
    3. Isokinetic test that fulfills criteria to throw
    4. Satisfactory clinical examination
    5. Completion of rehabilitation phases without difficulty
    Goals: Advanced strengthening exercises; initiate ITP; gradual return to throwing
    Beginning week 9:

Continue all strengthening exercises
Advanced Thrower's Ten program
Plyometrics program (1- and 2-hand program)
Beginning week 10:
Seated chest press machine
Initiate interval hitting program (at week 10)
Seated rowing
Biceps/triceps strengthening
Beginning weeks 11 to 16:
Initiate ITP phase 1: long toss (week 12)
Continue all exercises as in weeks 9 to 10
Beginning weeks 16 to 20:
Initiate interval throwing phase 2 (off the mound) when phase 1 is complete and athlete is ready
Continue Advanced Thrower's Ten program
Continue plyometrics
Continue ROM and stretching programs

V. Return to play phase (weeks 14+):
Goals: Gradual return to competitive throwing; continue all exercises and stretches
Week 20+:
Initiate gradual return to competitive throwing
Perform dynamic warm-ups and stretches
Continue Thrower's Ten Program
Return to competition when athlete is ready (physician decision)

Note: Each athlete may progress through ITP at different rates/pace.

Should complete 0 to 27.4M (90 feet) within 3 weeks of starting ITP and complete 36.6M (120 feet) within 8 weeks and then begin mound program.

organization of collagen tissue. Local modalities, including Cryotherapy, electrical stimulation, and class IV deep tissue laser, are used to control pain, control inflammation, speed healing of the incision, and increase nitrous oxide in the healing tissue. Pain-free, submaximal isometrics are used to initiate muscle activation and retard atrophy for all planes of elbow, forearm, wrist, and shoulder movements. Shoulder external rotation and internal rotation isometrics are performed with caution and must be completely pain free. Rhythmic stabilization and neuromuscular control drills for shoulder, elbow, and wrist along with seated scapular and postural exercises are also introduced early in the rehabilitation process.

The controlled mobility phase runs for a total of 3 weeks starting at the second week after surgery and focuses on a stepped restoration in elbow ROM, improved muscular strength/endurance, and normalizing joint arthrokinematics. Active-assisted, active, and passive ROM exercises, as well as more aggressive joint mobilizations, are incorporated for the elbow, forearm, and wrist with the primary goal to achieve full elbow extension and minimize the risk of developing an elbow flexion contracture. Strengthening exercises at this point are performed beginning with concentric and progressing to eccentric muscle contractions with the focus placed on a comprehensive strengthening program for the throwing athlete, such as the Thrower's Ten Program.[18]

The intermediate phase is from postoperative week 6 to 8 and emphasizes the maintenance of joint mobility, improving muscular strength, endurance, neuromuscular control of the elbow complex, and continuing with a functional progression of activity. Stretching, flexibility, and mobilizations are used to maintain full motion with a particular focus on elbow extension and forearm pronation flexibility. At 4 weeks, the athlete is progressed to the Advanced Thrower's Ten Program to place greater demands on the posterior shoulder and scapular muscles.[28]

Neuromuscular control manual resistance exercises are incorporated for the shoulder and elbow, proprioceptive neuromuscular facilitation, rhythmic stabilizations, and slow reversal hold techniques. Two-handed plyometrics are introduced 6 weeks following surgery progressing to 1-hand exercises 2 weeks later.

The fourth phase of UCL repair rehabilitation is the advanced phase, which runs from weeks 9 to 14, and is specifically designed to increase strength, power, endurance, and neuromuscular control to prepare for a return to sports using strengthening activities that emphasize high speed, eccentric contractions, and plyometrics. Elbow flexion exercises here emphasize high-speed eccentric control training elbow deceleration. Weight-machine exercises are begun 10 weeks after surgery and include seated chest press, seated rowing, and front latissimus dorsi pull-downs. A hitting program is permitted at week 10 and an ITP 11 weeks after surgery if the athlete meets the objective criteria for throwing. Pitchers are generally able to advance to throwing off of a mound 8 weeks after they begin the first phase of a throwing program.

The return to activity phase is the last part of the process and emphasizes a proper dynamic warmup, continued exercise loads, and managing the progression back to unrestricted activity and competitive throwing. The general timeframe to return to play following a UCL repair with Internal Brace is approximately 5 months. Functional testing can aid the return to play decision process. The authors use the prone ball drop test, developed by the senior author (K.E.W.), which uses a 1-kg (2-pound) PlyoBall with the patient prone, shoulder abducted to 90°, and elbow extended. The patient is instructed to perform as many ball drops and catches as possible in a 30-second timeframe, comparing successful catches bilaterally and seeking a goal of 110% for the throwing side (see **Fig. 9**).

At the authors' center, 350 UCL repairs with Internal Brace have been performed. Of these, 1-year follow-up data are available for 79 throwers, showing 98% of the 1-year follow-ups returned to their preinjury level of activity. Surgical repair of the UCL with Internal Brace is a viable option in athletes who meet specific findings at the time of surgery. The rehabilitation of this unique surgical procedure has been presented based on the authors' experience treating in excess of 350 athletes over the past 3 years. The average time required for an athlete to return to participation in their cohort is 7 months, which is approximately 5 months less than average return to play times after UCL reconstruction surgery. Long-term results of this surgery and rehabilitation program are still needed, but the authors' initial experience is extremely promising.

LATERAL COLLATERAL LIGAMENT COMPLEX RECONSTRUCTION

Lateral-sided instability of the elbow usually is the result of a sudden traumatic injury rather than a chronic repetitive injury. It results in varus instability and a posterolateral rotatory instability that can be promoted with elbow supination. For this reason, special attention to elbow rotation is emphasized during the rehabilitation.

Initially, the postoperative elbow is placed in a splint with 90° of flexion and mild pronation. The splint is removed at the end of the first week (the authors immobilize for 2–4 weeks, depending on the type of activity to which the patient will return), and a brace is used that incorporates an extension block of 30° and a flexion block of 100°. Extension is increased by 5° per week, and flexion is increased by 10° per week. Supination encourages the radial head to sublux laterally, potentially stretching the graft. Therefore, supination is restricted for 3 weeks. Active supination is allowed when the elbow passes 90° of flexion. Once supination is obtained at greater than 90° of elbow flexion, supination may be attempted in extension. Full motion about the elbow should be obtained by 6 weeks. Shoulder forward elevation and abduction may be treated aggressively for motion restriction, but internal and external rotation is limited to active motion only. Passive and active-assisted motion of the shoulder for rotation requires torque through the elbow and should be avoided until week 9.

Isometric strengthening exercises of the elbow and wrist are initiated once the splint has been removed. External and internal rotation strength exercises of the shoulder are avoided until 9 weeks after surgery, because these motions put the graft at risk. Light isotonic exercises may begin about the elbow and wrist at week 6. At week 9, an aggressive strengthening regimen may commence, including eccentric contraction exercises and plyometrics.

Nerve glides and scar massage are important to prevent pain from adherent scar after surgery. Scar massage should begin at 2 weeks, and nerve glides should commence once the appropriate motion has returned.

Tendinopathy

Medial epicondylitis and flexor-pronator tendinitis
Medial epicondylitis occurs because of changes within the musculotendinous flexor-pronator unit, characterized by microscopic or macroscopic tearing within the flexor carpi radialis or pronator teres near the origin on the medial epicondyle. Overhead throwers who exhibit flexor-pronator tendinitis also may have UCL pathologic condition that creates this secondary pathologic condition because of the underlying increased laxity. Furthermore, it may be beneficial to determine the number of episodes and the chronicity of medial epicondylar symptoms. Patients with long histories of medial epicondylitis may exhibit a chronic degeneration known as tendinosis or tendinopathy, not true tendinitis.

The treatment of tendinopathy is based on a careful examination to determine the exact pathologic condition present. Often, patients in whom tendinitis has been diagnosed only later discover that the tendon had undergone a degenerative process referred to as tendinosis.[46,47] The differential diagnosis of tendinosis may be made using MRI, ultrasonography, or tissue biopsy.

The treatment of tendinitis typically focuses on reducing inflammation and pain. This goal is accomplished through the reduction of activities, steroid injections, anti-inflammatory medications, cryotherapy, iontophoresis, light exercise, and stretching. Conversely, the treatment of tendinosis focuses on increasing the circulation to promote collagen synthesis and collagen organization. Such treatment would include heat, stretching, eccentric exercises, laser therapy, transverse massage, and soft tissue mobilization. These therapies are performed to increase the circulation and promote tissue healing. Dry needling has also been advocated for this pathologic condition to promote tendon healing.[48] The authors occasionally use piezo-wave (shock-wave) therapy on the tendon if they think the pathologic condition is tendinosis.

Platelet-rich plasma (PRP) therapy is a promising intervention in which a small sample of the athlete's own blood is separated, and the platelet-rich layer is injected into the site of injury. The proposed mechanism delivers humoral mediators and growth factors locally to induce a healing response. Other advantages of PRP therapy are that it is minimally invasive, provokes a local response only, and avoids an inflammatory response. Disadvantages can include the cost of treatment, a lack of supporting evidence, and increased staff time to withdraw and centrifuge the blood, and then reinject it into the site of pathologic condition. Early research on the clinical application of PRP to promote healing and an adaptive response is promising.[49,50] Substantial benefits of PRP were shown in patients with chronic lateral epicondylitis.[50] Basic science and controlled studies have yet to report the efficacy of such a treatment.

The nonsurgical approach for the treatment of epicondylitis (tendinitis and/or para-tendinitis) focuses on diminishing the pain and inflammation and then gradually improving muscular strength. The primary goals of rehabilitation are to control the applied loads and create an environment for healing. The initial treatment consists of warm whirlpool baths, iontophoresis, stretching exercises, and light strengthening exercises to stimulate a repair response. Therapeutic modalities often are used by rehabilitation specialists to reduce inflammation and promote healing. Very limited evidence supports using these modalities in isolation. Common modalities can include massage, cold laser therapy, iontophoresis, ultrasound, nitric oxide, and extracorporeal shock-wave therapy. When used in combination with exercise or with other modalities, however, studies have shown improved tissue quality and outcomes.[51–53] Conversely, patients with tendinosis are treated with transverse friction massage, forceful stretching, a focus on eccentric strengthening with gradually progressing loads, and warm modalities to promote tendon regeneration.

After the patient's symptoms have subsided, an aggressive stretching and strengthening program featuring high loads and low repetitions that emphasize eccentric contractions is initiated. Wrist flexion and extension activities should be performed, initially with the elbow flexed 30° to 45°. A gradual progression through plyometric and throwing activities precedes the initiation of the ITP.

LATERAL EPICONDYLITIS

A principal aspect of conservative treatment of lateral epicondylitis is therapy. Despite the misnomer, lateral epicondylitis is not a disease of inflammation, but rather a disease of degeneration. Usually little or no swelling is present; therefore, heat therapy should begin each treatment session. Stretching of the extensor mass with wrist flexion is an important component of treatment. This stretching may be done in conjunction with soft tissue mobilization. If the stretching and mobilization are well tolerated, isotonic eccentric strengthening exercises for the lateral extensor mass may be attempted. The patient also should perform shoulder and scapular flexibility and strengthening exercises during the rehabilitation program.

The treatment sequence the authors use for lateral epicondylitis for a tendon that exhibits degenerative changes is heat, soft tissue, eccentrics for the wrist extensors, strengthening for the shoulder rotator cuff, scapular muscles, piezo-wave therapy, laser, and a home program.

Conservative measures should be attempted for at least 6 months before surgical intervention is considered. Rehabilitation after surgical debridement primarily depends on whether the surgeon chooses to detach and reattach the extensor mass during surgery. If the extensor mass is detached during the procedure, active wrist extension and flexion should be prevented for 4 weeks. Although full passive motion is allowed, it should only be done gently and in the presence of the therapist for the first 4 weeks.

The posterior splint is removed at 10 to 14 days. Elbow flexion, extension, supination, and pronation are allowed immediately after removal of the splint. Care should be taken to perform supination and pronation gently. Cold therapy and electrical stimulation are instituted to reduce swelling and pain after sessions. Scar massage may begin at 2 to 3 weeks, and nerve glides may commence when adequate motion has been obtained. Full active motion at the elbow and wrist may begin at 4 weeks. If full motion already has been restored as a result of the passive motion instituted earlier, strengthening exercises may begin. Isometric exercises are succeeded by concentric exercises, which are followed by eccentric exercises. If the flexor mass was not detached, full motion of the elbow and wrist is allowed once the splint has been removed.

Ulnar Neuropathy

Ulnar nerve changes can result from tensile forces, compressive forces, or nerve insta-bility. Ulnar neuropathy occurs in 3 stages.[54] The first stage is characterized by an acute onset of radicular symptoms. During the second stage, a recurrence of symp-toms occurs as the athlete attempts to return to competition. The third stage is distin-guished by persistent motor weakness and sensory changes. If the athlete presents in the third stage of injury, nonsurgical management may not be effective.

A leading mechanism for tensile force on the ulnar nerve is valgus stress. This mech-anism may be coupled with an external rotation supination stress overload. The trac-tion forces are magnified further when underlying valgus instability from UCL injury is present. Ulnar neuropathy is often a secondary pathologic condition of UCL insuffi-ciency. Compression of the ulnar nerve is often due to hypertrophy of the surrounding soft tissues or the presence of scar tissue. The nerve also may be trapped between the 2 heads of the flexor carpi ulnaris. Repetitive flexion and extension of the elbow with an unstable nerve can irritate or inflame the nerve. In addition, the nerve may subluxate or rest on the medial epicondyle, rendering it vulnerable to direct trauma.

The nonsurgical treatment of ulnar neuropathy focuses on reducing ulnar nerve irri-tation, enhancing dynamic medial joint stability, and returning the athlete to competi-tion gradually. Using a night splint with the elbow flexed to 45° can help to restrict movement and prevent ulnar nerve irritation. NSAIDs can be prescribed as well as an iontophoresis disposable patch and cryotherapy. Throwing athletes are instructed to discontinue throwing activities for at least 4 weeks, depending on the severity and chronicity of symptoms. They will be progressed through the immediate motion and intermediate phases over 4 to 6 weeks, with emphasis on eccentric and dynamic sta-bilization drills. Plyometric exercises are used to facilitate further dynamic stabilization of the medial elbow. The athlete can begin an ITP when full pain-free ROM and muscle performance are achieved without neurologic symptoms.

Ulnar Nerve Transposition

An ulnar nerve transposition can be performed in a subcutaneous fashion using fascial slings. The clinician should use caution to avoid overstressing the soft tissue struc-tures involved in relocating the nerve while soft tissue healing occurs.[39] A posterior splint at 90° of elbow flexion is used for the first postoperative week to prevent exces-sive extension ROM and tension on the nerve. The splint is discontinued at the begin-ning of week 2, and light ROM activities are initiated. Full ROM usually is restored by weeks 3 to 4. Gentle isotonic strengthening is begun during week 3 to 4 and pro-gressed to the full Thrower's Ten Program by 4 to 6 weeks after surgery. Aggressive strengthening, including eccentric training, the Advanced Thrower's Ten Exercise Pro-gram, and plyometric training, is incorporated at week 8, and an ITP is begun at week 8 to 9 if all previously outlined criteria are met. A return to competition usually occurs be-tween weeks 12 and 16 postoperatively.

Osteochondritis Dissecans

Osteochondritis dissecans (OCD) of the elbow can develop as a result of the valgus strain on the elbow joint, which produces not only medial tension but also a lateral compressive force.[55] Lateral compression is observed as the capitellum of the humer-us is compressed against the radial head. Patients often report lateral elbow pain on palpation and valgus stress. Classification of the pathologic progression of OCD has been described in 3 stages.[56] Stage I describes patients without evidence of subchon-dral displacement or fracture, whereas stage II refers to lesions showing evidence of subchondral detachment or articular cartilage fracture. Stage III lesions involve detached osteochondral fragments, resulting in intraarticular loose bodies. Nonsurgical treatment is attempted for stage 1 patients only and consists of relative rest and immobilization until elbow symptoms have resolved.

Nonsurgical treatment includes 3 to 6 weeks of immobilization at 90° of elbow flexion. ROM activities for the shoulder, elbow, and wrist are performed 3 to 4 times a day. As symptoms resolve, a strengthening program is initiated with isometric exercises. Isotonic exercises are added after approximately 1 week of isometric exercise. Aggressive high-speed, eccentric, and plyometric exercises are included progressively to prepare the athlete for the start of an ITP.

If nonsurgical treatment fails or evidence of loose bodies exists, surgical intervention, including arthroscopic abrading and drilling of the lesion with fixation or removal of the loose bodies, is indicated.[56] Long-term follow-up studies regarding the outcome of patients undergoing surgery to drill or reattach the lesions have not reported favorable results, suggesting that prevention and early detection of symptoms may be the best form of treatment.[57]

Little Leaguer's Elbow

During the arm-cocking and acceleration phases of throwing, the medial epicondyle physis is subject to repetitive tensile and valgus forces that can lead to a spectrum of injuries to the medial epicondylar apophysis, ranging from microtrauma to the physis to fracture and displacement of the medial epicondyle through the apophysis. Pain in the medial elbow is common in adolescent throwers. These forces can result in microtraumatic injury to the physis, with potential fragmentation, hypertrophy, separation of the epiphysis, or avulsion of the medial epicondyle.

In the absence of an avulsion, a nonsurgical rehabilitation program like that used for the UCL is initiated. Initial emphasis is placed on the reduction of pain and inflammation and the restoration of motion and strength. Strengthening exercises are performed in a gradual fashion. First, isometrics are performed; then, light isotonic strengthening exercises are initiated. Young throwing athletes often exhibit poor core and scapular control, along with weakness of the shoulder musculature; therefore, core, leg, and shoulder strengthening are emphasized. In addition, stretching exercises are performed to normalize shoulder ROM, especially into internal rotation and horizontal adduction. No heavy lifting is permitted for 12 to 14 weeks. An ITP is initiated as tolerated when symptoms subside.

In the presence of a nondisplaced or minimally displaced avulsion, a brief period of immobilization for approximately 7 days is encouraged, followed by a gradual progression of ROM, flexibility, and strength. An ITP usually is allowed at week 6 to 8. If the avulsion is displaced, open reduction and internal fixation may be required.

Posterior Olecranon Osteophyte Excision

Surgical excision of posterior olecranon osteophytes is performed arthroscopically using an osteotome or motorized burr. Approximately 5 to 10 mm of the olecranon tip is removed, and a motorized burr is used to contour the coronoid, olecranon tip, and fossa to prevent further impingement during extreme flexion and extension.[58]

The rehabilitation program following arthroscopic posterior olecranon osteophyte excision is slightly more conservative in restoring full elbow extension secondary to postsurgical pain. ROM is progressed within the patient's tolerance, but by 10 days after surgery, the patient should exhibit at least 15° to 105°/110° of ROM, and 5° to 10° to 115° by day 14. Full ROM (0° to 145°) typically is restored by day 20 to 25 after surgery. The rate of ROM progression most often is limited by osseous pain and synovial joint inflammation, usually located at the top of the olecranon.

The strengthening program is similar to the previously discussed progression. Isometric exercises are performed for the first 10 to 14 days, and isotonic strengthening is performed from weeks 2 to 6. During the first 2 weeks following surgery, forceful triceps contractions can produce posterior elbow pain; therefore, the clinician should avoid initiating or reducing the force produced by the triceps muscle. The full Thrower's Ten Program is initiated by week 6. An ITP is included by week 10 to week 12. Emphasis again is placed on eccentric control of the elbow flexors and dynamic stabilization of the medial elbow.

The outcomes of elbow surgery in 72 professional baseball players have been reported.[59] Of these athletes, 47 exhibited a posterior olecranon osteophyte, and 18 of the athletes who underwent an isolated olecranon excision later required a UCL reconstruction.[59] These findings suggest that subtle medial instability can accelerate osteophyte formation.

ARTHROSCOPIC ARTHROLYSIS

Loss of motion is a difficult problem associated with injuries of the elbow. It can be a result of soft tissue contracture or heterotopic ossification (HO) associated with the injury. Often the motion cannot be regained through conservative measures alone, and surgical intervention is necessary. The surgeon should inform the therapist of what motion has been obtained in the operating room so that realistic goals can be set.

Motion and pain control are at the forefront of rehabilitation for this procedure. HO represents a difficult rehabilitation problem. It has been shown that passive stretching outside the painless arc of motion may cause the generation of ectopic bone in patients with burns or brain injuries.[57] Whether this literature, in a rather unique population, is relevant to other patients with HO is unclear; however, caution is advised, and aggressive passive motion exercises should not be performed. The goal is to obtain full motion by 4 weeks. The most beneficial means of achieving this goal has been the LLLD technique described earlier. As with all the motion exercises, the stretching should not cause pain.

With arthrolysis for soft tissue contractures, the clinician may be more aggressive with motion exercises. Although the risk of generating HO may be in question, other problems may arise with aggressive rehabilitation. Aggressive motion can create an inflammatory cascade and generate pain that could inhibit progress, which would be self-defeating. The goal of establishing full motion at 4 weeks does not change with soft tissue contractures.

As with the other protocols, pain should be treated with cryotherapy, high-voltage electrical stimulation, and gentle soft tissue mobilization. Heat and ultrasound may be used once the initial swelling from surgery has dissipated and are used before motion exercises to "warm up" the joint.

Strengthening exercises should begin after motion has been established. There are no contraindications to an aggressive approach to strengthening once motion has been restored. Isometric exercises are begun and progressed to plyometrics in the usual fashion.

Regardless of the origin of the contracture, stretching should be continued for 4 to 6 months after activities are resumed to prevent return of the contracture.

FRACTURES

The complexity of the fracture and the degree of stability after internal fixation can vary considerably in the elbow. Communication between the surgeon and all members of the rehabilitation team is essential to determine the aggressiveness of the rehabilitation process. Several different fractures about the elbow merit attention. The goal of rehabilitation after a fracture is to facilitate osseous healing, restore full motion and strength, and gradually return the individual to functional activities. With an elbow fracture (whether treated surgically or nonoperatively), the goal is to minimize immobilization to prevent loss of motion. Loss of motion is more common in adults than in children after an elbow fracture.

Radial Head and Neck Fractures

When fractures of the radial head and neck are nondisplaced, the injury may be treated conservatively, and motion should be initiated immediately. Unlimited passive and active motion is the priority, which is achieved through the use of stretching techniques, as well as through techniques for reducing swelling and pain, as has been mentioned earlier. The goal is to reestablish motion by 4 weeks. Strengthening about the elbow and wrist may begin once full motion has been established. Valgus stress should be avoided until the fracture has healed.

With displaced or angulated fractures, internal fixation may be necessary. In some cases, the fracture is beyond repair and requires replacement with a metal implant. With stable fixation or an implant, the elbow is placed in a posterior splint at 45° to 90° of elbow flexion for 10 days. Once the splint has been removed, motion exercises are initiated without limitation. Full flexion, extension, supination, and pronation should be obtained by 4 to 6 weeks. Often patients present with mechanical blocks to motion, which often results in soft tissue contractures. With these patients, the goals for motion may be more limited. Valgus stress is avoided in patients with internal fixation until the fracture has healed, but this is not necessary when a radial head prosthesis is used. Once full motion has been achieved, strengthening of the elbow and wrist may commence. If swelling and pain persist, cryotherapy and electrical stimulation may be used to limit these symptoms.

Olecranon Fractures

For most olecranon fractures, the treatment of choice is open reduction and internal fixation. Several fixation techniques yield a stable fracture, and rehabilitation should not have to be altered because of the type of fixation. Traditionally, a posterior splint is placed for 7 to 10 days to allow the soft tissues to heal. The length of immobilization depends on the patient's variables (ie, age, osseous status, health, desired goals, healing response). Once the splint has been removed, unlimited passive motion may begin. Active pronation, supination, and flexion are allowed, but active extension is avoided for 6 weeks. Full motion in all directions should be achieved by 6 weeks. Gentle active extension may be initiated, and strengthening of the elbow and wrist in all directions may begin at 8 weeks.

As with all fracture fixations at the elbow, cryotherapy and electrical stimulation should be used to reduce pain and swelling. Scar massage should be initiated at 2 weeks, and nerve glides should be used when possible.

Distal Humeral Fractures

Distal humeral fractures usually require open reduction and internal fixation. If the surgeon has difficulty with stability, a hinged external fixator that allows elbow flexion and extension may be used, although this is not common. After fixation, a splint is placed for 10 to 14 days. Once the splint has been removed, gentle passive motion at the elbow and wrist may begin. Pain and swelling are limiting factors in restoring motion to the elbow; therefore, cryotherapy and electrical stimulation are crucial to this process. The clinician must take care with cryotherapy to avoid nerve injury, because ulnar nerve transposition is a routine part of distal humeral fixation.

Active motion at the elbow and wrist may begin at 6 weeks. Once full motion has been established and bony healing is apparent, strengthening may begin. Strengthening should be limited to pain-free exercises. It begins with isotonic exercises and gradually progresses to plyometrics.

Coronoid Fractures and Elbow Dislocation

After dislocation of the elbow, the patient is temporarily immobilized to allow healing of the injured capsule. The length of immobilization varies, depending on the required use of the elbow for activities of daily living or work activities, the type of sport the patient plays, whether it is the dominant or nondominant elbow, the patient's age, and whether concomitant lesions are present. Coronoid fractures often put the patient at risk for future elbow instability. For this reason, the rehabilitation protocols for elbow dislocation and coronoid fractures are similar. The priority is to restore motion quickly while guarding against instability. The patient is placed in a posterior splint for 10 to 14 days in a position that allows no visible subluxation on radiographs. In the initial evaluation, the stable ROM is determined. The elbow will sublux with further extension; therefore, parameters are set so that the initial restrictions do not permit extension beyond this point. When the splint is removed, a dynamic elbow brace that prevents valgus and varus forces is used. This splint should also have a variable locking mechanism that blocks various degrees of extension. The clinician may work on flexion and pronation of the elbow without limitation. Passive extension may be increased by 10° every week until full extension is obtained. The patient should be closely watched for any evidence of subluxation. Often, with elbow dislocations, either the UCL or the lateral ulnar collateral ligament (LUCL) may rupture. If the LUCL ruptures, supination should be limited for at least 3 weeks after removal of the splint. The goal is to restore motion by 8 weeks.

Motion of the wrist should be instituted immediately. Upon removal of the splint, control of pain and swelling must be established immediately to aid in the restoration of motion. As mentioned earlier, cryotherapy and electrical stimulation are beneficial. Gentle soft tissue mobilization also may help.

Strengthening may begin at 8 weeks. If the expected motion has not been achieved, strengthening should be delayed until the desired motion is obtained. Strengthening is performed in the usual fashion.

If the patient's clinical picture requires operative intervention, rehabilitation should be dictated by the procedure performed. Lateral collateral ligament (LCL) reconstruction, UCL reconstruction, and radial head fixation are common surgical procedures. If a coronoid fracture is present and fixed, this should not change the protocol; the other fixations present should guide the treatment.

SUMMARY

The elbow joint is a common site of injury in athletes, especially in the overhead athlete, because of the repetitive forces occurring at the elbow that create repetitive microtraumatic injuries. Conversely, in athletes playing in collision sports, such as football, wrestling, soccer, and gymnastics, elbow injury often results from macrotraumatic forces to the elbow, leading to fractures, dislocations, and ligamentous injuries. Rehabilitation of the elbow, whether after injury or surgery, must follow a progressive and sequential order to ensure that the healing tissues are not overstressed. The rehabilitation program should limit immobilization and achieve full ROM early, especially elbow extension ROM. Furthermore, the rehabilitation program should restore strength and neuromuscular control progressively and should incorporate sport-specific activities gradually to successfully return the athlete to his or her previous level of competition as quickly and safely as possible. In addition, the rehabilitation of the elbow must include the entire kinetic chain (the scapula, shoulder, hand, core/hips, and legs) to ensure the athlete's return to high-level sports participation.

DISCLOSURE

Dr K.E. Wilk or an immediate family member serves as a paid consultant to LiteCure Medical; serves as an unpaid consultant to AlterG; and has received nonincome support (such as equipment or services, commercially derived honoraria, or other non–research-related funding) from Educational Grants from Bauerfeind, Performance Health, Joint Active Systems, and ERMI. Neither Mr C.A. Arrigo nor any immediate family member has received anything of value from or has stock or stock options held in a commercial company or institution related directly or indirectly to the subject of this article.

REFERENCES

1. Conte SA, Fleisig GS, Dines JS, et al. Prevalence of ulnar collateral ligament surgery in professional baseball players. Am J Sports Med 2015;43(7):1764–9.
2. Fleisig GS, Escamilla RF. Biomechanics of the elbow in the throwing athlete. Oper Tech Sports Med 1996;4(2):62–8.
3. Hodgins JL, Vitale M, Arons RR. Epidemiology of medial collateral ligament reconstruction: a 10-year study in New York State. Am J Sports Med 2016; 44(3):729–34.
4. Petty DH, Andrews JR, Fleisig GS, et al. Ulnar collateral ligament reconstruction in high school baseball players. Am J Sports Med 2004;32(5):1158–64.
5. Conte SA, Camp CL, Dines JS. Injury trends in Major League Baseball over 18 seasons. 1998-2015. Am J Orthop 2016;45(3):116–23.
6. Conte S, Requa RK, Garrick JG. Disability days in Major League Baseball. Am J Sports Med 2001;29(4):431–6.
7. Posner M, Cameron KL, Wolf JM, et al. Epidemiology of Major League Baseball injuries. Am J Sports Med 2011;39(8):1676–80.
8. Andrews JR, Craven WM. Lesions of the posterior compartment of the elbow. Clin Sports Med 1991;10(3):637–52.
9. Wilson FD, Andrews JR, Blackburn TA, et al. Valgus extension overload in the pitching elbow. Am J Sports Med 1983;11(2):83–8.
10. Wilk KE, Arrigo C, Andrews JR. Rehabilitation of the elbow in the throwing athlete. J Orthop Sports Phys Ther 1993;17(6):305–17.
11. Wright RW, Steger-May K, Wasserlauf BL, et al. Elbow range of motion in professional baseball pitchers. Am J Sports Med 2006;34(2):190–3.
12. Salter RB, Hamilton HW, Wedge JH, et al. Clinical application of basic research on continuous passive motion for disorders and injuries of synovial joints: a preliminary report of a feasibility study. J Orthop Res 1984;1(3):325–42.
13. Salter RB, Simmonds DF, Malcolm BW, et al. The biological effect of continuous passive motion on the healing of full-thickness defects in articular cartilage. An experimental investigation in the rabbit. J Bone Joint Surg Am 1980;62(8): 1232–51.
14. Green DP, McCoy H. Turnbuckle orthotic correction of elbow-flexion contractures after acute injuries. J Bone Joint Surg Am 1979;61(7):1092–5.

15. McClure PW, Blackburn LG, Dusold C. The use of splints in the treatment of joint stiffness: biologic rationale and an algorithm for making clinical decisions. Phys Ther 1994;74(12):1101–7.

16. Dines JS, Frank JB, Akerman M, et al. Glenohumeral internal rotation deficits in baseball players with ulnar collateral ligament insufficiency. Am J Sports Med 2009;37(3):566–70.

17. Crockett HC, Gross LB, Wilk KE, et al. Osseous adaptation and range of motion at the glenohumeral joint in professional baseball pitchers. Am J Sports Med 2002; 30(1):20–6.

18. Thomas SJ, Swanik CB, Higginson JS, et al. A bilateral comparison of posterior capsule thickness and its correlation with glenohumeral range of motion and scapular upward rotation in collegiate baseball players. J Shoulder Elbow Surg 2011;20(5):708–16.

19. Wilk KE, Andrews JR, Arrigo C. Preventive and rehabilitative exercises for the shoulder and elbow. 6th edition. Birmingham (AL): American Sports Medicine Institute; 2001.

20. Moseley JB Jr, Jobe FW, Pink M, et al. EMG analysis of the scapular muscles during a shoulder rehabilitation program. Am J Sports Med 1992;20(2):128–34.

21. Townsend H, Jobe FW, Pink M, et al. Electromyographic analysis of the glenohumeral muscles during a baseball rehabilitation program. Am J Sports Med 1991;19(3):264–72.

22. Reinold MM, Wilk KE, Fleisig GS, et al. Electromyographic analysis of the rotator cuff and deltoid musculature during common shoulder external rotation exercises. J Orthop Sports Phys Ther 2004;34(7):385–94.

23. Kibler WB. The role of the scapula in athletic shoulder function. Am J Sports Med 1998;26(2):325–37.

24. Paine RM. The role of the scapula in the shoulder. In: Andrews JR, Wilk KE, editors. The athlete's shoulder. New York: Churchill Livingstone; 1994. p. 495–512.

25. Wilk KE, Arrigo CA. An integrated approach to upper extremity exercises. Orthop Phys Ther Clin North Am 1992;1:337–60.

26. Tucker WS, Armstrong CW, Gribble PA, et al. Scapular muscle activity in overhead athletes with symptoms of secondary shoulder impingement during closed chain exercises. Arch Phys Med Rehabil 2010;91(4):550–6.

27. Wilk KE, Yenchak AJ, Arrigo CA, et al. The Advanced Throwers Ten Exercise Program: a new exercise series for enhanced dynamic shoulder control in the overhead throwing athlete. Phys Sportsmed 2011;39(4):90–7. The authors describe the Advanced Thrower's Ten Exercise Program.

28. Carpenter JE, Blasier RB, Pellizzon GG. The effects of muscle fatigue on shoulder joint position sense. Am J Sports Med 1998;26(2):262–5.

29. Andrews JR, Jobe FW. Valgus extension overload in the pitching elbow. In: Andrews JR, Zarins B, Carson WB, editors. Injuries to the throwing arm. Philadelphia: Saunders; 1985. p. 250–7.

30. Swanik KA, Lephart SM, Swanik CB, et al. The effects of shoulder plyometric training on proprioception and selected muscle performance characteristics. J Shoulder Elbow Surg 2002;11(6):579–86.

31. Fortun CM, Davies GJ, Kernozck TW. The effects of plyometric training on the shoulder internal rotators. Phys Ther 1998;78(51):S87.

32. Wilk KE, Voight ML, Keirns MA, et al. Stretch-shortening drills for the upper extremities: theory and clinical application. J Orthop Sports Phys Ther 1993; 17(5):225–39.

33. Voight ML, Hardin JA, Blackburn TA, et al. The effects of muscle fatigue on and the relationship of arm dominance to shoulder proprioception. J Orthop Sports Phys Ther 1996;23(6):348–52.

34. Murray TA, Cook TD, Werner SL, et al. The effects of extended play on professional baseball pitchers. Am J Sports Med 2001;29(2):137–42.

35. Fleisig GS, Bolt B, Fortenbaugh D, et al. Biomechanical comparison of baseball pitching and long-toss: implications for training and rehabilitation. J Orthop Sports Phys Ther 2011;41(5):296–303.

36. Wooden MJ, Greenfield B, Johanson M, et al. Effects of strength training on throwing velocity and shoulder muscle performance in teenage baseball players. J Orthop Sports Phys Ther 1992;15(5):223–8.

37. Escamilla RF, Ionno M, deMahy MS, et al. Comparison of three baseball-specific 6-week training programs on throwing velocity in high school baseball players. J Strength Cond Res 2012;26(7):1767–81.

38. Davidson PA, Pink M, Perry J, et al. Functional anatomy of the flexor pronator muscle group in relation to the medial collateral ligament of the elbow. Am J Sports Med 1995;23(2):245–50.

39. Andrews JR, Jelsma RD, Joyce ME, et al. Open surgical procedures for injuries of the elbow in throwers. Oper Tech Sports Med 1996;4(2):109–13.

40. Dines JS, ElAttrache NS, Conway JE, et al. Clinical outcomes of the DANE TJ technique to treat ulnar collateral ligament insufficiency of the elbow. Am J Sports Med 2007;35(12):2039–44.

41. Rohrbough JT, Altchek DW, Hyman J, et al. Medial collateral ligament reconstruction of the elbow using the docking technique. Am J Sports Med 2002;30(4):541–8.

42. Bernas GA, Ruberte Thiele RA, Kinnaman KA, et al. Defining safe rehabilitation for ulnar collateral ligament reconstruction of the elbow: A biomechanical study. Am J Sports Med 2009;37(12):2392–400.

43. Cain EL Jr, Andrews JR, Dugas JR, et al. Outcome of ulnar collateral ligament reconstruction of the elbow in 1281 athletes: results in 743 athletes with minimum 2-year follow-up. Am J Sports Med 2010;38(12):2426–34.

44. Dugas JR, Walters BL, Beason DP, et al. Biomechanical comparison of ulnar collateral ligament repair with internal bracing versus modified Jobe reconstruction. Am J Sports Med 2016;44(3):734–41.

45. Wilk KE, Arrigo CA, Bagwell MS, et al. Repair of the ulnar collateral ligament of the elbow: rehabilitation following internal brace surgery. J Orthop Sports Phys Ther 2019;49(4):253–61.

46. Kraushaar BS, Nirschl RP. Tendinosis of the elbow (tennis elbow). Clinical features and findings of histological, immunohistochemical, and electron microscopy studies. J Bone Joint Surg Am 1999;81(2):259–78.

47. Nirschl RP, Ashman ES. Tennis elbow tendinosis (epicondylitis). Instr Course Lect 2004;53:587–98.

48. Suresh SP, Ali KE, Jones H, et al. Medial epicondylitis: is ultrasound guided autologous blood injection an effective treatment? Br J Sports Med 2006;40(11):935–9 [discussion: 939].

49. de Mos M, van der Windt AE, Jahr H, et al. Can platelet-rich plasma enhance tendon repair? A cell culture study. Am J Sports Med 2008;36(6):1171–8.

50. Mishra A, Pavelko T. Treatment of chronic elbow tendinosis with buffered platelet-rich plasma. Am J Sports Med 2006;34(11):1774–8.

51. Gum SL, Reddy GK, Stehno-Bittel L, et al. Combined ultrasound, electrical stimulation, and laser promote collagen synthesis with moderate changes in tendon biomechanics. Am J Phys Med Rehabil 1997;76(4):288–96.
52. Reddy GK, Gum S, Stehno-Bittel L, et al. Biochemistry and biomechanics of healing tendon: part II. Effects of combined laser therapy and electrical stimulation. Med Sci Sports Exerc 1998;30(6):794–800.
53. Stergioulas A, Stergioula M, Aarskog R, et al. Effects of low-level laser therapy and eccentric exercises in the treatment of recreational athletes with chronic achilles tendinopathy. Am J Sports Med 2008;36(5):881–7.
54. Alley RM, Pappas AM. Acute and performance related injuries of the elbow. In: Pappas AM, editor. Upper extremity injuries in the athlete. New York: Churchill Livingstone; 1995. p. 339–64.
55. Andrews JR, Whiteside JA. Common elbow problems in the athlete. J Orthop Sports Phys Ther 1993;17(6):289–95.
56. Morrey BF. Osteochondritis dessicans. In: DeLee JC, Drez D, editors. Orthopedic sports medicine. Philadelphia: Saunders; 1994. p. 908–12.
57. Bauer M, Jonsson K, Josefsson PO, et al. Osteochondritis dissecans of the elbow. A long-term follow-up study. Clin Orthop Relat Res 1992;284:156–60.
58. Martin SD, Baumgarten TE. Elbow injuries in the throwing athlete: diagnosis and arthroscopic treatment. Oper Tech Sports Med 1996;4(2):100–8.
59. Andrews JR, Timmerman LA. Outcome of elbow surgery in professional baseball players. Am J Sports Med 1995;23(4):407–13.

Orthobiologics in Elbow Injuries

Cleo D. Stafford II, MD, MS[a], Ricardo E. Colberg, MD[b],*, Hunter Garrett, MD[c]

KEYWORDS

- Orthobiologics • Elbow injuries • Platelet-rich plasma • Tendinopathy
- Cartilage injuries • Ligament injuries

KEY POINTS

- Several orthobiologic options exist for various injuries in the elbow.
- Level 1 evidence is present for the use of platelet-rich plasma for lateral epicondylopathy.
- Orthobiologics are safe alternatives to traditional nonsurgical options for elbow injuries.

INTRODUCTION
What Is Regenerative Medicine

Regenerative medicine is a relatively young field of medicine in which a patient's own growth factors and cells are used to promote or enhance tissue healing.[1] The products used in regenerative medicine are referred to as orthobiologics. It is an evolving field with many indications in specialties including, but not limited to, cardiology, plastic surgery, orthopedics, and sports medicine. The first orthobiologic described in the literature was platelet-rich plasma (PRP) in 1970[2] and subsequently used in vivo in 1987 intraoperatively during cardiac surgery.[3] The applications of PRP have since advanced within orthopedics especially over the last decade. PRP is now routinely used to treat tendon, ligament, and cartilage injuries.[4]

In the search for an orthobiologic product that could potentially have a higher concentration of growth factors, mesenchymal stem cells (MSCs) have been studied for their healing potentials. MSCs can be obtained from bone marrow, adipose tissue, and from the amniotic membrane of a placenta, among other tissues.[5] They have a very strict cellular expression; thus, they are difficult to isolate in culture.[6] Yet, they are believed to have vast orthopedic potentials due to their ability to stimulate growth

[a] Department of Orthopaedics and Rehabilitation Medicine, Emory University School of Medicine, 49 Jessie Hill Junior Drive Southeast 3rd Floor, Atlanta, GA 30303, USA; [b] Andrews Sports Medicine and Orthopedic Center, American Sports Medicine Institute, 805 St Vincent's Drive Suite 100, Birmingham, AL 35205, USA; [c] American Sports Medicine Institute, 805 St Vincent's Drive Suite 100, Birmingham, AL 35205, USA
* Corresponding author.
E-mail address: rcolberg@gmail.com
Twitter: @CleoStaffordMD (C.D.S.)

Clin Sports Med 39 (2020) 717–732
https://doi.org/10.1016/j.csm.2020.02.008
0278-5919/20/© 2020 Elsevier Inc. All rights reserved.

and reproduce of osteoblasts, adipocytes, and chondrocytes.[7] However, recent evidence has uncovered that these cells may not necessarily have the multipotent or differentiation potential as once thought. These cells now seem to create the environment where other cells named pericytes are recruited and have been shown to stimulate cells in the surrounding environment to replicate.[8] Given this information, MSCs have been renamed as medicinal signaling cells[9] (MSCs) and referred to as such throughout this article.

Furthermore, the use of PRP and MSC in regenerative medicine is still in its infancy. Nonetheless, its future role in orthopedics and sports medicine will continue evolving, with further research looking to understand the risks and benefits of using orthobiologics to heal injured tissues.

How Do Orthobiologics Work?

Orthobiologic products have a series of growth factors and bioactive proteins that contain the capacity of enhancing the healing process of an acute injury. The goal of this enhancement is to accelerate the return to regular activities and sports. In addition, physicians can use techniques such as percutaneous tenotomy and the trophic effects of these growth factors to activate the healing process of a chronically injured tissue that did not fully heal, even injuries in a chronic, degenerative, painful state.[1] In order to understand how these regenerative medicine products work, it is of the utmost importance to have a solid grasp of the inflammatory, proliferative, and maturation/remolding phases of wound healing[10] (**Fig. 1**).

For the purpose of this article, the authors use a soft tissue wound as an example. The inflammatory phase typically occurs within the first 72 hours. Platelets and white blood cells travel to the injured site to control bleeding, release growth factors that stimulate healing, and clean up necrotic debris, respectively. This phase can be initiated by injecting PRP into a chronically injured tissue, with or without including the white blood cells in the PRP product. During the proliferative phase (typically between days 3 and 42), the growth factors released by platelets attract fibroblasts and vascular proliferative cells to the injured site and stimulate them to ultimately form a new extracellular matrix of disorganized collagen fibrin. This causes contraction of soft tissue at the injury site. The third phase is the maturation or remodeling phase (occurring between 42 days and 6 months). During this phase, the scar size decreases and strength increases, reaching its peak at 6 months after the injury. Any alteration to these phases may ultimately change the outcome of the injury and delay the healing process. This may be stress induced such as returning to activity too soon or by the inappropriate use of medications that impair wound healing.[10] Following a rehabilitation protocol that respects these three phases by protecting the tissue when needed and strengthening it when ready is paramount in achieving the optimal outcome after a treatment when using an orthobiologic.[10]

Key Growth Factors and Signaling Cells

Platelets typically are active 5 to 9 days and are vital for proper wound healing.[11] Platelet alpha granules contain approximately 300 bioactive substances that help prepare surrounding tissue and cells for the proliferative and remodeling phases.[12] Injury and exposure to extracellular proteins cause activation of these platelets, leading to stimulation of the release of growth factors.[13] The most important platelet-derived factors for wound healing are platelet-derived growth factor (PDGF), vascular endothelial growth factor (VEGF), fibroblast growth factor (FGF), insulin-like growth factor, and transforming growth factor beta (TGF-beta)[1] (**Table 1**). TGF-beta has been proved to recruit MSCs to the site of injury and promote chondrogenesis.[1,14,15] VEGF is

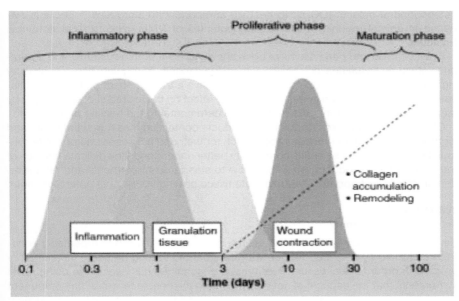

Fig. 1. Three phases of wound healing.

primarily responsible for angiogenesis, which is directly related to tissue site repair. PDGF, connective tissue growth factor, and epidermal growth factor (EGF) also work in conjunction with VEGF to accomplish the angiogenesis. Previous studies involving the use of VEGF and TGF-beta have shown improved revascularization and graft strengthening of the anterior cruciate ligament using Achilles tendon graft in animal model.[16] Other studies have looked at the relationship of FGF-2 on the surrounding vasculature causing an improvement in chrondrogenesis.[17] This is only a subset of a few of the important growth factors that play a role in controlled healing.

Another very important and powerful growth factor is a subset of TGF-beta called bone morphogenic proteins (BMPs). BMPs have the potential to induce large

Table 1
Fundamental growth factors for regenerative medicine

Growth Factor	Biological Actions
IGF-1	Anabolic effects including protein synthesis, enhancing collagen, and matrix synthesis in the early inflammatory phase.
PDGF($\alpha\beta$)	Assists in proliferation of growth factors by attracting stem cells and progenitor cells to stimulate tissue remodeling.
TGF (α-β)	A proinflammatory immunosuppressant that aids in cell migration, expression of collagen, and helps control angiogenesis and fibrosis.
VEGF	Promotes angiogenesis and neovascularization in the late inflammatory phase.
FGF	Promotes angiogenesis and neovascularization and seems to help in the regulation of cell migration and stimulate endothelial cells to produce granulation tissue during the late inflammatory phase.

Adapted from Kumar V, Abbas A, Fausto N. Tissue renewal and repair: regeneration, healing, and fibrosis. In: Robbins and Cotran Pathologic Basis of Disease (7th Edition). Elsevier Saunders, PA, USA, 87–118 (2005; with permission.

osteochondral defects (OCDs) to heal via an endochondralprocess.[18] There is evidence in animal models of the healing potential of BMP used to treat nonunion fractures.[19]

Finally, MSCs and pericytes have been shown to have both a systemic and a paracrine effect on tissue healing.[20,21] They have the capacity to regulate tissue healing by signaling bioactive proteins and other cells to have a trophic effect on the injured tissues.[22] They also have an immunomodulatory effect on the injured site, specifically by suppressing inflammatory cells that may be detrimental to the healing process.[22,23]

Clinical applications of orthobiologic products containing these growth factors and signaling cells are under further investigation for their optimal doses and possible synergistic effects. As our scientific community better understands the delicate balance of the orthobiologic products, we will be able to standardize treatments and rehabilitation protocols that appropriately stimulate tissue healing in the most optimal manner.

TERMINOLOGY
Percutaneous Tenotomy

Percutaneous tenotomy is a procedure in which a needle is used to repeatedly penetrate a chronically diseased tendon with the goal of creating an acute inflammatory process in order to heal tissue. Over time, the technique has evolved to using novel instruments that are capable of not only providing the needle fenestration component but also removing the disease tissue. A microdebrider coblation instrument uses a radiofrequency energy that is passed through an electrically conductive fluid, such as saline, to create a controlled, stable plasma field. The instrument precisely removes tissue at a relatively low temperature, resulting in minimal thermal damage to surrounding soft tissues.[24] In addition to the coblation instrument, an ultrasonic water jet stream device has also been used to emulsify and remove the diseased tissue via an inflow-outflow circuit.[25]

Autologous Blood Injection

Autologous blood injection (ABI) is a procedure in which autologous blood is extracted from the patient's peripheral venous system and injected into the injured tissue. The objective is to provide cellular and humoral mediators found in blood in order to restart the healing cascade.[26,27]

Platelet-Rich Plasma

PRP is an autologous blood product that has been concentrated via centrifugation. The end product contains a combination of powerful growth factors that has showed promising results in treating tendinopathic conditions.[28] It has also been shown to be effective in treating osteoarthritis pain, among other conditions.[29]

Bone Marrow Aspirate Concentrate

Bone marrow aspirate concentrate (BMAC) refers to preparations of bone marrow that have been aspirated and then centrifuged to concentrate the sample. This preparation has been shown to provide growth factors and immunomodulators without the need for laboratory culturing and processing.[30]

Adipose-Derived Medical Signaling Cells

Adipose-derived tissue is another source being used in orthopedics for its MSC capabilities. The MSCs associated with adipose tissue are typically a part of an aqueous portion of enzymatic derived lipoaspirate; however, because of Food and Drug Administration regulations, only minimal manipulation of this product is allowed.[31] The most common way of obtaining MSCs from the lipoaspirate occurs through nonenzymatic isolation, more specifically mechanical agitation. The product of this isolation is a stromal vascular fraction that contains growth factors similar to its hematopoietic counterparts.

Amniotic-Derived Products

Amniotic-derived products are collected from placentas of consenting women who have been screened for various diseases including human immunodeficiency virus, hepatitis, and syphilis.[32] Following screening, the placenta is cleansed with antibiotic solution to cover the most common bacteria and fungi. Then, the amniotic membrane is separated and processed. The amniotic membrane is thought to contain an extracellular matrix that can be used as scaffold for cellular proliferation and migration.[33] Recent literature has challenged these products being considered MSCs, given the lack of colony-forming units and plastic adherence of the cells in these preparations and the fact that most of the cells die during the preparation process.[34]

PATHOLOGIES
Lateral Epicondylopathy/Common Extensor Tendinopathy

The full pathogenesis of lateral epicondylopathy is covered in another chapter in this edition; however, it is commonly referred to as "tennis elbow" and is the tendinopathy of the common extensor tendon in the elbow. It is typically seen in patients who perform strong gripping or repetitive wrist flexion and extension movements.[35] Lateral epicondylopathy has a prevalence of 1% in the general population and as high as 50% among the recreational tennis players.[36,37] For many years, it has been described as an inflammation within the tendon or tendinitis; however, histologic studies have shown that there is a paucity in inflammatory cells.[38] These studies revealed a degenerative process of the tendon where increased concentration of angiofibroplastic hyperplasia is present.[39] This degenerative process occurs when the rate of injury has surpassed the rate of healing within a tendon leading to disarray of the normal architecture of the tissue.

Percutaneous needle tenotomy

There have been several studies evaluating percutaneous tenotomy for lateral epicondylopathy with promising results.[40] One of the first investigations was done by McShane and colleagues[41] where 58 subjects underwent ultrasound-guided percutaneous tenotomy followed by corticosteroid injection, and 80% of that cohort rated the procedure as being excellent or good at an average of 28 months following the procedure. The investigators concluded that the procedure was effective and safe, given no adverse events occurred during the study. McShane and colleagues[42] then performed a follow-up study where 57 patients underwent the same ultrasound-guided procedure without subsequent steroid injection, and 92.3% of the patients rated the procedure as either excellent or good with a response rate of 91.2% response rate and average follow-up time of 22 months. The investigators concluded that percutaneous tenotomy without a steroid injection was an effective and safe procedure for lateral epicondylopathy based on the patients' perception of the procedure and no reported adverse events. **Fig. 2** shows an ultrasound image of a percutaneous tenotomy for lateral epicondylosis.

As mentioned earlier, other instruments have been studied that are capable of both completing the percutaneous tenotomy and also removing the diseased tissue. Koh and colleagues[25] published initial results using an ultrasonic water jet stream device where 20 patients underwent the procedure. Nineteen of the twenty (95%) patients

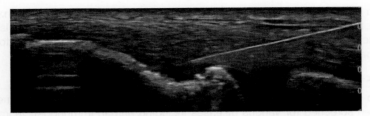

Fig. 2. Ultrasound image of a percutaneous tenotomy for lateral epicondylosis.

in the study expressed either being very satisfied or somewhat satisfied with the procedure at 1-year follow-up. Seng and colleagues[43] performed a follow-up study of the same cohort where subjects maintained their pain reduction and functional improvements. Ultrasound findings at 36 months following the procedure also revealed decreased tendon thickness and hypervascularity. Lastly, Barnes and colleagues[44] completed a prospective study evaluating the use of the same percutaneous ultrasonic tenotomy procedure in 19 patients with either lateral or medial epicondylopathy. At 12 months following the procedure, the average improvement of the visual analog scale (VAS) and Disabilities of the Arm, Shoulder and Hand (DASH) assessment score maintained statistical significance when compared with baseline scores. The investigators reported no complications, and the average procedure time was less than 15 minutes.

A microdebrider coblation device has similarly been shown to achieve successful outcomes in treating lateral epicondylopathy. Meknas and colleagues[24] carried out a prospective, randomized controlled trial in which 24 patients were randomized into 2 treatment groups: extensor tendon surgical release and repair and percutaneous tenotomy using the device. The patients in the tenotomy group had better outcomes than the surgery group with regard to VAS for pain and grip strength, which persisted for 18 months.

Autologous blood injection
The earliest study documenting this technique was performed by Edwards and Calandrucio where 28 patients who had failed other nonsurgical treatments (physical therapy, splinting, nonsteroidal antiinflammatory drugs [NSAIDs], and steroid injections) were injected at the point of maximum tenderness with 2 mL of autologous blood mixed with either 1 mL of 2% lidocaine HCL or 0.5% bupivacaine HCL.[45] The patients were followed-up to an average of 9.5 months after their injection, and 79% of the patients experienced complete relief. Since this initial study, there have been several studies comparing ABI with other modalities.[26] Chou and colleagues[26] performed a meta-analysis of randomized controlled trials using ABI for lateral epicondylopathy and determined that ABI is more effective than corticosteroid injections (CSI) in reducing pain scores but not as effective as PRP in decreasing pain scores. Arirachakaran and colleagues[46] performed a systematic review and network meta-analysis of PRP versus ABI versus CSI in the treatment of lateral epicondylitis and concluded that ABI may provide more improvement in pain VAS and DASH assessment when compared with CSI, but not when compared with PRP. In addition, ABI was shown to have a higher risk of complications versus the other 2 injections. Houck and colleagues[47] completed a systematic review of overlapping meta-analysis of treatments of lateral epicondylopathy and reached similar conclusions to Arirachakaran and colleagues. Furthermore, they determined that the study performed by Arirachakaran and colleagues seemed to have the highest level of evidence.

Platelet-rich plasma

One of the initial studies documenting PRP use in lateral epicondylopathy was performed by Mishra and Pavelko.[35] They injected 20 patients (15 with PRP and 5 with anesthetic) who experienced lateral elbow pain for at least 3 months with a VAS score of 60 out of 100 or higher, in addition to failing conservative treatments, including home exercise program, bracing, NSAIDs, and steroid injection. The PRP group showed a 93% reduction in their pain score compared with baseline and 94% returned to sporting activities at an average follow-up of 25.6 months. Mishra and colleagues then conducted a double-blind randomized controlled trial where they compared the use of leukocyte-rich PRP to needle fenestration (with anesthetic) in 230 patients. A successful outcome was defined as a greater than 25% improvement from baseline on VAS with resisted wrist extension. At 24 weeks postprocedure 83.9% of PRP patients experienced successful outcome as compared with 68.3% of the needle fenestration group. Since these studies, there have been several investigations evaluating PRP utilization for this condition.[46,47] The aforementioned papers highlight the ability of PRP to produce long-term improvement when compared with steroid injections and without the complications of ABI. In addition, PRP has been shown to improve the architecture of the diseased tendon.[48] This improvement in tendon architecture correlates with decrease pain and improved resisted wrist extension.[48] Lastly, PRP for this condition has demonstrated the capacity to reduce the need for surgical intervention.[49] Hastie and colleagues[49] performed a retrospective review in which they looked at the need for arthroscopic release of the common extensor tendon 4 years before implementing PRP into their institution and compared it with that 4 years after implementing PRP. They found a statistically significant decrease in the number of patients requiring surgical intervention; the number of surgical patients went from 12.75 per year to 4.25 per year after including PRP in their treatment algorithm for lateral epicondylopathy.

Bone marrow aspirate concentrate

There is limited but favorable literature involving the use of bone marrow aspirate concentrate for elbow epicondylopathy.[50] Moon and colleagues[51] explored the use of BMAC injections of the common extensor or common flexor tendons following elbow arthroscopy for epicondylopathy. The outcomes of the study included VAS and Mayo elbow performance scores (MEPS) at 8 weeks and 6 months after the procedure and sonographic appearance of the tendon pre- and postprocedure. All patients showed improvement in their VAS, although not statistically significant. However, their improvement in their MEPS was shown to be statistically significant. In addition, all participants had normal-appearing tendon echotexture postprocedure. The second study evaluating BMAC injections for common extensor tendinopathy was performed by Singh and colleagues[52] where 30 patients were injected. The main outcome was patient-rated tennis elbow evaluation score (PRTEE). They noted that the mean decrease in the PRTEE score was statistically significant at 2, 6, and 12 weeks. The investigators determined that BMAC injections were an effective treatment of common extensor tendinopathy in the short and medium term.

Adipose tissue

Currently only one published article exists dealing with the use of adipose MSC for the use for elbow epicondylopathy. Lee and colleagues[53] injected 12 participants' hypo-echoic areas in the common extensor tendon with allogenic adipose-derived MSCs. Of the 12 patients, 6 patients received 10^6 cells in 1 mL, and the remaining 6 patients received an injection of 10^7 cells in 1 mL. All patients had their injections mixed with fibrinogen to create a fibrin matrix for the adipose tissue. These investigators evaluated the safety of the procedure by tracking adverse outcomes and the efficacy by measuring VAS, modified mayo elbow performance index (MEPI), and musculoskeletal ultrasound evaluation at 6, 12, 26, and 52 weeks postinjection. The investigators observed that the VAS progressively decreased over the entire postinjection period and the MEPI improved as well; however, both these outcomes plateaued after 6 weeks. No statistical difference in improvement of VAS or MEPS was found between the 2 groups. In addition, the investigators noted progressive decrease in the hypoechoic defect in both groups over the postprocedure period. Lastly, no significant adverse events were noted in either group.

Medial Epicondylopathy/Common Flexor Tendinopathy

This degenerative process is the second most common tendinopathy at the elbow.[54] It occurs at the common flexor tendon originating from the medial epicondyle. It is 3- to 6-fold less common than lateral epicondylopathy; however, it has similar pathogenesis to its lateral elbow counterpart.[54]

Percutaneous tenotomy

There are no studies exclusively evaluating the treatment of the common flexor tendon with this technique. However, it has been evaluated in conjunction with other elbow tendon pathologies. As mentioned previously, Barnes and colleagues[44] evaluated the use of an ultrasound-guided percutaneous ultrasonic tenotomy procedure on common flexor and common extensor tendinopathy. Of the 19 patients evaluated, 7 of them had their common flexor tendon treated. There was a statistically significant improvement in VAS, MEPS, and DASH scores at 6 months and 12 months in all patients (medial and lateral epicondyle tendons); however, the investigators did not report the individual results for the common flexor and common extensor tendon patients. Boden and colleagues[55] conducted a retrospective review of 62 patients who underwent either PRP or ultrasound-guided percutaneous ultrasonic tenotomy procedure performed for their elbow epicondylopathy, with 10 patients having medial epicondylopathy. The patients completed a postprocedure outcome survey with the primary outcomes being VAS, Quick DASH, and EuroQol-5D scores. PRP and ultrasound-guided percutaneous ultrasonic tenotomy procedure both demonstrated clinical and statistical improvement in the VAS, Quick DASH, and EuroQol-5D scores with an average follow-up of 10 months in the percutaneous ultrasonic tenotomy group and 17 months in the PRP group. There was no statistically significant difference between the 2 treatment groups. The investigators concluded that both techniques are effective, minimally invasive nonsurgical treatment options for medial and lateral epicondylopathy. Lastly, Stover and colleagues[56] performed a retrospective chart review on 131 patients who underwent ultrasound-guided percutaneous tenotomy for common extensor, common flexor, or triceps tendinopathy. The outcomes measured included pain, quality of life, satisfaction with outcome, and complications at short-term (2 weeks, 6 weeks, and 12 weeks) and long-term (up to 4 years) follow-up. Of the 131 patients, 19 underwent treatment of their common flexor tendinopathy. In that group, pain decreased from 93% at baseline to 0% at long term follow-up. The common flexor group also demonstrated improvement in physical function and long-term follow-up, and there were no reported complications. The investigators concluded that the ultrasound-guided percutaneous tenotomy for elbow tendinopathies can reduce pain and improve physical function.

Autologous blood injection

Suresh and colleagues[57] conducted a prospective study where 20 patients received needle fenestration and 2 ABI injections 4 weeks apart. The outcomes measured for the study were VAS score, modified Nirschl score, and sonographic changes in the tendon (hypoechoic changes, neovascularity, and interstitial tears) at 4 weeks and 10 months. Seventeen of the twenty patients had favorable outcomes. Of that cohort, their improvement in VAS at 4 weeks and 10 months was statistically significant. In addition, the decrease in modified Nirschl score was statistically significant at both times when compared with preprocedure scores. With regard to the sonographic changes, all 17 patients showed a decrease in their hypoechoic changes and neovascularity; however, only 11 of the 17 patients achieved complete resolution of their interstitial tears.

Platelet-rich plasma

There are no studies exclusively evaluating PRP for medial epicondylopathy. The study with the largest number of patients to receive PRP for this issue was performed by Varshney and colleagues.[58] This randomized control trial compared the use for PRP versus steroid injections for elbow epicondylopathy. Of the 83 patients in the analysis; 20 patients had medial epicondylopathy. Overall, the investigators concluded that PRP was superior to steroid injections at reducing pain and increasing elbow function starting at 6 months. However, there was no distinction made between lateral and medial epicondylopathy in the results.

Ulnar Collateral Ligament Injury

The full pathogenesis of this injury is discussed elsewhere in this issue. Briefly, ulnar collateral ligament (UCL) injuries occur from acute trauma including elbow dislocations or as an overuse injury resulting in the chronic degeneration of the ligament and eventual tears. The latter is a serious injury typically occurring in overhead athletes, particularly baseball pitchers.[59] It occurs from repetitive valgus stress across the medial elbow, specifically, the anterior band of the medial UCL.[59]

Platelet-rich plasma

Several retrospective studies exist in the literature evaluating the use of PRP for UCL injuries with promising results.[60] The first published study performed by Podesta and colleagues[61] consisted of 34 patients receiving a single ultrasound-guided leukocyte-rich PRP injection (**Fig. 3**) for MRI-confirmed UCL partial thickness tear followed by a specific postinjection rehabilitation protocol and interval throwing program. The outcomes for the study included return to play at 12 weeks, Kerlan-Jobe Othropedic Clinic Shoulder and Elbow questionnaire (KJOC), DASH, and dynamic ultrasound evaluation of humeral-ulnar joint space measurement with applied valgus stress. The improvement in postinjection KJOC, DASH, and dynamic ultrasound evaluation were all statistically significant with an average follow-up time of 70 weeks. Lastly, 30 of the 34 patients were able to return to their previous level of competition. Deal and colleagues[62] conducted a retrospective study of 25 patients who received a PRP injection for this injury. In the study, all subjects' physical examination findings were consistent with UCL insufficiency and MRI-confirmed grade 2 partial thickness injury. On MRI confirmation, patients were placed in a varus-forcing hinged elbow brace followed by 2 ultrasound-guided autologous nonactivated leukocyte-rich PRP injections spaced 2 weeks apart. Following the injections, the patients completed a supervised rehabilitation protocol and progressed to a return to throwing program when they were able to wean out of the hinged brace when they were pain free on examination. Four weeks after starting the postinjection protocol, a new MRI was

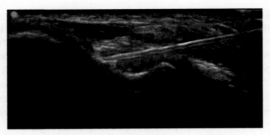

Fig. 3. PRP injection of a proximal ulnar collateral ligament injury.

performed to evaluate for the reconstitution of the ligament. All 25 patients showed reconstitution of the ligament with 20 of the athletes showing complete reconstitution. In addition, 96% of the athletes were able to return to the same or higher level of competition with an average return-to-competition time of 82 days.

Elbow Osteochondral Defect

OCDs of the elbow joint are the third most common location for OCDs to occur in the body after knee and ankle joints.[63] A high incidence of OCD lesions among youth baseball pitchers are typically the result of excessive or repetitive stress from pitching mechanics leading to this condition.[64]

Platelet-rich plasma

No published evidence exists for the use of PRP in elbow OCDs; however, there are investigations of its use for OCDs in other joints. In ankle cartilage issues, several investigations used PRP alone or combined with surgical intervention, which have shown encouraging results.[65] Mei-Dan and colleagues[66] performed a randomized controlled trial where 30 patients with osteochondral lesions of the talus were injected with either PRP or hyaluronic acid intraarticularly for 3 consecutive weeks. All patients in the study showed a statistically significant improvement in their VAS and Ankle-Hindfoot Scale scores at 4, 12, and 28 weeks; however, the PRP group showed greater statistically significant improvement than the hyaluronic acid injection group at all time points. Akpancar and Gül[67] performed a retrospective study comparing PRP and prolotherapy for osteochondral lesions of the talus. The investigators used periarticular and intraarticular injections in their approach as opposed to just intraarticularly. An activating agent was not used in their PRP injection, which is a different technique when compared with Mei-Dan and colleagues'. All 49 patients in the study showed statistically significant improvement in pain and function scores, and 90.9% of the PRP patients rated their outcomes as excellent or good compared with 88.8% in the prolotherapy group.

Bone marrow aspirate concentrate

Similar to PRP, there are no currently published studies evaluating BMAC for elbow OCDs; however, there is evidence supporting the use of BMAC for chondral injuries in the knee joint.[68] It has been used as an adjuvant in surgical procedures, as well as implanted using scaffolds into the defect.[68,69] Gobbi and Whyte performed a prospective study where 50 patients with grade IV cartilage injury underwent a microfracture procedure or implantation of activated BMAC within a hyaluronic acid scaffold.[70] At 2 years postprocedure, both groups showed statistically significant improvement in their patient-reported outcome scores. In the BMAC group, 100% of the patients were classified as being normal or nearly normal according to the International Knee

Documentation Committee (IKDC) objective score versus only 64% in the microfracture group. At 5-year follow-up, 28% of the patients in the microfracture group remained at normal or nearly normal in the IKDC objective score, whereas the whole BMAC group maintained their improvement.

Adipose tissue–derived medicinal signaling cells

There are no published studies discussing the use of adipose tissue for treatment of OCDs, but there has been promising evidence of its use in treatment of chondral injuries of the ankle and knee.[71] In a prospective comparative study conducted by Koh and colleagues,[72] the use of adipose-derived tissue combined with fibrin glue after microfracture was compared with microfracture alone for isolated knee cartilage defects in 80 patients. At 24 months postprocedure, in the adipose-derived tissue group, 65% of the patients achieved complete cartilage coverage of their lesion on MRI compared with 45% in the microfracture group. In addition, the adipose-derived tissue group revealed a significantly better signal intensity of the cartilage on repeat MRI, with 80% of the patients having normal or near normal intensity. Lastly, the adipose-derived tissue group, when compared with the microfracture group, showed significantly greater improvements in their mean Knee Injury and Osteoarthritis Outcome Score and symptom subscores.

Elbow Osteoarthritis

Primary osteoarthritis of the elbow is an uncommon condition. It typically occurs in patients involved in heavy labor or sports with the ulnohumeral joint being predominately affected.[73] Posttraumatic osteoarthritis occurs from a variety of insults to the area, especially with fractures that extend intraarticularly resulting in cartilage damage.[73] It can also occur as part of a systemic inflammatory arthropathy condition.

Platelet-rich plasma

As with elbow OCDs, no currently published studies exist evaluating the use of the PRP for elbow osteoarthritis. There is extensive evidence of its use in knee osteoarthritis. Dai and colleagues[74] completed a meta-analysis of 10 randomized controlled trials with a total of 1069 patients evaluating the efficacy of PRP for knee osteoarthritis. The investigators concluded that PRP, when compared with other injectables such as hyaluronic acid and saline, may have more benefit in pain relief and functional improvement in patients with symptomatic knee osteoarthritis at 1-year postprocedure with no increased risk of adverse events. Shen and colleagues[75] completed a more recent systematic review and meta-analysis of 14 randomized controlled trials including 1423 patients comparing the efficacy and safety of PRP with that of other injectables. They reached similar conclusions to Dai in which PRP was likely more efficacious in pain relief and self-reported functional improvement of knee osteoarthritis when compared with other injections such as corticosteroids, hyaluronic acid, saline placebo, and ozone.

Bone marrow aspirate concentrate

There are no published studies using BMAC for elbow osteoarthritis, but there are some studies with encouraging results for its use in knee osteoarthritis.[20,68,76] Kim and colleagues[76] evaluated the combination of BMAC and adipose tissue injections for knee degenerative joint disease. Forty-one patients were injected with BMAC and followed-up for 1 year after the injection where an average of 50% improvement was achieved in pain scores and functional scales, with better outcomes in mild-to-moderate osteoarthritic knees. Shapiro and colleagues[20] performed a single-blind controlled trial using BMAC for knee osteoarthritis. In the study, 25 patients with bilateral knee pain from bilateral osteoarthritis were randomized to receive BMAC into one knee and saline placebo into the other; therefore each patient became his or her own control. All patients showed significant improvement in VAS and Osteoarthritis Research Society International measurements at 1 week, 3 months, and 6 months. However, there was no statistically significant difference between the BMAC- and saline placebo–injected knee. Chahla and colleagues[68] performed a systematic review of the utilization of BMAC for osteoarthritis and chondral lesions of the knee joint. Of the studies evaluated, they concluded BMAC may be effective; however, given the heterogeneity of the studies, they were not able to make direct comparisons and formal conclusions.

Adipose-derived medicinal signaling cells

Similar to PRP and BMAC, there are currently no published studies on its use in elbow osteoarthritis, but there is some available evidence on its use for knee osteoarthritis. Jo and colleagues[77] performed an investigation where 18 patients were randomized to receive low-, medium-, and high-dose adipose-derived stem cells. All 3 groups improved in pain and functional scores with the low- and medium-dose groups plateauing at 1 year and the high-dose group plateauing at 2 years postinjection. Di Matteo and colleagues[78] completed a systematic review of 13 studies where they elucidated adipose tissue in the form of stromal vascular fraction had no serious adverse events. It also showed significant improvement in range of movement, pain, and articular function during daily activities. Similar to BMAC, they also noted that, provided the level of bias of the studies, they could not give a final recommendation on its use.

SUMMARY

Orthobiologics continue to be innovative techniques that are increasingly used in orthopedic issues of the elbow. There is level I evidence for its use for lateral epicondylopathy. There is also encouraging evidence for other pathologies in the elbow. Given the heterogenicity of the current literature, more randomized controlled trials with standardized reporting are needed in order to determine how these procedures can treat the pathology and the functionality of those affected.

DISCLOSURE

The authors have nothing to disclose.

REFERENCES

1. Nguyen RT, Borg-Stein J, McInnis K. Applications of platelet-rich plasma in musculoskeletal and sports medicine: an evidence-based approach. PM R 2011;3(3):226–50.
2. Weibrich G, Hansen T, Kleis W, et al. Effect of platelet concentration in platelet-rich plasma on peri-implant bone regeneration. Bone 2004;34(4):665–71.
3. Ferrari M, Zia S, Valbonesi M. A new technique for hemodilution, preparation of autologous platelet-rich plasma and intraoperative blood salvage in cardiac surgery. Int J ArtifOrgans 1987;10:47–50.
4. Bashir J, Sherman A, Lee H, et al. Mesenchymal stem cell therapies in the treatment of musculoskeletal diseases. PM R 2014;6(1):61–9.
5. Caplan AI. Mesenchymal stem cells. J Orthop Res 1991;9:641–50.

6. Dominici M, Le Blanc K, Mueller I, et al. Minimal criteria for defining multipotent-mesenchymal stromal cells. The International Society for Cellular Therapy position statement. Cytotherapy 2006;8(4):315–7.

7. Malanga G, Nakamura R. The role of regenerative medicine in the treatment of sports injuries. Phys Med RehabilClin N Am 2014;25(4):881–95.

8. Caplan AI. All MSCs are pericytes? Cell Stem Cell 2008;3:229–30.

9. Caplan AI. Mesenchymal stem cells: time to change the name! Stem CellsTransl Med 2017;6:1445–51.

10. Mautner K, Malanga G, Colberg R. Optimization of ingredients, procedures and rehabilitation for platelet-rich plasma injections for chronic tendinopathy. Pain Manag 2011;1(6):523–32.

11. Sampson S, Gerhardt M, Mandelbaum B. Platelet-rich plasma injection grafts for musculoskeletal injuries: a review. Curr Rev Musculoskelet Med 2008;1(3–4):165–74.

12. Golebiewska EM, Poole AW. Platelet recreation: from homeostasis to wound healing and beyond. Blood Rev 2015;29(3):153–62.

13. Mehta S, Watson JT. Platelet-rich concentrate: basic science and current clinical application. J OrthopTrauma 2008;22(6):432–8.

14. Huang Q, Goh JC, Hutmacher DW, et al. In vivo mesenchymal cell recruitment by a scaffold loaded with transforming growth factor beta -1 and the potential for in situ chondrogenesis. TissueEng 2002;8:469–82.

15. Park JS, Yang HJ, Wood DG, et al. Chondrogenic differentiation of mesenchymal stem cells embedded in a scaffold by long term release of TGF-beta3complexed with chondroitin sulfate. J Biomed Mater Res A 2010;92:806–16.

16. Wei X, Mao Z, Hou Y, et al. Local administration of TGF- 1/VEGF gene-transduced bone mesenchymal stem cells for Achilles allograft replacement of the anterior cruciate ligament in rabbits. BiochemBiophys Res Commun 2011;406:204–10.

17. Hellingman C, Koevoet W, Kops N, et al. Fibroblast growth factor receptors in in vitro and in vivo chondrogenesis: relating tissue engineering using adult mesenchymal stem cells to embryonic development. TissueEng Part A 2010; 16:545–56.

18. Ketenjian AY, Jafri AM, Aresenis C. Studies on the mechanism of callus cartilage differentiation and calcification during fracture healing. OrthopClin North Am 1978;9(1):43–65.

19. Evans CH, Liu FJ, Glatt V, et al. Use of genetically modified muscle and fat grafts to repair defects in bone and cartilage. EurCell Mater 2009;18:96–111.

20. Shapiro SA, Kazmerchak SE, Heckman MG, et al. A prospective, single-blind, placebo-controlled trial of bone marrow aspirate concentrate for knee osteoarthritis. Am J Sports Med 2017;45(1):82–90.

21. Kuroda K, Kabata T, Hayashi K, et al. The paracrine effect of adipose-derived stem cells inhibits osteoarthritis progression. BMCMusculoskeletDisord 2015;16(1):236.

22. Caplan AI. Adult mesenchymal stem cells for tissue engineering versus regenerative medicine. JCell Physiol 2007;213(2):341–7.

23. Franquesa M, Hoogduijn MJ, Bestard O, et al. Immunomodulatory effect of mesenchymal stem cells on B cells. Front Immunol 2012;3:212.

24. Meknas K, Odden-MilandÅ, Mercer JB, et al. Radiofrequency microtenotomy: a promising method for treatment of recalcitrant lateral epicondylitis. Am J Sports Med 2008;36(10):1960–5.

25. Koh JS, Mohan PC, Howe TS, et al. Fasciotomy and surgical tenotomy for recalcitrant lateral elbow tendinopathy: early clinical experience with a novel device for minimally invasive percutaneous microresection. Am J Sports Med 2013;41(3): 636–44.

26. Chou LC, Liou TH, Kuan YC, et al. Autologous blood injection for treatment of lateral epicondylosis: a meta-analysis of randomized controlled trials. PhysTherSport 2016;18:68–73.

27. Kazemi M, Azma K, Tavana B, et al. Autologous blood versus corticosteroid local injection in the short-term treatment of lateral elbow tendinopathy: A randomized clinical trial of efficacy. Am J Phys Med Rehabil 2010;89:660–7.

28. Mautner K, Colberg RE, Malanga G, et al. Outcomes after ultrasound-guided platelet-rich plasma injections for chronic tendinopathy: a multicenter, retrospective review. PM R 2013;5:169–75.

29. Smith PA. Intra-articular autologous conditioned plasma injections provide safe and efficacious treatment for knee osteoarthritis: an FDA-sanctioned, randomized, double-blind, placebo-controlled clinical trial. Am J Sports Med 2016; 44(4):884–91.

30. Murray I, Robinson P, West Ch, et al. Reporting standards in clinical studies evaluating bone marrow aspirate concentrate: a systematic review. Arthroscopy 2018;34:1366.e5.

31. Bora P, Majumdar AS. Adipose tissue-derived stromal vascular fraction in regenerative medicine: a brief review on biology and translation. Stem Cell Res Ther 2017;8(1):145.

32. Duerr R, Ackermann J, Gomoll A. Amniotic-derived treatments and formulations. ClinSports Med 2019;38:45–59.

33. Rocha SCM, Baptista CJM. Biochemical Properties of Amniotic Membrane. Springer: Amniotic Membrane; 2015. p. 19–40.

34. Panero A, Hirahara A, Andersen W, et al. Are amniotic fluid products stem cell therapies? a study of amniotic fluid preparations for mesenchymal stem cells with bone marrow comparison. Am J Sports Med 2019;47. 036354651982903.

35. Mishra A, Pavelko T. Treatment of chronic elbow tendinosis with buffered platelet-rich plasma. Am J Sports Med 2006;34:1774–8.

36. Shiri R, Viikari-Juntura E, Varonen H, et al. Prevalence and determinants of lateral and medial epicondylitis: a population study. Am J Epidemiol 2006;164(11): 1065–74.

37. Hume PA, Reid D, Edwards T. Epicondylar injury in sport: epidemiology, type, mechanisms, assessment, management, and prevention. Sports Med 2006; 36(2):151–70.

38. Bishai SK, Plancher KD. The basic science of lateral epicondylitis: update for the future. Tech Orthop 2006;21:250–5, 23.

39. Ahmad Z, Siddiqui N, Malik SS, et al. Lateral epicondylitis: a review of pathology and management. Bone Joint J 2013;95-B(9):1158–64.

40. Mattie R, Wong J, McCormick Z, et al. Percutaneous needle tenotomy for the treatment of lateral epicondylitis: a systematic review of the literature. PM R 2017;9(6):603–11.

41. McShane JM, Nazarian LN, Harwood MI. Sonographically guided percutaneous needle tenotomy for treatment of common extensor tendinosis in the elbow. J Ultrasound Med 2006;25:1281–9.

42. McShane JM, Shah VN, Nazarian LN. Sonographically guided percutaneous needle tenotomy for treatment of common extensor tendinosis in the elbow: is a corticosteroid necessary? J Ultrasound Med 2008;27:1137–44.

43. Seng C, Mohan PC, Koh SB, et al. Ultrasonic percutaneous tenotomy for recalcitrant lateral elbow tendinopathy: sustainability and sonographic progression at 3 years. Am J Sports Med 2016;44(2):504–10.

44. Barnes DE, Beckley JM, Smith J. Percutaneous ultrasonic tenotomy for chronic elbow tendinosis: a prospective study. J ShoulderElbow Surg 2015;24(1):67–73.
45. Edwards SG, Calandruccio JH. Autologous blood injections for refractory lateral epicondylitis. J Hand Surg Am 2003;28:272–8.
46. Arirachakaran A, Sukthuayat A, Sisayanarane T, et al. Platelet-rich plasma versus autologous blood versus steroid injection in lateral epicondylitis: systematic review and network meta-analysis. J OrthopTraumatol 2016;17(2):101–12.
47. Houck DA, Kraeutler MJ, Thornton LB, et al. Treatment of lateral epicondylitis with autologous blood, platelet-rich plasma, or corticosteroid injections: A systematic review of overlapping meta-analyses. Orthop J Sports Med 2019;7(3). https://doi.org/10.1177/2325967119831052.
48. Khattab EM, Abowarda MH. Role of ultrasound guided platelet-rich plasma (PRP) injection in treatment of lateral epicondylitis. Egypt J Radiol Nucl Med 2017;48:403–13.
49. Hastie G, Soufi M, Wilson J, et al. Platelet rich plasma injections for lateral epicondylitis of the elbow reduce the need for surgical intervention. J Orthop 2018;15(1):239–41.
50. Imam MA, Holton J, Horriat S, et al. A systematic review of the concept and clinical applications of bone marrow aspirate concentrate in tendon pathology. SICOT J 2017;3:58.
51. Moon YL, Jo SH, Song CH, et al. Autologous bone marrow plasma injection after arthroscopic debridement for elbow tendinosis. Ann Acad Med Singapore 2008;37(7):559–63.
52. Singh A, Gangwar DS, Singh S. Bone marrow injection: a novel treatment for tennis elbow. J Nat SciBiol Med 2014;5(2):389–91.
53. Lee SY, Kim W, Lim C, et al. Treatment of lateral epicondylosis by using allogeneic adipose-derived mesenchymal stem cells: a pilot study. Stem Cells 2015;33:2995–3005.
54. Donaldson O, Vannet N, Gosens T, et al. Tendinopathies around the elbow part 2: medial elbow, distal biceps and triceps tendinopathies. Shoulder Elbow 2014;6(1):47–56.
55. Boden AL, Scott MT, Dalwadi PP, et al. Platelet-rich plasma versus TENEX in the treatment of medial and lateral epicondylitis. J ShoulderElbow Surg 2019;28(1):112–9.
56. Stover D, Fick B, Chimenti R, et al. Ultrasound-guided tenotomy improves physical function and decreases pain for tendinopathies of the elbow: a retrospective review. J ShoulderElbow Surg 2019. https://doi.org/10.1016/j.jse.2019.06.011.
57. Suresh S, Ali KE, Jones H, et al. Medial epicondylitis: is ultrasound guided autologous blood injection an effective treatment? Br J Sports Med 2006;40(11):935–9.
58. Varshney A, Maheshwari R, Juyal A, et al. Autologous platelet-rich plasma versus corticosteroid in the management of elbow epicondylitis: a randomized study. Int J ApplBasic Med Res 2017;7(2):125–8.
59. Dugas J, Chronister J, Cain EL, et al. Ulnar collateral ligament in the overhead athlete—a current review. Sports Med Arthrosc Rev 2014;22:169–82.
60. Cascia N, Picha K, Hettrich CM, et al. Considerations of conservative treatment after a partial ulnar collateral ligament injury in overhead athletes: a systematic review. Sports Health 2019;11(4):367–74.
61. Podesta L, Crow SA, Volkmer D, et al. Treatment of partial ulnar collateral ligament tears in the elbow with platelet-rich plasma. Am J Sports Med 2013;41:1689–94.

62. Deal JB, Smith E, Heard W, et al. Platelet-rich plasma for primary treatment of partial ulnar collateral ligament tears: MRI correlation with results. Orthop J Sports Med 2017;5. 2325967117738238.

63. Weiss JM, Nikizad H, Shea KG, et al. The incidence of surgery in osteochondritisdissecans in children and adolescents. Orthop J Sports Med 2016;4(3). 2325967116635515.

64. Bruns J, Werner M, Habermann CR. Osteochondritisdissecans of smaller joints: the elbow. Cartilage 2019. https://doi.org/10.1177/1947603519847735.

65. Vannini F, Di Matteo B, Filardo G. Platelet-rich plasma to treat ankle cartilage pathology-from translational potential to clinical evidence: a systematic review. J ExpOrthop 2015;2:2.

66. Mei-Dan O, Carmont MR, Laver L, et al. Platelet-rich plasma or hyaluronate in the management of osteochondral lesions of the talus. Am J Sports Med 2012;40(3): 534–41.

67. Akpancar S, Gül D. Comparison of platelet rich plasma and prolotherapy in the management of osteochondral lesions of the talus: a retrospective cohort study. Med SciMonit 2019;25:5640–7.

68. Chahla J, Dean CS, Moatshe G, et al. Concentrated bone marrow aspirate for the treatment of chondral injuries and osteoarthritis of the knee: a systematic review of outcomes. Orthop J Sports Med 2016;4. 2325967115625481.

69. Southworth TM, Naveen NB, Nwachukwu BU, et al. Orthobiologics for focal articular cartilage defects. ClinSports Med 2019;38:109–22.

70. Gobbi A, Whyte GP. One-stage cartilage repair using a hyaluronic acid-based scaffold with activated bone marrow-derived mesenchymal stem cells compared with microfracture: five-year follow-up. Am J Sports Med 2016;44(11):2846–54.

71. McIntyre JA, Jones IA, Han B, et al. Intra-articular mesenchymal stem cell therapy for the human joint: a systematic review. Am J Sports Med 2018;46(14): 3550–63.

72. Koh YG, Kwon OR, Kim YS, et al. Adipose-derived mesenchymal stem cells with microfracture versus microfracture alone: 2-year follow-up of a prospective randomized trial. Arthroscopy 2016;32:97–109.

73. Biswas D, Wysocki RW, Cohen MS. Primary and posttraumatic arthritis of the elbow. Arthritis 2013;2013. https://doi.org/10.1155/2013/473259.

74. Dai WL, Zhou AG, Zhang H, et al. Efficacy of platelet-rich plasma in the treatment of knee osteoarthritis: a meta-analysis of randomized controlled trials. Arthroscopy 2017;33(3):659–70.e1.

75. Shen L, Yuan T, Chen S, et al. The temporal effect of platelet-rich plasma on pain and physical function in the treatment of knee osteoarthritis: systematic review and meta-analysis of randomized controlled trials. J OrthopSurg Res 2017;12:16.

76. Kim JD, Lee GW, Jung GH, et al. Clinical outcome of autologous bone marrow aspirates concentrate (BMAC) injection in degenerative arthritis of the knee. Eur J OrthopSurgTraumatol 2014;24(8):1505–11.

77. Jo CH, Chai JW, Jeong EC, et al. Intra-articular injection of mesenchymal stem cells for the treatment of osteoarthritis of the knee: a 2-year follow-up study. Am J Sports Med 2017;45(12):2774–83.

78. Di Matteo B, Vandenbulcke F, Vitale ND, et al. Minimally manipulated mesenchymal stem cells for the treatment of knee osteoarthritis: a systematic review of clinical evidence. StemCellsInt 2019;2019:1735242.

Moving?

Make sure your subscription moves with you!

To notify us of your new address, find your **Clinics Account Number** (located on your mailing label above your name), and contact customer service at:

Email: journalscustomerservice-usa@elsevier.com

800-654-2452 (subscribers in the U.S. & Canada)
314-447-8871 (subscribers outside of the U.S. & Canada)

Fax number: 314-447-8029

Elsevier Health Sciences Division
Subscription Customer Service
3251 Riverport Lane
Maryland Heights, MO 63043

*To ensure uninterrupted delivery of your subscription, please notify us at least 4 weeks in advance of move.

Printed and bound by CPI Group (UK) Ltd, Croydon, CR0 4YY

08/05/2025

01864692-0004